Bladder Diseases: Assessment and Therapeutics

Bladder Diseases: Assessment and Therapeutics

Editor: William Miller

AMERICAN
MEDICAL PUBLISHERS
www.americanmedicalpublishers.com

AMERICAN
MEDICAL PUBLISHERS
www.americanmedicalpublishers.com

Cataloging-in-Publication Data

Bladder diseases : assessment and therapeutics / edited by William Miller.
p. cm.
Includes bibliographical references and index.
ISBN 978-1-63927-936-4
1. Bladder--Diseases. 2. Bladder--Diseases--Diagnosis. 3. Bladder--Diseases--Treatment.
4. Bladder--Examination. I. Miller, William.
RC919 .B53 2023
616.62--dc23

American Medical Publishers,
41 Flatbush Avenue,
1st Floor, New York,
NY 11217, USA

ISBN 978-1-63927-936-4 (Hardback)

Contents

Preface

Human body contains a hollow organ in the lower abdomen known as the bladder. The function of the bladder is to store urine. Bladder diseases are a group of medical conditions or diseases that affect the bladder. There are several forms of bladder diseases including cystitis, bladder cancer, overactive bladder, urinary incontinence (UI) and interstitial cystitis. UI are problems associated with the loss of bladder control. Some symptoms of UI include an inability to control urine, strong urge to urinate, bed-wetting, and leaking urine during routine activities such as lifting, bending, coughing or exercising. Interstitial cystitis is a chronic condition in which a person experiences painful urinary symptoms such as pressure, discomfort and tenderness or pain in the areas of bladder, pelvis and lower abdomen. The diagnosis of bladder diseases is completed with the help of urine tests and X-rays. Doctors also examine the bladder wall and urethra with an instrument known as cystoscope. Usually, the treatment of bladder diseases involves the use of medications. However, some severe cases are treated with the help of surgery. This book provides a detailed explanation of the assessment methods and therapeutics for bladder diseases. It will also provide interesting topics for research, which the interested readers can take up. The book will serve as a valuable source of reference for students studying these diseases.

This book is a comprehensive compilation of works of different researchers from varied parts of the world. It includes valuable experiences of the researchers with the sole objective of providing the readers (learners) with a proper knowledge of the concerned field. This book will be beneficial in evoking inspiration and enhancing the knowledge of the interested readers.

In the end, I would like to extend my heartiest thanks to the authors who worked with great determination on their chapters. I also appreciate the publisher's support in the course of the book. I would also like to deeply acknowledge my family who stood by me as a source of inspiration during the project.

Editor

Transurethral resection of a bladder trigone leiomyoma: A rare case report

Athanasios Zachariou[1*], Maria Filiponi[1], Fotios Dimitriadis[2], Aris Kaltsas[1] and Nikolaos Sofikitis[1]

Abstract

Background: Bladder leiomyomas are rare and benign tumors of the bladder. They account for 0.43% of all bladder tumors, and only 250 cases have been reported in English literature. Based on the size and localization of the lesion, their symptoms vary considerably. Women seem to be more affected, and obstructive symptoms predominate. Surgical treatment is almost always highly effective, leaving a low recurrence rate.

Case presentation: We present a clinical case of a 52-year old man with macroscopic hematuria and obstructive lower urinary tract symptoms due to a large bladder trigone leiomyoma. CT and MRI showed a well-defined large bladder leiomyoma and cystoscopy established the initial findings. The patient underwent successful transurethral resection of the lesion, and pathology findings confirmed the diagnosis.

Conclusions: This case report demonstrates that transurethral resection of a large bladder trigone leiomyoma is a feasible and successful procedure. Long term follow-up proves that there is neither scarring distortion of the bladder trigone area nor damage in the ureteral orifices, even though there was a thorough removal of the trigone wall.

Keywords: Bladder, Trigone, Leiomyoma, Obstruction, Transurethral resection

Background

Leiomyoma describes a benign growth of smooth muscle tissue. These tumors can occur anywhere in the body where smooth muscle is found, but are frequently located in the uterus (commonly called fibroids) or the gastrointestinal tract. Bladder leiomyoma is a rare, benign tumor with an incidence rate of about 0.43% among all types of bladder tumors [1]. Approximately 250 cases have been reported to date to English literature, including patients who had leiomyoma in a urethral location [2]. Some of the leiomyomas observed in the bladder are diagnosed accidentally, and these patients could have a variety of clinical presentations such as obstructive symptoms from the lower urinary tract, irritative symptoms, hematuria, and dysuria. Surgery is the standard treatment, and the surgical approach depends on tumor size and location at the bladder wall. Small and easily accessible tumors can be treated with transurethral resection of the bladder tumor, while an unfavorable location may require segmental resection or laparoscopic partial cystectomy [3].

Here we report a case of a large bladder trigone leiomyoma in a 52-year-old Caucasian male who presented with complaints of lower urinary tract obstruction, sporadic hematuria, and dysuria. To our knowledge, this case is one of the few reported cases of bladder trigone leiomyoma mimicking the median prostate lobe and distorting the left ureteric orifice. Our primary concern was that scar tissue following the procedure could further change the bladder trigone area, thus exacerbating patient's dysuria.

Case presentation

A 52-year-old man presented at our clinic with gross macroscopic hematuria, and a 12-month history of the lower urinary tract symptoms. He reported frequency,

*Correspondence: zahariou@otenet.gr
[1] Urology Department, Medical School, University of Ioannina, 3 Spyridi Street, 38221 Vólos, Greece
Full list of author information is available at the end of the article

urgency, nocturia, straining at voiding, dribbling at the end of urination and inability to empty the bladder. He had diagnosed with a urinary tract infection 3 months earlier. Although he had received antibiotic therapy, his urinary complaints persisted. As prescribed by a General Practitioner, his treatment was tamsulosin 0.4 mg/daily, for 2 months with limited success for the reported symptoms.

During the initial evaluation, no abnormalities were found on physical examination or in routine laboratory studies. Ultrasound of the lower urinary tract revealed a smooth endovesical bladder lesion in the bladder trigone area which mimicked the median prostate lobe as well as mild prostate hyperplasia (prostate volume 43 cc). The tumor presented peripheral hyperechogenicity. There was also mild hydronephrosis in the left kidney with no indication of kidney stone.

Given that asymptomatic macroscopic hematuria requires extensive investigation and the questions concerning the existence of a prostate median lobe, the patient was scheduled for computed tomography (CT). CT confirmed the presence of a solid, well-delineated mass measuring 41 × 24 mm that appeared to arise from the bladder trigone wall, independent from prostate, without any evidence of distant metastasis (Fig. 1). There was an obstructed and mildly dilated left pelvicalyceal system due to the bladder tumor displacing the left ureteric orifice. Urine cytology showed unremarkable squamous and urothelial cells and was negative for malignancy. MRI revealed a well-defined intramural mass (Figs. 2, 3).

The patient underwent cystoscopy, which revealed a protruding mass in bladder trigone next to bladder neck with normal covering urothelium. There was a distortion in the area of the left ureteric orifice, which

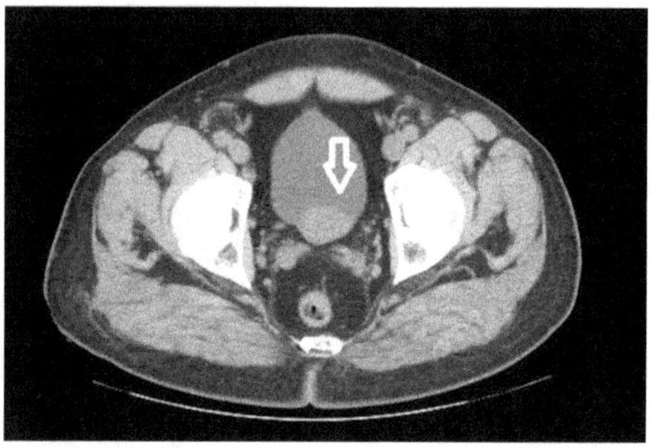

Fig. 1 CT confirmed the presence of a solid, well-delineated mass measuring 41 × 24 mm that appeared to arise from the bladder trigone wall

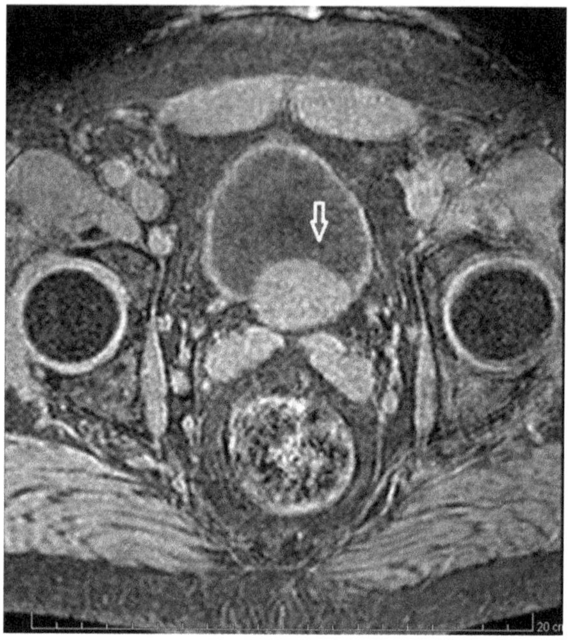

Fig. 2 MRI revealed a well-defined 41 × 24 mm intramural mass

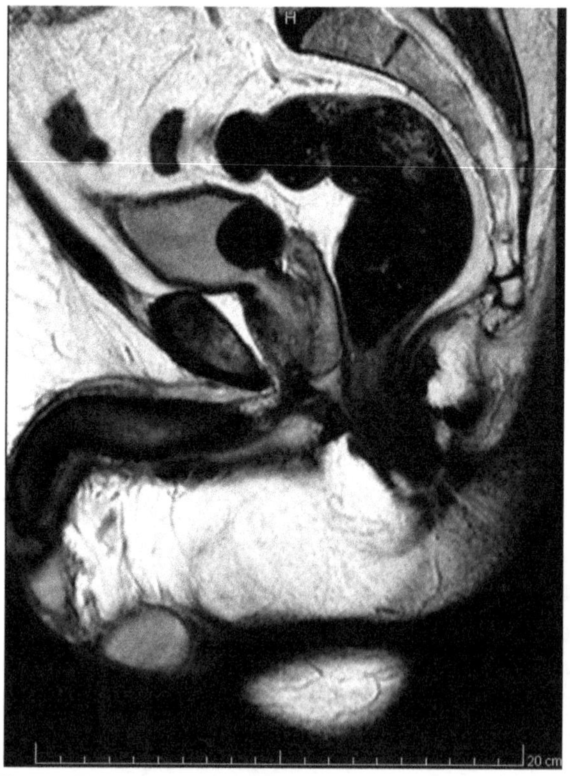

Fig. 3 MRI sagittal view of leiomyoma

was displaced by the mass posterior to its normal position (Fig. 4).

The patient underwent an uneventful TURBT. After the resection, a yellowish well-defined adipose tissue was revealed in the region of the bladder trigone. There are specific anatomical variations of the bladder trigone; muscularis propria bundles are nearer to the suburothelium and become smaller in caliber towards the surface. Adipose tissues can be seen in between muscularis propria bundles, which may continue extravesically or extend superficially to the lamina propria. Conversely, the outer boundary of muscularis propria with perivesical soft tissues (a landmark for staging extravesical invasion) is irregular and not well defined.

Special care was taken as regards the left ureteric orifice. Both ureteric orifices were seen to be intact. There was a significant concern about the future formation of scar tissue in the trigone area that could distort normal anatomy. The catheter was removed on the second postoperative day and the patient was discharged without any problem. Pathology proved that the lesion was a benign submucosal leiomyoma. The material consisted of interlacing fascicles of spindle-shape cells. The cells displayed no pleomorphism and contained bland-looking central spindle nuclei and eosinophilic cytoplasm. Microscopic examination of the whole tissue fragments did not reveal mitotic activity or coagulative necrosis. Immunohistochemical analysis showed an extended and robust cytoplasmic expression of smooth muscle actin (SMA) stain applied to the tissue.

Six months after surgery, an ultrasound revealed no recurrence of the tumor. A 12 month ultrasound follow-up also confirmed that the patient had no remaining lesions. Since a benign condition had already been confirmed, a usual postoperative evaluation involves the ultrasound scan. However, our concerns about a probable scarring in the blabber trigone area and distortion of ureteral orifices made a postoperative cystoscopy necessary.

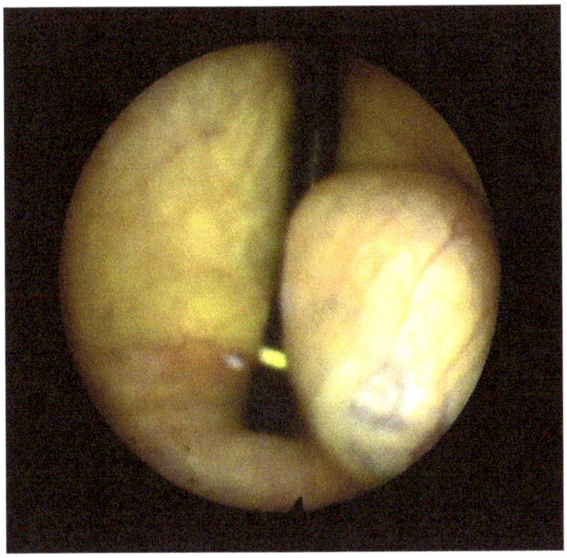

Fig. 4 Appearance of bladder trigone leiomyoma in cystoscopy

Discussion and conclusions

Bladder leiomyoma is a rare, benign, mesenchymal tumor of the bladder, with an incidence rate lower than 0.5% among all types of bladder tumors. It was first described by Kretschmer et al. in 1931 [4]. During the period 2012–2017, He et al. [5] recorded data from 21 patients in 20 reports in the English literature. The incidence of bladder leiomyoma in women is twice as high as that in men. Furthermore, middle-aged patients of approximately 50 years old present the most considerable adverse symptoms among all age groups [5].

The etiology of leiomyomas is still unknown, and multiple theories try to explain their origin. Blum's irritative theory suggests that the reason is the presence of chronic inflammatory stimuli over the bladder wall and the detrusor smooth muscle. Some speculate that leiomyoma may arise from perivascular inflammation or chromosomal alterations [1]. Piegel's disontogenic theory claims that its origin comes from embryogenic rests of Muller and Wolffian ducts [6]. Finally, Lips-Chutz's theory proposes that the background of leiomyoma is secondary to an endocrine disorder, with estrogen and progesterone having a primary role. This theory supports peak incidence in females when fertile, and the presence of steroidal ovarian receptors on the tumor [7].

Leiomyomas are classified according to three different locations, i.e., endovesical, intramural, and extravesical. Endovesical is the most common location, and it corresponds to 63–86% of cases, while intramural leiomyomas are present in 3–7% and extravesical in 11–30% [6, 8].

Patients with bladder leiomyomas can be asymptomatic, but the majority of them present with obstructive symptoms (49%), irritative symptoms (38%) and hematuria (11%) [6]. Larger lesions have more symptoms, although there is a report of a bladder leiomyoma smaller than 1.4 cm in diameter that caused pain and urinary retention [9]. The location of the leiomyoma mainly attributes to the phenomenon. A leiomyoma located in the bladder trigone, like our case, may cause more severe obstructive symptoms compared with a lesion located in the bladder wall.

Traditional detection methods of bladder leiomyoma include ultrasound, CT, MRI, and cystoscopy. Ultrasound findings include homogenous, smooth lesions with peripheral hyperechogenicity [10, 11]. CT imaging is used to determine the size and extent of the tumor. Solid tumors of the bladder wall, with densities of around 30 HU and bladder displacement are the typical CT findings in bladder leiomyomas. MRI imaging is better than CT for detecting the origin and distinguishing the boundary of the tumor. Leiomyomas on MRI have a medium-signal intensity on T1-WI and homogenous low signal intensity on T1-WI, with a smooth peripheral mimicking a uterine leiomyoma. After injecting gadolinium contrast medium, contrast enhancement is variable, and degenerated areas lack enhancement [12–14]. In any case, all imaging techniques can never exclude a malignancy; therefore, only histological studies can provide an accurate diagnosis.

Leiomyomas are grossly clear-bordered, thin-capsuled solid masses with yellow-colored sectional surface. Microscopically, leiomyoma is made of intersecting smooth muscle fascicles surrounding vascular structures lined with normal endothelium and arranged as bundles extending in various directions. No mitotic activity, hemorrhage or necrosis foci are observed in these lesions. Immunohistochemically, they have positive staining with smooth muscle actin (SMA), muscle-specific actin (MSA), desmin, h-caldesmon, and vimentin. They are negative with keratins and epithelial membrane antigens (EMA). Detrusor muscle invasion is the most significant factor in differential diagnosis with leiomyosarcoma [15, 16]. Lake et al. [17] described in 1981, the only case of a leiomyoma with malignant degeneration.

The treatment of leiomyomas is determined primarily by their size, anatomic location, and relationship with the bladder wall [6]. Surgery is indicated because of the potential growth capacity of these tumors [18]. Given the benign nature of these lesions, the operation must be as conservative as possible. Treatment options include transurethral resection and open surgical excision (enucleation or/with partial cystectomy) [6]. Transurethral resection is the treatment of choice for small tumours. There are few publications reporting transurethral resections for the treatment of patients with broad bladder neck leiomyomas [19–21]. There are no relevant records about postoperative scar tissue formation in the bladder trigone area after a long term follow-up.

In some exceptional cases, specific operations were developed, such as vaginal resection for bladder leiomyoma [22]. Other minimally invasive techniques, such as laparoscopic cystotomy or robotic extramucosal excision, are also suitable [23]. In our case, the patient mainly experienced obstructive symptoms due to the specific location and the size of the leiomyoma. Therefore, transurethral resection was suitable despite the large size and the anatomic position of the leiomyoma and a successful outcome was achieved.

Recurrence after surgical removal is rare, and recurrent cases have been successfully managed with repeat enucleation or transurethral resection [24]. Having in mind that there are no guidelines regarding the follow-up of these cases, the clear suggestion is to avoid exposing the patients to invasive or radiologic investigations to detect small asymptomatic recurrences postoperatively [3].

This case report demonstrates that transurethral resection of a large bladder trigone leiomyoma is a feasible, safe and effective procedure. Long term follow-up proves that there is neither scarring distortion in the bladder trigone nor damage in the ureteral orifices, even though there was a thorough removal of trigone wall.

Abbreviations

CT: Computed tomography; EMA: Epithelial membrane antigens; MRI: Magnetic resonance imaging; MSA: Muscle-specific actin; SMA: Smooth muscle actin; T1-WI: T1 weighted images; T2-WI: T2 weighted images.

Acknowledgements

Not applicable.

Authors' contributions

AZ drafted the manuscript and reviewed the literature. MF, FD, AK helped with the draft. NS revised the manuscript. All authors read and approved the final

Author details

[1] Urology Department, Medical School, University of Ioannina, 3 Spyridi Street, 38221 Vólos, Greece. [2] 1st Urology Department, Medical School, Aristotle University of Thessaloniki, Thessaloníki, Greece.

References

1. Cornella JL, Larson TR, Lee RA, Magrina JF, Kammerer-Doak D. Leiomyoma of the female urethra and bladder: report of twenty-three patients and review of the literature. Am J Obstet Gynecol. 1997;176:1278–85.
2. Dodia B, Mahajan A, Amlani D, et al. Leiomyoma of urinary bladder in middle-aged female. J Obstet Gynaecol India. 2017;67:147–9.
3. Haddad RG, Murshidi MM, Abu Shahin N, Murshidi MM. Leiomyoma of urinary bladder presenting with febrile urinary tract infection: a case report. Int J Surg Case Rep. 2016;27:180–2.
4. Kretschmer JL. Leiomyoma of the bladder with a report of a case and a review of the literature. J Urol. 1931;24:26–57.
5. He L, Li S, Zheng C, Wang C. Rare symptomatic bladder leiomyoma: case report and literature review. J Int Med Res. 2018;4:1678–84.
6. Goluboff ET, O'Toole K, Sawczuk IS. Leiomyoma of bladder: report of case and review of literature. Urology. 1994;43:238–41.
7. Furuhashi M, Suganuma N. Recurrent bladder leiomyoma with ovarian steroid hormone receptors. J Urol. 2002;167:1399–400.
8. Knoll LD, Segura JW, Scheilhauer BW. Leiomyoma of the bladder. J Urol. 1986;136:906–13.
9. Aggarwal RS, Mishra VV, Jasani AF. Incidence and prevalence of female sexual dysfunction in infertile females. Middle East Fertil Soc J. 2013;18:187–90.
10. Saunders SE, Conjeski JM, Zaslau S, Williams J. Leiomyoma of the urinary bladder presenting as urinary retention in the female. Can J Urol. 2009;16:4762–4.
11. Katz RB, Waldbaum RS. Benign mesothelial tumors of the bladder. Urology. 1975;5:236–8.
12. Fernandez A, Dehesa TM. Leiomyoma of the urinary bladder floor: diagnosis by transvaginal ultrasound. Urol Int. 1992;48:99.

13. Wenz W, Sommerkamp H, Dinkel E. Leiomyoma of the bladder. Urol Radiol. 1986;8:114–7.
14. Melicow MM. Tumors of the urinary bladder. J Urol. 1937;37:117.
15. Chen M, Lipson SA, Hricak H. MR imaging evaluation of benign mesenchymal tumors of the urinaryy bladder. AJR Am J Roentgenol. 1997;168:399–403.
16. Goldman HB, McAchran SE, MacLennan GT. Leiomyoma of the urethra and bladder. J Urol. 2007;177:1890.
17. Lake MH, Kossow AS, Bokinsky G. Leiomyoma of the bladder and urethra. J Urol. 1981;125:742–3.
18. Jimenez Aristu JI, Lozano Urunuela F, de Pablo CA, et al. Leiomyoma of the bladder. Report of a case. Actas Urol Esp. 2001;25:223–5.
19. Goktug GH, Ozturk U, Sener NC, Tuygun C, Bakirtas H, Imamoglu AM. Transurethral resection of a bladder leiomyoma: a case report. Can Urol Assoc J. 2014;8(1–2):E111–3.
20. Gok A. Transurethral resection of a large urinary bladder leiomyoma: a rare case report. Urol J. 2017;14(4):4052–4.
21. Wu S. Imaging findings of atypical leiomyoma of the urinary bladder simulating bladder cancer: a case report and literature review. Med Ultrason. 2013;15(2):161–3.
22. Nagai N, Katayama Y, Iguchi M, Esa A. A case of urinary retention due to a female paraurethral leiomyoma. Hinyokika Kiyo. 1988;34:696–700.
23. Murota T, Komai Y, Danno S, Fujita I, Kawakita M, Matsuda T. Endoscopic partial cystectomy for bladder leiomyoma using retroperitoneoscopic and transurethral procedures. Int J Urol. 2002;9:190–2.
24. Park JW, Jeong BC, Seo SI, Jeon SS, Kwon GY, Lee HM. Leiomyoma of the urinary bladder: a series of nine cases and review of the literature. Urology. 2010;76:1425–9.

2

Bladder neck reconstruction in girls' pelvic fracture bladder neck avulsion and urethral rupture

Rong Lv[1], Chongrui Jin[1], Huiquan Shu[1], Lin Wang[1,2] and Yinglong Sa[1,3*]

Abstract

Background: Girls' pelvic fracture bladder neck avulsion and urethral rupture is rare however it causes great morbidity. The management is complex and not standard yet. We report our experience and a technique of bladder neck reconstruction with anterior bladder wall flap.

Methods: We retrospectively analysed data of 5 girls with pelvic fracture bladder neck avulsion and urethral rupture admitted to our institution from July 2017 to October 2019. They all came to our institution with a suprapubic tube. Patients' trauma was all initially treated at other hospitals, 4 had suprapubic cystotomy and 1 had urethral realignment. One girl also had three other urethroplasties at other hospitals. We took pubectomy, posterior urethroplasty and bladder neck reconstruction with anterior bladder wall flap in these 5 girls. Post-operative assessments included voiding cystourethrography, uroflowmetry and urethroscopy after urethral catheter removal. Verbal consent to participate was obtained from the parent or legal guardian of the children.

Results: Operation time ranged from 120 to 180 min. Follow-up time is 12 to 27 months. Uroflowmetry showed that maximum urine flow rate improved significantly. Cystourethrography indicated good continuity of the urethra. Two girls had urinary incontinence postoperatively but were continent 3 months later. One patient developed vesical-abdominal fistula and got repaired by surgery 6 months later. She was continent ever since. Other complications were not observed during the follow-up period.

Conclusions: Our method of bladder neck reconstruction using bladder flap as a patch is feasible and provides good continence, especially for those with serious bladder neck avulsion and urethral rupture caused by extensive trauma and those who had posttraumatic urethral distraction needed second repair.

Keyword: Female pediatric urethral injury, Bladder neck reconstruction, Urinary continence, Pediatric pelvic trauma

Background

Comparing to male urethra, female urethra with an average length of 4 cm is much shorter and less fixed in the pelvic, thus the chance of getting injured is low. Although pelvic fracture urethral and bladder injuries in girls are rare, the management is complex. Unlike male patients, there is no standard treatment for female pelvic fracture urethral injury and the surgical management in published literature remains controversial because the morbidity of postoperative incontinence and stricture were still high. Hence in this article, we introduced 5 cases of girls with intensive bladder neck avulsion and urethral rupture associated with pelvic fracture and elaborated our surgical technique of bladder flap bladder neck reconstruction.

*Correspondence: yinglongsa@126.com
[1] Department of Urology, Shanghai Jiao Tong University Affiliated Sixth People's Hospital, Shanghai, China
Full list of author information is available at the end of the article

Methods

Clinical materials

From July 2017 to October 2019, 5 girls with bladder neck avulsion and urethral rupture caused by traumatic pelvic fracture were admitted to our institution and accepted surgery. Their clinical characteristics were listed in Table 1. Their mean age is 7.4 years old. Trauma was caused by motor vehicle accident in 4 cases, pedestrian-car accident in 1 case. All the patients were initially treated at other hospitals when the trauma happened, hence the type and extent of urinary injury weren't available. Their urinary injuries were dealt with suprapubic cystotomy in 4 and 1 had urethral realignment. Their pelvic fractures were managed with external fixation in 3 cases and internal fixation in 2 cases. The interval between the trauma and our surgery ranged from 6 months to 9 years. They all came to our institution with a suprapubic tube. One girl had posterior urethra end-to-end anastomosis, percutaneous nephrolithotomy and posterior urethroplasty using bladder mucosa at other hospitals.

Preoperative evaluations

we evaluated patient medical history, physical examination and routine laboratory investigations before the operation. Blood urea and serum creatinine in patients were normal and USG abdomen showed bilateral normal kidneys. Voiding cystourethrography showed completely atresia of bladder neck and urethral distraction (Fig. 1a). Vesicovaginal fistula was found in one girl (Fig. 1c, d). Urethroscopy entered the urethra for around 2 cm and was blocked. Suprapubic cystoscopy showed the bladder neck was obliterate, ureteric orifices were normal and vesicovaginal fistula was found in one patient. Vaginoscopy under anesthesia was also done to rule out urethrogenital fistula.

Surgical technique

All patients were administered by general anesthesia and were under lithotomy position. The surgery was accomplished by combined vaginal and transpubic approach through a lower midline abdominal incision. Then a 2 cm around segment of pubic bone was cut using a Gigli saw to get enough surgical field of the bladder neck and proximal urethra, then the atresic bladder neck which was obstructed by fibrosis was showed. Under the guidance of a urethral dilator, we could see that remain distal urethra length is 1–2 cm and the defect between the atresic bladder neck and the obstructed proximal urethra is 0.5–1.5 cm. The obstructed urethra and bladder neck were incised longitudinally under the guidance of urethral dilator and periurethral fibrous tissue was excised. The process of bladder neck reconstruction is rather like a modified Y–V plasty. A T-shaped incision was made at the anterior bladder wall so as to obtain two 1.5–3 cm long, 1–2 cm width well vascularized flaps. We reserved the dorsal part of bladder neck and proximal urethra. Then the bladder wall flaps are flipped downwards as a patch to augment the ventral part of bladder neck and proximal urethra. Fat tissues were wrapped around the new urethra and bladder neck to eliminate the cavity around the urethra. A 6–14 Fr silicone Foley catheter and a suprapubic catheter were placed after bladder closure (Fig. 2). A drainage tube was left in the pelvis.

Postoperative management

Prophylactic antibiotics were used for 3 days. The pelvic drainage tube was removed 3 days after the surgery. The urethral silicone catheter was left indwelled for 3 weeks and the suprapubic catheter was removed 1 weeks after the removal of urethral catheter. Postoperative evaluations included voiding cystourethrography, uroflowmetry and urethroscopy after urethral catheter removal.

Results

Operation time ranged from 120 to 180 min. Follow-up time is 12 to 27 months. Uroflowmetry showed that maximum urine flow rate improved significantly, ranging from 16.5 to 20 ml/s, and mean value is 17 ml/s.

Table 1 Clinical information of patients

	Age	Etiology	Condition history	Operation history	Complications
Case 1	13 years old	Motor vehicle accident	9 years	Suprapubic cystotomy, posterior urethra end-to-end anastomosis, percutaneous nephrolithotomy and posterior urethroplasty using bladder mucosa	None
Case 2	9 years old	Pedestrian-car accident	7 months	Urethral realignment	Vesicovaginal fistula; urinary incontinence
Case 3	8 years old	Motor vehicle accident	1 year	Suprapubic cystotomy	None
Case 4	21 months	Motor vehicle accident	6 months	Suprapubic cystotomy	None
Case 5	5 years old	Motor vehicle accident	2 years	Suprapubic cystotomy	None

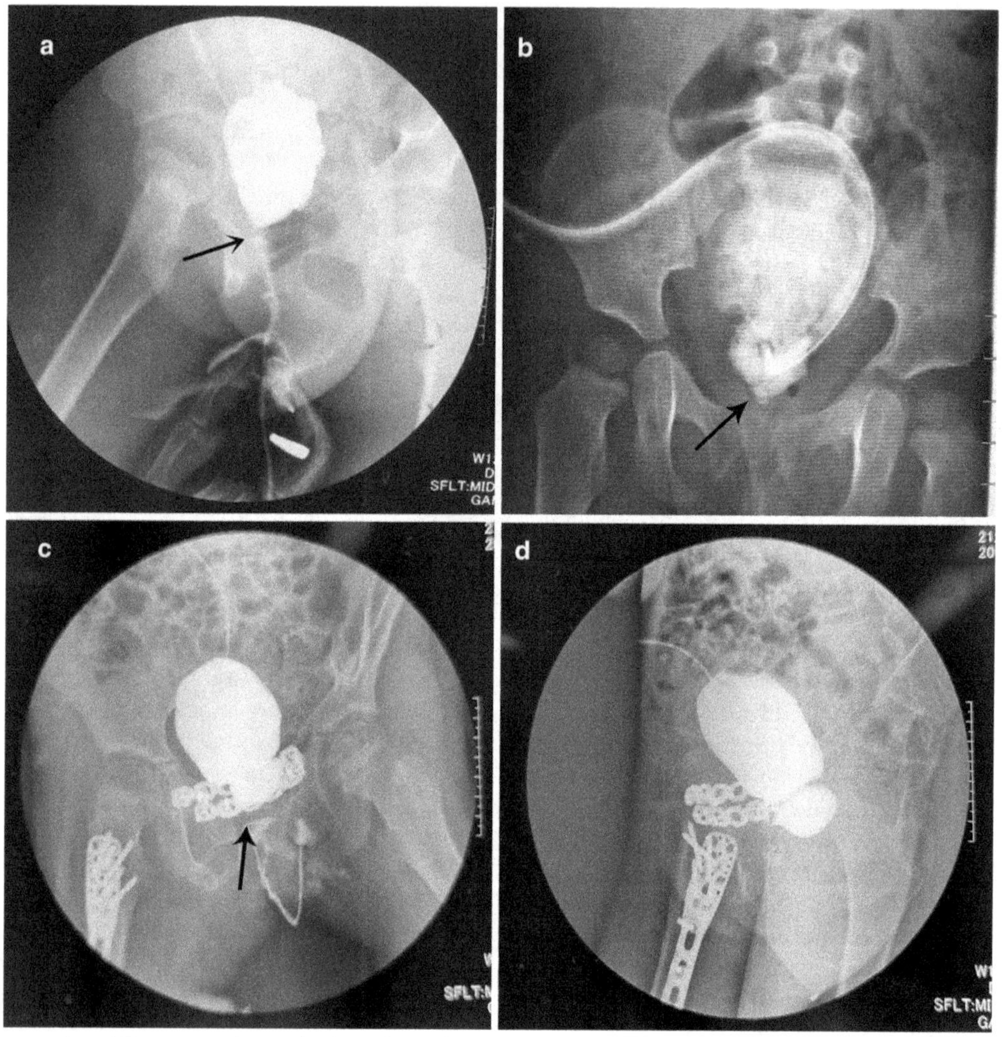

Fig. 1 **a–c** Preoperative voiding cystourethrography showed completely atresia of bladder neck; **d** preoperative voiding cystourethrography showed vesicovaginal fistula

Cystourethrography indicated good continuity of the urethra (Fig. 3). Two girls had urinary incontinence postoperatively but were continent 3 months later. One patient developed vesical-abdominal fistula due to multiple surgical experiences and poor healing of abdominal incision. The fistula got repaired by surgery 6 months later and she was continent ever since. Other complications were not observed during the follow-up period.

Discussion

Female urethral injuries caused by pelvic fracture is a rare occurrence because the female urethral is short and has a good mobility in the pelvic. As for children, the skeletally immature pelvis is more plastic and flexible because there is a more percentage of cartilage, a more porous cortical bone, and the pubic symphysis and sacroiliac joints are more elastic [1], hence the pelvic absorbs higher energy during trauma. Also, girl's bladder neck and urethra are more vulnerable because the relative higher position in the pelvis [2], which may explain why the proportion of girls urethral injuries is higher than female adults in the current literature [3]. Although rare, the management of female pelvic fracture urethral injuries is complex and there is no guideline yet.

For the diagnosis of bladder and urethral injury in those patients, their genitourinary injuries were often ignored in the emergency room during the primary trauma, unless there were symptoms of hematuria and vaginal bleeding, cause patient's vitals and life-threatening risks were put in the first place. Black et al. [4] report in their study that nearly 25% of these patients were diagnosed with urinary injuries accidentally during

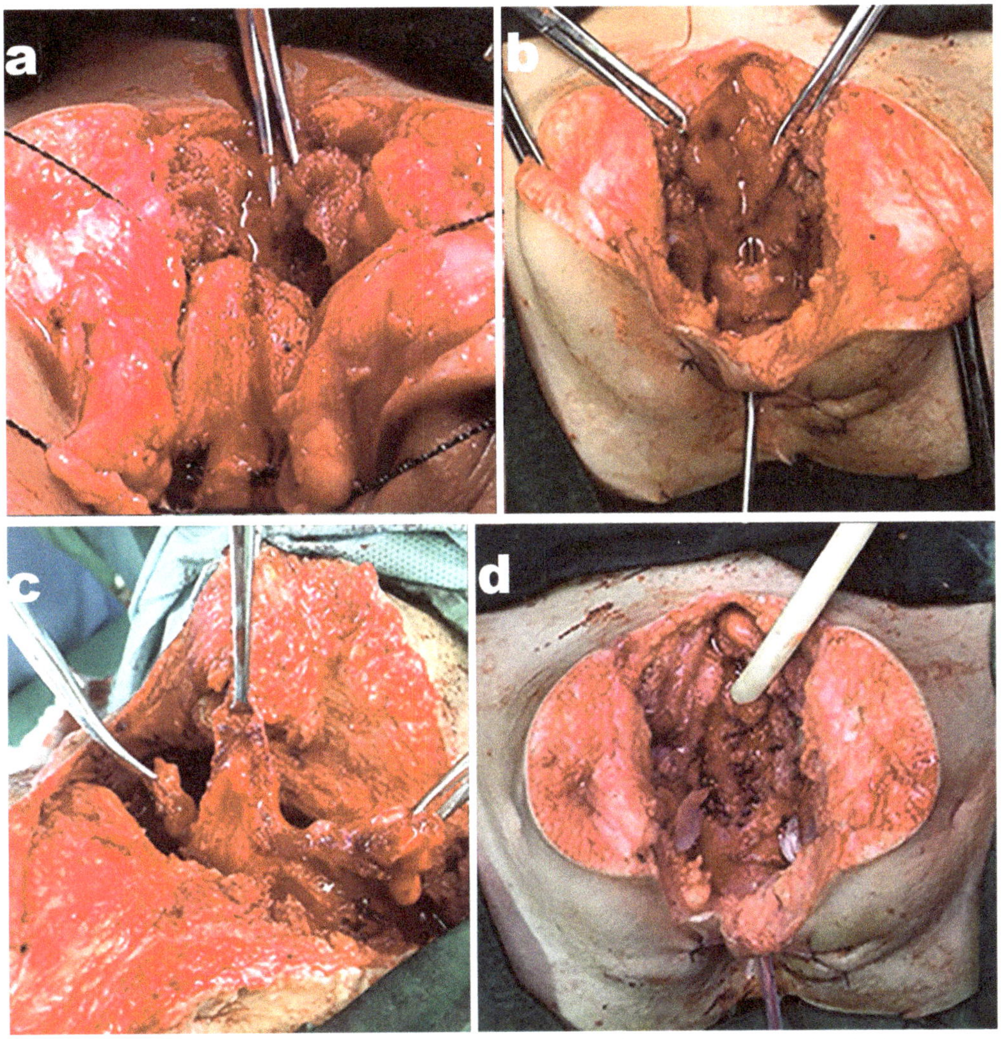

Fig. 2 **a** Pubectomy with Gigli saw; **b** the defect between the atresic bladder neck and the obstructed proximal urethra is 1 cm; **c** acquiring the bladder flap from the anterior bladder wall; **d** reconstruction of the bladder neck and proximal urethra

surgical exploration. Hence we recommend a careful physical examination in the emergency room, and unstable patients might need lower genitourinary tract imaging [5]. Even diagnosed, most patients were dealt with suprapubic cystotomy. In our cases, all the patients had suprapubic cystotomy after the trauma happened, preoperative cystourethrography showed bladder neck atresia and urethral distraction. We also advise that urethroscopy is needed to know the lesions of bladder and rule out genitourinary fistula. Because of partial healing and fibrosis of their urethral injury, the bladder neck is completely atresic, and the restoration of urinary tract continuity and continence became rather tricky.

Casselman et al. [6] reported the first case of traumatic complete disruption of the female membranous urethra in the English literature in 1977, the patient was a 2.5 years old girl with an approximately 1 cm avulsion of urethra at the urogenital diaphragm, Casselman drawn down the bladder and the urethra and anastomosed, but after 8 weeks the girl had urethral stricture and the problem was solved by urethral dilation. Direct anastomosis of the urethra would most likely lead to stricture, the missing part of urethra needs to be replaced. Vaginal flap and buccal mucosal graft urethroplasty were more reported and used for female urethral reconstruction, while these techniques are more suitable for female urethral stricture and small urethral loss. For long urethral defect or proximal urethral injuries bladder wall flaps can be adopted for urethroplasty [7–9].The female urethral replacement is mainly accomplished by anterior bladder wall (Tanagho) tube or tubularization of vaginal mucosa [10]. Tanagho was first to bring up the technique of reconstructing bladder neck with tubular anterior bladder flap in 1981 [11]. Nayyar et al. [12] reported their technique

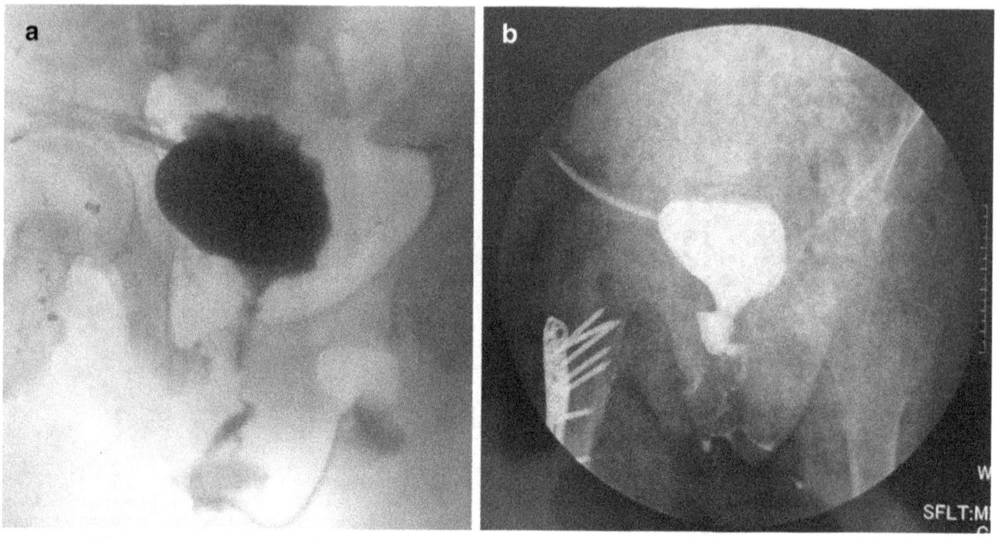

Fig. 3 Post-operative voiding cystourethrography showed good continuity of urethra and a wide bladder neck

of a novel anterior bladder tube for the treatment of traumatic bladder neck contracture based on Tanagho technique. Their report included 3 female patients with good results, which also need further followup and more literature report. For surgical access, we took the combined vaginal and transpubic access, it is recognized that combined vaginal-partial transpubic access is a dependable method for female pediatric patients with complicated bladder neck and urethral trauma after pelvic fracture [13]. These pediatric female patients all came to our institution with suprapubic catheter, the intervals since their primary trauma are mostly over 6 months, the bladder neck is obliterated by scar tissues and the urethra is atresic, hence the transpubic access provides the maximum operation field and we took total pubectomy to get access to the bladder neck. With combined vaginal approach, the distal urethra is located and urethrovaginal fistulas were repaired. Through the T shape incision of the anterior bladder, two well-vascularized and free flaps are acquired. Giving that the fundus of bladder neck is generally existed in those patients, we used the bladder flap to augment the ventral part of bladder neck and then anastomosed it with distal urethra. Thus, the bladder neck and proximal urethra were expanded, decreasing the chance of further stricture.

Controversy also exist in the surgical repair timing. Black et al. [4] indicated that the bladder neck injury should be repaired primarily because it is crucial in continence. Patel et al. [3] did a systematically review of the literature about female urethral injuries associated with pelvic fracture, their results showed that patients who had primary alignment were more likely to have urethral stenosis and fistula. From our perspective, patients who had extensive urethra injury often accomplished by serious damage of other organs, the principle is to deal with life-threatening risks first, so the patients were mostly managed with suprapubic cystotomy and deferred repair [14].

The mechanism of female continence is not completely clarified yet. It is generally thought that the female urinary continence mechanism is mainly made of the urinary sphincter complex, bladder trigone and the pelvic floor. The urinary sphincter complex includes the inner smooth muscle layer and the external striated muscle layer. The smooth muscle layer mainly locates at the level of bladder neck and the external striated sphincter muscle covers from the bladder neck to proximal urethra. Hence the bladder neck is of great importance in urinary continence. The urethral smooth muscle is under sympathetic control while the striated muscle is mostly under voluntary control. The running of autonomic nerve fibers is near lateral vaginal walls. The innervation of striated muscle transverses the pelvic and enters the caudal third of the urethra laterally [15–21]. The bladder musculature has 3 different muscular layers and forms the internal urethral sphincter at bladder neck. Bladder and urethral muscles have β-adrenergic inhibitory receptors and α-adrenergic excitatory receptors, which can lead to the relaxation and contraction of these muscles [16, 22, 23]. The muscular distribution and neuroreceptors of bladder is thought to promote continence in bladder flap urethral reconstruction [11]. In Tanagho technique and existed studies adopting the method of bladder wall flap urethroplasty, the stenosis bladder neck was transected and the fibrous tissues were completely excised, which we think might sacrifice some function of the bladder neck [10, 11, 14, 24]. An intact bladder neck is crucial to continence, not only because it is where the detrusor locate at and it's sphincteric, but also because it is where the autonomic nerve and somatic nerve converge. In our surgical procedure, we just incised the atresia bladder neck and used the bladder flap as a patch to expand it. More importantly the dorsal part of bladder neck was preserved, which we thought might favor for continence because more nerve fibers and the intactness of bladder neck might get saved in this way.

Conclusions

Our method of bladder neck reconstruction using bladder flap as a patch is feasible and provides good continence, especially for those with serious bladder neck avulsion and urethral rupture caused by extensive trauma and those who had posttraumatic urethral distraction needed second repair.

Acknowledgements

The authors wish to express their gratitude to all the participants for their sincere cooperation.

Authors' contributions

YLS. contributed primarily to the Conception, Design; RL., LW., HQS., CRJ contributed to the performing of the research; RL. contributed to interpreting the data and writing the manuscript. All authors have read and approved the manuscript.

Author details

Department of Urology, Shanghai Jiao Tong University Affiliated Sixth People's Hospital, Shanghai, China. [2] Department of Urology, Shanghai Children's Hospital, Shanghai Jiao Tong University, Shanghai, China. [3] Shanghai Eastern Institute of Urologic Reconstruction, Shanghai, China.

References:

1. de la Calva C, Jover N, Alonso J, Salom M. Pediatric pelvic fractures and differences compared with the adult population. Pediatr Emerg Care. 2018.
2. Delaney KM, Reddy SH, Dayama A, Stone ME Jr, Meltzer JA. Risk factors associated with bladder and urethral injuries in female children with pelvic fractures: an analysis of the National Trauma Data Bank. J Trauma Acute Care Surg. 2016;80(3):472–6.
3. Patel DN, Fok CS, Webster GD, Anger JT. Female urethral injuries associated with pelvic fracture: a systematic review of the literature. BJU Int. 2017;120(6):766–73.
4. Black PC, Miller EA, Porter JR, Wessells H. Urethral and bladder neck injury associated with pelvic fracture in 25 female patients. J Urol. 2006;175(6):2140–4.
5. Tarman GJ, Kaplan GW, Lerman SL, McAleer IM, Losasso BE. Lower genitourinary injury and pelvic fractures in pediatric patients. Urology. 2002;59(1):123–6.
6. Casselman RC, Schillinger JF. Fractured pelvis with avulsion of the female urethra. J Urol. 1977;117(3):385–6.
7. Agochukwu-Mmonu N, Srirangapatanam S, Cohen A, Breyer B. Female urethral strictures: review of diagnosis, etiology, and management. Curr Urol Rep. 2019;20(11):74.
8. Waterloos M, Verla W. Female urethroplasty: a practical guide emphasizing diagnosis and surgical treatment of female urethral stricture disease. Biomed Res Int. 2019;2019:6715257.
9. Faiena I, Koprowski C, Tunuguntla H. Female urethral reconstruction. J Urol. 2016;195(3):557–67.
10. Wadie BS, Elhifnawy A, Khair AA. Reconstruction of the female urethra: versatility, complexity and aptness. J Urol. 2007;177(6):2205–10.
11. Tanagho EA. Bladder neck reconstruction for total urinary incontinence: 10 years of experience. J Urol. 1981;125(3):321–6.
12. Nayyar R, Jain S, Sharma K, Pethe S, Kumar P. A novel anterior bladder tube for traumatic bladder neck contracture in females: initial results. Urology. 2020;139:201–6.
13. Podesta ML, Jordan GH. Pelvic fracture urethral injuries in girls. J Urol. 2001;165(5):1660–5.
14. Hemal AK, Dorairajan LN, Gupta NP. Posttraumatic complete and partial loss of urethra with pelvic fracture in girls: an appraisal of management. J Urol. 2000;163(1):282–7.
15. Ashton-Miller JA, DeLancey JO. Functional anatomy of the female pelvic floor. Ann N Y Acad Sci. 2007;1101:266–96.
16. Unger CA, Tunitsky-Bitton E, Muffly T, Barber MD. Neuroanatomy, neurophysiology, and dysfunction of the female lower urinary tract: a review. Female Pelvic Med Reconstr Surg. 2014;20(2):65–75.
17. Mistry MA, Klarskov N, DeLancey JO, Lose G. A structured review on the female urethral anatomy and innervation with an emphasis on the role of the urethral longitudinal smooth muscle. Int Urogynecol J. 2019.
18. Yucel S, Baskin LS. An anatomical description of the male and female urethral sphincter complex. J Urol. 2004;171(5):1890–7.
19. Colleselli K, Stenzl A, Eder R, Strasser H, Poisel S, Bartsch G. The female urethral sphincter: a morphological and topographical study. J Urol. 1998;160(1):49–54.
20. Huisman AB. Aspects on the anatomy of the female urethra with special relation to urinary continence. Contrib Gynecol Obstet. 1983;10:1–31.
21. Wiseman OJ, Swinn MJ, Brady CM, Fowler CJ. Maximum urethral closure pressure and sphincter volume in women with urinary retention. J Urol. 2002;167(3):1348–52.
22. DeLancey JO. Structural aspects of the extrinsic continence mechanism. Obstet Gynecol. 1988;72(3 Pt 1):296–301.
23. Andersson KE, Arner A. Urinary bladder contraction and relaxation: physiology and pathophysiology. Physiol Rev. 2004;84(3):935–86.
24. Venn SN, Greenwell TJ, Mundy AR. Pelvic fracture injuries of the female urethra. BJU Int. 1999;83(6):626–30.

3

Proteomic analysis of bladder biopsies from interstitial cystitis/bladder pain syndrome patients with and without Hunner's lesions reveals differences in expression of inflammatory and structural proteins

Elijah P. Ward[1], Sarah N. Bartolone[1], Michael B. Chancellor[1,2], Kenneth M. Peters[1,2] and Laura E. Lamb[1,2*]

Abstract

Background: Interstitial cystitis/bladder pain syndrome is a bladder disease usually characterized by pain, urgency, and frequency. Interstitial cystitis is currently classified into two subtypes, with and without Hunner's lesions. However, the underlying etiology of interstitial cystitis and its subtypes are largely unknown.

Methods: To better understand the biological changes in the bladder of interstitial cystitis/bladder pain syndrome patients, we directly analyzed bladder tissue of interstitial cystitis patients, both those with Hunner's lesions and those without. Proteins in the bladder biopsies were analyzed using nanoscale high-performance liquid chromatography-tandem mass spectrometry. Disease subgroups were compared and significantly expressed proteins were mapped using STRING to determine protein associations and functions.

Results: We found that patients with Hunner's lesions had significant increases in inflammatory and endoplasmic reticulum stress proteins, with a decrease in cellular adhesive proteins, compared to patients without Hunner's lesions. These patients also exhibited a decrease in proteins associated with the Rap1 signaling pathway, which regulates cell proliferation and wound healing. When comparing diseased and non-disease-apparent tissue in patients with Hunner's lesions, diseased tissue exhibited a decrease in ubiquitination proteins.

Conclusions: In summary, there are significant differences in protein expression found in the bladders of interstitial cystitis patients with and without Hunner's lesions, indicating a disturbance in proteins associated with cellular adhesion, proliferation, protein processing, and wound healing.

Keywords: Interstitial cystitis, Proteomics, HPLC, Urinary bladder

Background

Interstitial cystitis (IC) is a disease of the bladder that can be characterized by urinary frequency, urgency, pelvic pressure, and pain in the absence of a urinary tract infection. The projected incidence of IC varies, ranging from 45 per 100,000 to as many as 307 per 100,000 individuals [1, 2]. However, the incidence may be higher than estimated as IC is commonly misdiagnosed. The

*Correspondence: Laura.Lamb@Beaumont.org
[1] Department of Urology, Beaumont Health System, 3811 W. 13 Mile Road, Suite 504, Royal Oak, MI 48073, USA
Full list of author information is available at the end of the article

pathogenicity of IC is currently unknown, though multiple theories have been proposed [3]. There are two IC/BPS subtypes, the first is IC/BPS with Hunner's lesions (HIC; also known as Hunner's ulcers), representing 5–10% of IC/BPS patients [4]. HIC is diagnosed via cystoscopy and is characterized by areas of increased inflammation and cellular degradation. HIC patients often have more severe symptoms, including increased pain, sensitivity, and changes in bladder permeability [5]. The second subtype is IC/BPS without Hunner's lesions (NHIC). NHIC is difficult to diagnose given the lack of clear physiological changes; patients may or may not have areas of submucosal glomerulations, or small areas of submucosal bleeding in the bladder wall distinct from Hunner's lesions. As a result, diagnosis is mainly based on exclusion of other conditions with similar symptoms [6].

While IC/BPS is a widely studied urological condition, the molecular differences between healthy patients, NHIC and HIC remain poorly understood. Several studies have illustrated that IC bladders, compared to healthy bladders, display decreased cellular proliferation and cell permeability [7, 8]. Additionally, biomarker studies have identified distinct differences between HIC and NHIC bladders; urine from HIC patients have higher concentrations of inflammatory cytokines and urothelial breakdown products [9]. The differences between diseased and non-disease-apparent (NDA) areas within one bladder also remains unknown. Therefore, the goal of our study is to use nanoscale high performance liquid chromatography coupled to tandem mass spectrometry (nHPLC-MS/MS) on bladder biopsies of diseased and NDA tissue to identify distinct protein differences between NHIC and HIC. This method is highly sensitive, which is beneficial when working with limited sample volume, such as bladder biopsies. This is the first time nHPLC-MS/MS has been used to examine IC bladders directly. Using this innovative approach, we found that HIC patients exhibit increased inflammatory proteins and decreased cellular adhesion proteins in the urothelium, as well as increased ER stress, suggesting a possible difference in disease etiology between HIC and NHIC.

Methods

Sample collection and storage

This study was approved by the institutional IRB (IRB# 2009-218) and written consent for all participants was obtained. Disease state was determined during cystoscopy by a trained urologist. Bladder samples were obtained from 4 female patients with HIC and 4 female patients with NHIC during routine medical cystoscopy. Two biopsies were collected from each patient: one from a diseased site (glomerulations in NHIC patients, Hunner's lesions in HIC patients), and another from an adjacent non-disease-apparent (NDA) site as determined by an experienced urologist. 5 mm × 5 mm samples of bladder tissue were snap-frozen and stored at −80 °C. Patients were asked to complete the validated Interstitial Cystitis Symptom Index and Problem Index (ICSI/ICPI) to measure lower urinary tract symptoms (LUTS) and impact on patient quality of life (QOL) [10]. ICSI scores range from 0 to 19 and ICPI scores range from 0 to 16, with higher scores representing more severe symptoms and impact [3].

Sample processing

Deidentified samples were sent to MSBioworks for processing and analysis. Samples were blinded and randomized to the researchers. Samples were washed in 1 × PBS and mechanically disrupted in a Bullet Blender (NextAdvance) with 1.6 mm stainless steel beads in 100μL of modified RIPA lysis buffer (2% SDS, 150 mM NaCl, 50 mM Tris pH 8, 1X Roche complete protease inhibitor). Samples were incubated at 60 °C for 30 min, then clarified by centrifugation. The protein concentration of each extract was determined by Qubit fluorometry (Invitrogen). 10 μg of each sample was processed by SDS-PAGE using a 10% Bis–Tris NuPage mini-gel (Invitrogen) in the MES buffer system. The migration window (2 cm lane) for each sample was excised into ten equally sized bands, each was processed by in-gel digestion with trypsin using a ProGest robot (DigiLab). Samples were first washed with 25 mM ammonium bicarbonate, followed by acetonitrile. Samples were reduced with 10 mM dithiothreitol at 60 °C, followed by alkylation with 50 mM iodoacetamide at room temperature. Digestion was performed with trypsin at 37 °C for 4 h. Finally, samples were quenched with formic acid and the supernatant was analyzed via nHPLC-MS/MS.

Liquid chromatography and mass spectrometry

Sample supernatants were analyzed by nHPLC-MS/MS with a NanoAcquity HPLC system (Waters) linked to a Q Exactive mass spectrometer (ThermoFisher). Digested proteins were loaded on a Luna C18 resin (Phenomenex) trapping column and eluted over a Luna C18 resin 75 μm analytical column at a flow rate of 350 nL/min. The mass spectrometer was operated in data-dependent mode, with the Orbitrap operating at 70,000 FWHM for MS and 17,500 FWHM for MS/MS. The fifteen most abundant ions were selected for MS/MS.

Data processing and statistical analysis

Data was analyzed using Mascot with the following parameters: the database used was SwissProt Human (concatenated forward and reverse plus common contaminants), with the enzyme set to Trypsin/P. Fixed modifications were set to Carbamidomethyl (C), while variable modifications included Acetyl (N-term), Deamidation (N,Q), Oxidation (M), and Pyro-Glu (N-term Q). Mass values were monoisotopic. Peptide and Fragment Mass Tolerances were 10 ppm and 0.02 Da, respectively. 2 max missed cleavages were allowed. After Mascot processing, data was parsed into Scaffold for validation and filtering. Data were filtered using a 1% protein and peptide false discovery rate (FDR) while requiring at least 2 unique peptides per protein. To determine approximate relative abundance of proteins within a given sample and between samples, normalized spectral abundance factor (NSAF) was calculated based on the following equation:

$$NSAF = (SpC/MW)/\Sigma(SpC/MW)_N$$

where SpC = Spectral Counts, MW = Protein Molecular Weight (in kDa), and N = Total Number of Proteins. Significant proteins were determined by comparing average NSAF values for diseased and adjacent NDA tissues to generate fold change values, as well as a T-test for significance. Proteins were considered significant if they had a fold change difference ≥ 4 and a p value ≤ 0.05. Interactions and relationships between these proteins were mapped using STRING. Proteins were connected by function and interaction, with interactions predicted by experimental data, database searches, text mining, and co-expression.

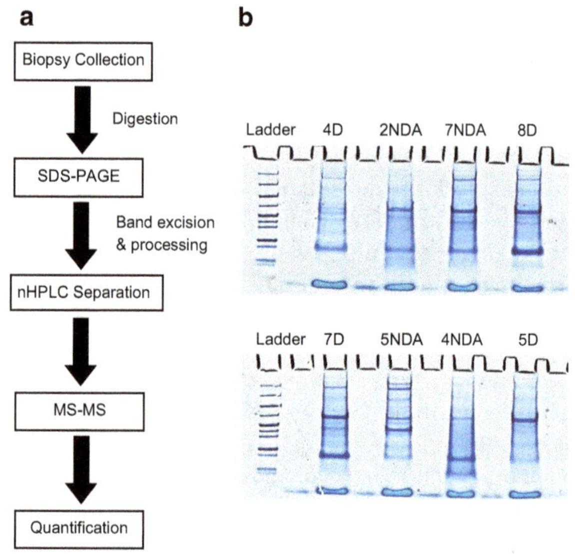

Fig. 1 Experimental workflow of IC bladder biopsies. **a** Patient biopsies were digested and separated by SDS-PAGE before analysis via nHPLC-MS/MS. Data was searched using Mascot, and a list of detected proteins was created for each sample. Significant proteins were mapped for associations and shared function via STRING. **b** 10 μg of digested bladder tissue was loaded onto an SDS-PAGE and separated. Bands were excised and digested prior to nHPLC-MS/MS. Samples were blinded and randomized to avoid bias. Patient number corresponds to patient number in Table 1. D = Disease tissue biopsy; NDA = Non-disease apparent tissue biopsy

STRING mapping

Significant proteins were uploaded to STRING [11] (string-db.org) and mapped to predict protein–protein interactions, represented by colored lines between protein nodes. These relationships include known interactions determined by experiments (purple) and database mining (teal), predicted interactions via gene neighborhood (green), co-occurrence (blue), or gene fusion (red), or from text mining (yellow), co-expression (black), or protein homology (light blue).

Table 1 Patient demographics

Patient #	Age	Gender	IC subtype	ICSI score	ICPI score
1	60	F	HIC	19	16
2	79	F	HIC	15	16
3	71	F	HIC	N/A	N/A
4	55	F	HIC	18	15
5	36	F	NHIC	10	9
6	63	F	NHIC	19	16
7	43	F	NHIC	11	13
8	53	F	NHIC	15	12

Results

Our group was interested in understanding the differences in protein expression between bladder biopsies from HIC and NHIC patients These biopsies were processed and analyzed via nHPLC-MS/MS (Fig. 1), resulting in 2,625 unique proteins identified between all patient samples. Patients also completed the ICSI and ICPI questionnaires, with HIC patients reporting higher average scores than NHIC patients (Table 1). This is consistent with what has been previously reported. When comparing protein of interest between subgroups, we focused on proteins that showed a fold change of $\geq 4\times$ and a significant difference between groups (e.g. $p \leq 0.05$).

Diseased areas in HIC patients exhibit decreased expression of ubiquitination proteins compared to NDA areas in HIC patients

First, we compared diseased areas of HIC tissue to NDA areas of HIC bladders to determine protein differences. 18 proteins were found to be significantly altered when comparing NDA to diseased HIC tissues. Three of these proteins were linked to ubiquitination (Table 2).

Table 2 Diseased Hunner's IC biopsies compared to non-disease-apparent Hunner's IC biopsies

Accession ID	Gene name	Description	Fold change	*p* value ($p \leq 0.05$)
		Ubiquitination (down-regulated) *3 of 18 significant proteins*	NDA HIC/diseased HIC	
P68036	*UBE2L3*	Ubiquitin-conjugating enzyme E2 L3	7.565	0.0119
P63279	*UBE2I*	SUMO-conjugating enzyme UBC9	7.288	0.0347
Q7Z6Z7	*HUWE1*	E3 ubiquitin-protein ligase	6.997	0.0040

Diseased areas in NHIC patients show minimal changes in protein composition when compared to NDA areas

Comparing diseased areas of NHIC bladder tissue to NDA areas revealed 13 proteins were significant. These proteins function in various stages of peptide and lipid metabolism, as well as partial function in cytoskeleton organization.

Areas of disease in HIC patients show increased expression of inflammatory proteins and decreased expression of cellular adhesion proteins compared to areas of disease in NHIC patients

Next, we compared diseased areas of HIC patients with diseased areas of NHIC patients. 34 proteins were found to be significantly increased when comparing diseased HIC tissue to diseased NHIC tissue. STRING's protein mapping (Fig. 2) revealed that ten of these proteins are involved in immune response and are associated with inflammatory diseases, such as asthma and type I diabetes mellitus, while nine of these proteins are associated with protein processing in the endoplasmic reticulum (ER) (Table 3). In addition, five proteins involved in collagen formation and cellular adhesion were significantly decreased in HIC patients compared to NHIC patients (Table 3).

NDA areas in HIC patients exhibit decreased expression of protein metabolism and Rap1 signaling proteins compared to NDA areas in NHIC patients

Finally, we sought to compare NDA tissues of HIC patients with NDA tissue of NHIC patients. 50 proteins were found to be significantly altered when comparing NDA NHIC tissue to NDA HIC tissue. STRING's protein mapping (Fig. 3) revealed nine proteins involved in protein metabolism and four proteins linked to the Rap1 signaling pathway, which is involved in cell proliferation and adhesion, as well as three proteins involved in the immune response (Table 4).

Discussion

To better understand the underlying mechanisms of disease in IC, we sought to determine differences in protein expression between patients with HIC and NHIC. To accomplish this, we collected tissue biopsies from diseased and non-disease apparent areas (NDA) of the bladder from four female patients with HIC and four female patients with NHIC. The tissue samples were processed, and nHPLC-MS/MS was used to analyze the protein compositions. We found significant differences in protein expression in bladder biopsies between patients with HIC and NHIC. Diseased HIC tissues showed a decrease in proteins involved in ubiquitination compared to NDA HIC tissues. Diseased NHIC compared to NDA NHIC tissues showed few differences, mainly in lipid and peptide metabolism. Diseased HIC patient tissues, when compared to diseased NHIC tissues, showed an increase in proteins involved with ER stress and inflammatory response, with a decrease in cell adhesion proteins. Finally, NDA HIC patient tissues also showed a decrease in immune cell adhesion proteins compared to NDA NHIC tissues.

Within the same patient and bladder, the diseased HIC tissue samples had decreased expression of ubiquitination pathway proteins compared to NDA HIC tissue samples. Ubiquitination is a posttranslational modification and plays an important role in regulation of multiple protein pathways, including membrane trafficking and protein turnover involving the ER [12]. Ubiquitination is also important for wound healing and angiogenesis, as well as protein metabolism [13]. This data suggests that the diseased areas of HIC bladders are impaired in their ability to identify and label misfolded or damaged proteins for intracellular proteolysis by the proteasome, which may result in the accumulation of damaged proteins, abnormal protein aggregation, and/or inappropriate association with other proteins. This could subsequently influence oxidative and ER stress, inflammation, and apoptosis, as is common for other chronic conditions, especially neurodegenerative disorders, including Alzheimer's, Parkinson's and Huntington's diseases [14].

Comparing diseased and NDA NHIC biopsies revealed 13 significant proteins. These proteins function primarily in peptide (ADE2) and lipid (APOC-III) metabolism, as well as cytoskeletal formation and organization (Spectrin alpha chain). These results imply that there is not as extreme a difference between areas in the same bladder

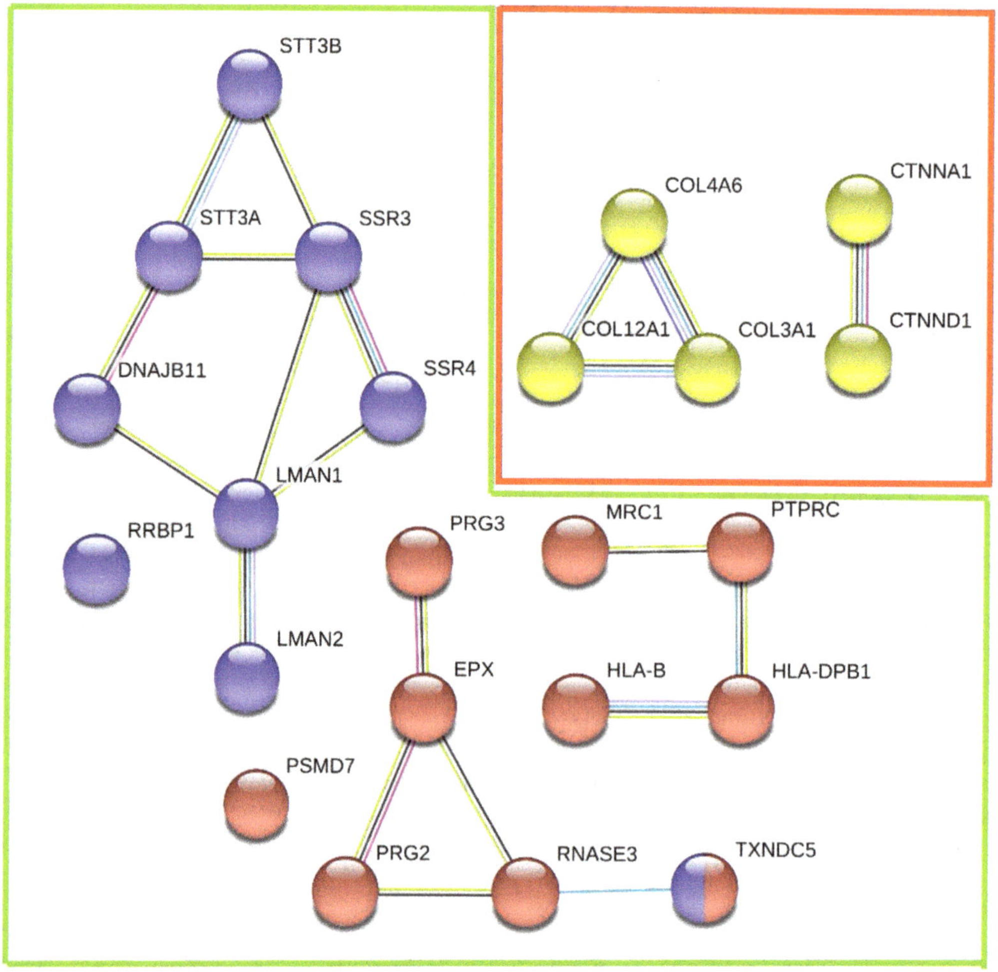

Fig. 2 Diseased HIC samples exhibited increased expression of immune response and ER stress proteins, with a decrease in cellular adhesion proteins. Association map for proteins differentially expressed in diseased Hunner's IC biopsies compared to diseased non-Hunner's IC biopsies. Nodes in the green box represent proteins with increased expression in diseased HIC tissue, while nodes within the red outline represent proteins with decreased expression. Red nodes represent proteins with an immune response function, blue represents ER protein processing/stress response, and yellow represent cellular adhesive proteins. Lines between nodes indicate reported associations as detailed in "Methods" section

of NHIC patients, compared to differences seen in HIC patients. There is also no overlap in significant protein expression between the two comparison groups, which could imply a difference in disease etiology.

Comparing areas of disease in HIC patients to NHIC patients, there was a significant increase in proteins associated with inflammation in HIC. The upregulation of inflammatory proteins may indicate an increased immune response within Hunner's lesions. These proteins have various functions in the mediation of immune processes, including Eosinophil Peroxidase and Tyrosine-Phosphatase C, which had a fold change of 74.7 and 45.9, respectively. These proteins are indicative of increased eosinophil and leukocyte activity. Other immune cell proteins increased in HIC tissue are known to be expressed by monocytes. This increased expression of immune cells is consistent with prior research, as the literature suggests that HIC may have an immune response component [15, 16].

Diseased HIC bladder tissue also showed an increase in proteins involved with ER stress when compared to diseased NHIC tissues. ER stress is a cellular response to improperly folded proteins or high cellular secretory load and may lead to cell death. An increase in the concentration of ER stress proteins in the biopsies of HIC patients may suggest impaired protein processing, which can lead to inflammation and apoptosis. A study in rats with protamine/lipopolysaccharide-induced IC noted an increase in ER stress biomarkers post-procedure, suggesting a link between IC and ER stress [13]. Diseased HIC tissues

Table 3 Diseased Hunner's IC biopsies compared to diseased non-Hunner's IC biopsies

Accession ID	Gene Name	Description	Fold change ($FC \geq 4$)	*p* value ($p \leq 0.05$)
		Immune and inflammatory response (up-regulated) *10 of 34 significant proteins*	Diseased HIC/diseased NHIC	
P11678	*EPX*	Eosinophil peroxidase	74.7	0.0184
P08575	*PTPRC*	Tyrosine phosphatase C	45.9	0.0163
P12724	*RNASE3*	Eosinophil cationic protein	19.6	0.0072
P13727	*PRG2*	Bone marrow proteoglycan precursor	13.6	0.0046
P01889	*HLA-B*	HLA class I histocompatibility antigen, B-41	10.5	0.0011
P51665	*PSMD7*	26S proteasome non-ATPase regulatory subunit	9.16	0.0481
P04440	*HLA-DPB1*	HLA class II histocompatibility antigen, DP beta 1 chain	6.77	0.0079
Q8NBS9	*TXNDC5*	Thioredoxin domain-containing protein 5	5.55	0.0065
P22897	*MRC1*	Mannose-receptor C-type 1	5.91	0.0303
Q9Y2Y8	*PRG3*	Proteoglycan 3	4.46	0.0038
		ER protein processing & ER stress (up-regulated) *9 of 34 significant proteins*		
Q8TCJ2	*STT3B*	Dolichyl-diphosphooligosaccharide-protein glycosyltransferase subunit STT3B	22.2	0.026
Q9UNL2	*SSR3*	Translocon-associated protein subunit gamma	13.6	0.0135
Q2P2E9	*RRBP1*	Ribisome-binding protein 1	11.2	0.0119
Q9UBS4	*DNAJB11*	DnaJ Homolong subfamily B member 11	11.1	0.0008
P46977	*STT3A*	Dolichyl-diphosphooligosaccharide-protein glycosyltransferase subunit STT3A	8.79	0.0248
P49257	*LMAN1*	Protein ERGIC-53	5.97	0.0244
Q8NBS9	*TXDNC5*	Thioredoxin domain-containing protein 5	5.55	0.0065
Q12907	*LMAN2*	Vesicular integral-membrane protein VIP36	5.27	0.0028
P51571	*SSR4*	Translocon-associated protein subunit delta	4.04	0.0091
		Cellular adhesion (down-regulated) *5 of 42 significant proteins*	Diseased NHIC/Diseased HIC	
Q14031	*COL4A6*	Collagen alpha-6(IV)	12.6	0.0144
P35221	*CTNNA1*	Catenin alpha-1	9.54	0.0005
O60716	*CTNND1*	Catenin delta-1	5.69	0.0288
P02461	*COL3A1*	Collagen alpha-1(III)	4.62	0.0039
Q99715	*COL12A1*	Collagen alpha-1(XII)	4.46	8.13e-5

also showed decreased expression of cellular adhesive proteins, including multiple collagen (collagen alpha-1, collagen alpha-6) and catenin (catenin alpha-1, catenin delta-1) subtypes. These results could imply a weakening of the urothelial lining of the bladder and loss of the barrier function, exposing underlying cell layers to irritants and possibly explaining in part the pain symptoms of patients. Increased ER stress proteins and decreased cellular adhesion proteins in HIC bladders further suggest that the diseased areas of HIC patients are more disrupted and compromised than the diseased areas of NHIC, and also why focal treatment of these areas in HIC can lead to at least temporary symptom relief.

NDA bladder biopsies of HIC patients showed decreased expression of proteins involved in peptide metabolism and protein processing when compared to NDA biopsies from NHIC patients. These patients also showed a decrease in proteins related to Rap1 signaling. The Rap1 signaling pathway controls cell proliferation, cell-to-cell adhesion, and cellular junction formation. The decreased expression of these proteins suggests a weakened cell-to-cell connection in the urothelium of HIC patients and possibly an impaired wound healing response, consistent with the chronic course of IC.

The limitations of this study include the limited number of patient samples, the exclusion of male samples, and the lack of healthy controls. The small number of patient samples reflects the difficultly of obtaining human bladder biopsy samples, which requires an invasive procedure and has some risks including infection and pain. The majority of IC patients are females, therefore we focused on female samples to eliminate gender as a variable. There were several advantages of this study. While other groups have analyzed protein concentrations in

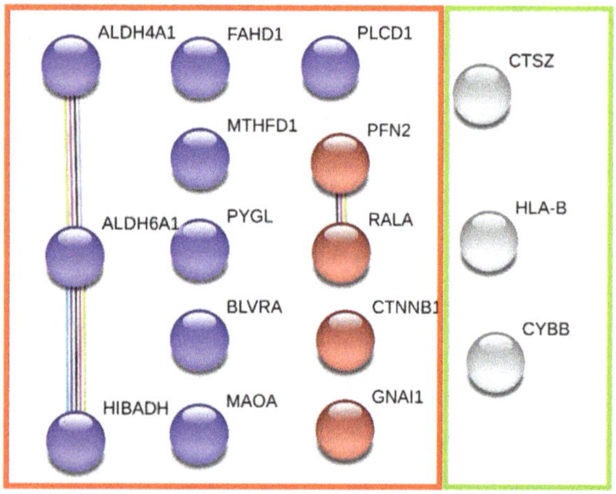

Fig. 3 NDA HIC tissues exhibited increased expression of immune response proteins, with decreased protein expression for Rap1 signaling and general metabolism. Association map for proteins differentially expressed in NDA Hunner's IC biopsies compared to NDA non-Hunner's IC biopsies. Nodes in the green box were increased in NDA HIC samples, while nodes in the red box were decreased. White nodes represent immune response proteins, while blue and red nodes represent protein metabolism and Rap1 signaling proteins, respectively. Lines between nodes indicate reported associations as detailed in "Methods" section

bladder tissue from IC patients [17], this is the first time nHPLC-MS/MS has been used for proteomic analysis of IC bladder tissues; nHPLC-MS/MS uses significantly less material compared to normal HPLC, which is important considering how precious these bladder biopsy samples are [18]. This study also directly examined human bladder tissue samples of IC patients, rather than examining human urine or experimental animal models of interstitial cystitis.

Conclusions

Interstitial cystitis is a disease with unknown etiology. We sought to understand the differences in protein expression in the bladder tissue of patients with two IC subtypes, Hunner's IC and Non-Hunner's IC. To do this, we collected biopsies from four female HIC patients and four female NHIC patients, processed the biopsies, and analyzed them using nHPLC-MS/MS. In the same bladder, diseased HIC tissues showed a decrease in ubiquitination proteins compared to NDA tissues. When comparing between IC subtypes, HIC patients showed significantly increased inflammatory response and ER stress proteins, with a decrease in cellular adhesive proteins and proteins associated with the Rap1 signaling pathway, which regulates cellular adhesion and wound healing. These results indicate that the bladder cells of

Table 4 Non-disease-apparent Hunner's IC biopsies compared to non-disease-apparent Non-Hunner's IC biopsies

Accession ID	Gene name	Description	Fold change (FC ≥ 4)	*p* value ($p \leq 0.05$)
		Immune and inflammatory response (up-regulated) *3 of 11 significant proteins*	NDA HIC/NDA NHIC	
P30479	*HLA-B*	Human leukocyte antigen B	15.6	0.0039
P04839	*CYBB*	Cytochromeb-245 beta chain	8.11	0.0136
Q9UBR2	*CTSZ*	Cathepsin Z	7.88	0.0037
		Protein metabolism (down-regulated) *9 of 50 significant proteins*	NDA NHIC/NDA HIC	
P30038	*ALDH4A1*	Delta-1-pyrroline-5-carboxylate dehydrogenase	17.9	0.0252
P06737	*PYGL*	Glycogen phosphorylase	8.13	0.0316
P31937	*HIBADH*	3-Hydroxyisobutyrate dehydrogenase	7.73	0.0073
P53004	*BLVRA*	Biliverdin reductase A	5.57	0.0316
P51178	*PLCD1*	1-Phosphatidylinositol 4,5-bisphosphate phosphodiesterase delta 1	5.18	0.0093
Q02252	*ALDH6A1*	Methylmalonate-semialdehyde dehydrogenase	4.66	0.0265
Q6P587	*FAHD1*	Acylpyruvase FAHD1	4.61	0.0235
P21397	*MAOA*	Amine oxidase [Flavin-containing] A	4.61	0.0117
P11586	*MTHFD1*	C-1-tetrahydrofolate synthase	4.28	0.0107
		Rap1 Signaling (down-regulated) *4 of 50 significant proteins*	NDA NHIC/NDA HIC	
P11233	*RALA*	Ras-related protein Ral-A	7.11	0.0026
P35080	*PFN2*	Profilin-2	6.49	0.0124
P63096	*GNAI1*	Guanine nucleotide-binding protein G(i) subunit alpha-1	4.23	0.0266
P35222	*CTNNB1*	Catenin beta-1	4.04	0.0118

HIC patients are significantly more disrupted than those of NHIC patients, with increased protein misfolding and decreased cellular adhesion leading to an inflammatory response and painful lesions in the bladder wall which heal slowly. These results are important, as they may lead to a greater understanding of the underlying causes of IC, as well as potential new therapeutic targets for HIC or NHIC.

Abbreviations

D: Disease; IC/BPS: Interstitial cystitis/bladder pain syndrome; HIC: Hunner's interstitial cystitis; NHIC: Non-Hunner's interstitial cystitis; nHPLC-MS/MS: Nano high performance liquid chromatography linked to tandem mass spectrometry; NDA: Non-disease apparent; ICSI: Interstitial Cystitis Symptom Index; ICPI: Interstitial Cystitis Problem Index; MS: Mass spectrometry; MS/MS: Tandem mass spectrometry; NSAF: Normalized spectral abundance factor; ER: Endoplasmic reticulum; HLA: Human leukocyte antigen.

Acknowledgements

The authors would like to thank Dr. Bernadette Zwaans for her critical review of the manuscript and the Beaumont BioBank for sample storage.

Authors' contributions

EW analyzed and interpreted proteomic data, and was the primary contributor in writing the manuscript. SB assisted in analyzing and interpreting proteomic data, and was a contributor in writing the manuscript. MC was a contributor in writing the manuscript. KP planned the study and collected the samples. LL was a contributor in writing the manuscript. All authors read and approved the final manuscript.

Author details

[1] Department of Urology, Beaumont Health System, 3811 W. 13 Mile Road, Suite 504, Royal Oak, MI 48073, USA. [2] Oakland University William Beaumont School of Medicine, Rochester, MI, USA.

References

1. Temml C, Wehrberger C, Riedl C, Ponholzer A, Marszalek M, Madersbacher S. Prevalence and correlates for interstitial cystitis symptoms in women participating in a health screening project. Eur Urol. 2007;51(3):803–8 (**discussion 809**).
2. Parsons JK, Kurth K, Sant GR. Epidemiologic issues in interstitial cystitis. Urology. 2007;69(4 Suppl):5–8.
3. Sant GR. Etiology, pathogenesis, and diagnosis of interstitial cystitis. Rev Urol. 2002;4(Suppl 1):S9–15.
4. Peeker RFM. Toward a precise definition of interstitial cystitis: further evidence of differences in classic and nonulcer disease. J Urol. 2002;167(6):2470–2.
5. Slobodov G, Feloney M, Gran C, Kyker KD, Hurst RE, Culkin DJ. Abnormal expression of molecular markers for bladder impermeability and differentiation in the urothelium of patients with interstitial cystitis. J Urol. 2004;171(4):1554–8.
6. Wein AJ, Hanno PM, Gillenwater JY. Interstitial cystitis: an introduction to the problem. In: Hanno PM, Staskin DR, Krane RJ, Wein AJ, editors. Interstitial cystitis. London: Springer; 1990. p. 3–15.
7. Keay S, Zhang CO, Kagen DI, et al. Concentrations of specific epithelial growth factors in the urine of interstitial cystitis patients and controls. J Urol. 1997;158(5):1983–8.
8. Keay S, Zhang CO, Shoenfelt JL, Chai TC. Decreased in vitro proliferation of bladder epithelial cells from patients with interstitial cystitis. Urology. 2003;61(6):1278–84.
9. Maeda D, Akiyama Y, Morikawa T, et al. Hunner-type (classic) interstitial cystitis: A distinct inflammatory disorder characterized by pancystitis, with frequent expansion of clonal B-cells and epithelial denudation. PLoS ONE. 2015;10(11):e0143316.
10. Brookes ST, Donovan JL, Wright M, Jackson S, Abrams P. A scored form of the Bristol Female Lower Urinary Tract Symptoms questionnaire: data from a randomized controlled trial of surgery for women with stress incontinence. Am J Obstet Gynecol. 2004;191(1):73–82.
11. Szklarczyk D, Gable AL, Lyon D, et al. STRING v11: protein-protein association networks with increased coverage, supporting functional discovery in genome-wide experimental datasets. Nucleic Acids Res. 2019;47(D1):D607–13.
12. Goder V. Roles of ubiquitin in endoplasmic reticulum-associated protein degradation (ERAD). Curr Protein Pept Sci. 2012;13(5):425–35.
13. Wu S, Yao M. Advances in the research of mechanism of protein ubiquitination in wound healing. Zhonghua Shao Shang Za Zhi. 2016;32(2):119–21.
14. Huang Q, Figueiredo-Pereira ME. Ubiquitin/proteasome pathway impairment in neurodegeneration: therapeutic implications. Apoptosis. 2010;15(11):1292–311.
15. Duh K, Funaro MG, DeGouveia W, et al. Crosstalk between the immune system and neural pathways in interstitial cystitis/bladder pain syndrome. Discov Med. 2018;25(139):243–50.
16. Gamper M, Viereck V, Eberhard J, et al. Local immune response in bladder pain syndrome/interstitial cystitis ESSIC type 3C. Int Urogynecol J. 2013;24(12):2049–57.
17. Shie JH, Liu HT, Kuo HC. Increased cell apoptosis of urothelium mediated by inflammation in interstitial cystitis/painful bladder syndrome. Urology. 2012;79(2):484.e487-413.
18. Gama MR, Collins CH, Bottoli CB. Nano-liquid chromatography in pharmaceutical and biomedical research. J Chromatogr Sci. 2013;51(7):694–703.

4

The role of antibody expression and their association with bladder cancer recurrence: A single-centre prospective clinical-pilot study in 35 patients

Peter Ella-Tongwiis[1,2], Rebecca May Lamb[4], Alexander Makanga[3], Iqbal Shergill[1,2,5] and Stephen Fôn Hughes[1,2*]

Abstract

Background: Bladder cancer (BC) is the 10th most common cancer in the UK, with about 10,000 new cases annually. About 75–85% of BC are non-muscle invasive (NMIBC), which is associated with high recurrence and progression rates (50–60% within 7–10 years). There are no routine biomarkers currently available for identifying BC patients at increased risk of developing recurrence. The focus of this research study was to evaluate antibody expression in BC patients and their association with cancer recurrence.

Methods: 35 patients scheduled for TURBT were recruited after written informed consent. Ethical approval for the project was granted via IRAS (REC4: 14/WA/0033). Following surgical procedure, tissues were preserved in 10% buffered formalin and processed within 24 h in FFPE blocks. 7 sections (4 µm each) were cut from each block and stained for CD31, Human epidermal growth factor receptor-2 (HER-2), S100P, Cyclooxygenase-2 (COX-2), VEGFR-3 thrombomodulin and CEACAM-1 using immunohistochemistry. Clinical outcome measures (obtained via cystoscopy) were monitored for up to 6 months following surgical procedure.

Results: There was significantly increased expression of CD31 ($p<0.001$), HER-2 ($p=0.032$), S100P ($p<0.001$), COX-2 ($p<0.001$), VEGFR-3 ($p<0.001$) and decreased expression of thrombomodulin ($p=0.010$) and CEACAM-1 ($p<0.001$) in bladder tumours compared to normal bladder tissues. HER-2 expression was also significantly associated with cancer grade ($p=0.003$), especially between grade 1 and grade 2 ($p=0.002$) and between grade 1 and grade 3 ($p=0.004$). There was also a significant association between cancer stage and HER-2 expression ($p<0.001$). Although recurrence was significantly associated with cancer grade, there was no association with antibody expression.

Conclusion: Findings from the present study may indicate an alternative approach in the monitoring and management of patients with BC. It is proposed that by allowing urological surgeons access to laboratory markers such as HER-2, Thrombomodulin and CD31 (biomarker profile), potentially, in the future, these biomarkers may be used in addition to, or in combination with, currently used scoring systems to predict cancer recurrence. However, verification and validation of these biomarkers are needed using larger cohorts.

Keywords: Immunohistochemistry, Recurrence, Biomarkers, Bladder

*Correspondence: Stephen.hughes6@wales.nhs.uk

[1] North Wales Clinical Research Centre, Betsi Cadwaladr University Health Board (BCUHB), Wrexham Maelor Hospital, Wrexham, Wales, UK

Full list of author information is available at the end of the article

Background

Globally, there were approximately 549,393 new bladder cancer (BC) diagnoses in 2018 of which about 90% are Transitional cell carcinomas (TCC) [1]. An estimated 80% of TCC are Non-Muscle Invasive (NMIBC) while about 20% are Muscle Invasive BC (MIBC). High recurrence rates in NMIBC means patients are exposed to frequent hospital visits with increased risks of infection and post-operative complications. The Transurethral Resection of the Bladder Tumour (TURBT) is still the main procedure for treatment and diagnosis of BC. Insufficient resection has been associated with an increased risk of early recurrence [2].

Although there is intense ongoing BC-related research, no routinely used biomarkers exist for predicting recurrence following TURBT. Cyclooxygenase-2 (COX-2) plays important roles in the inflammatory response [3] with high expression of COX-2 being reported in high grade and high stage colorectal cancer [4] and endometrial carcinoma [5].

Thrombomodulin is a 74 kDa membrane receptor expressed on endothelial cells with important roles in physiological coagulation, inflammation and cancer promotion [6, 7]. The effects of Thrombomodulin activity in cancer have been linked to its roles in anticoagulation, anti-inflammation and tissue adhesion and proliferation [8].

The S100 proteins are associated with cellular processes such as regulation of cell cycle, growth, transcription and differentiation [9]. It is thought that, when secreted, S100P may have paracrine or autocrine signalling effects [10], while cellular expression of S100P may interact with growth factors and receptors leading to several effects such as proliferation [9]. The association between S100P and cellular processes such as cell survival, proliferation, tumour invasion and angiogenesis have been studied by various researchers [9, 11–13].

As an oncogene, HER2 over-amplification causes tumourigenesis due to activation of signalling pathways such as MAPK [14, 15]. HER2 gene amplification and higher protein expression occurs in about 25% of people with metastatic breast cancer [16].

Even though VEGFR-3 expression is usually located on endothelial cells within the lymphatic system [17] and has been mainly involved in lymphangiogensis [18]. Some studies have observed that any inhibition of VEGFR-3 activity, reduces Angiogenic sprouting and vascular network formation [19]. Due to the high recurrence rates in BC, measurement of VEGF and their receptors may provide useful for predicting recurrence and progression.

Decreased expression, down regulation or loss of CEACAM-1 expression in tumour cells has previously been reported [20, 21]. In hepatocellular carcinoma, loss of CEACAM-1 expression is significantly associated with high grade and poor survival [22].

CD31 plays various roles in angiogenesis, leucocyte migration and activation of integrins [23, 24] and may be secreted, membrane bound or localised intracellularly. Increased CD31 expression has also been associated with worst cancer specific survival [25] and poor prognosis [26].

Findings from the present study may indicate an alternative approach in the monitoring and management of patients with BC. It is proposed that by allowing urological surgeons access to laboratory markers such as HER-2, Thrombomodulin and CD31 (biomarker profile), potentially, in the future, these biomarkers may be used in addition to, or in combination with, currently used scoring systems to predict cancer recurrence. However, verification and validation of these biomarkers are needed using larger cohorts.

Methods

Ethical approval and subject recruitment

Permission for this research study was granted by the Research Ethics Service (REC reference 14/WA/0033). Subjects recruited for this research attended the Betsi Cadwaladr University Health Board (BCUHB) Wrexham Maelor Hospital, North Wales for elective procedures for the treatment/management of BC (Table 1). 35 patients (average age = 74, males = 29 and females = 6) prospective patients scheduled for a Transurethral Resection of the Bladder tumour (TURBT) for the treatment of BC,

Table 1 Demographic and clinical characteristics of recruited subjects

Age (years)	
Mean	74
Median	75
Range	43–95
Sex	
Male	29
Female	6
Cancer stage	
pTa	22
pT1	6
pT2	5
Cancer grade	
Grade 1	9
Grade 2	11
Grade 3	13
Cancer recurrence	
Recurrence	14
No recurrence	21

were recruited into this research study after informed consent.

Tissue preservation, processing and microtomy

Formalin Fixed, Paraffin Embedded (FFPE) tissue blocks of recruited patients were retrieved from storage at the histopathology department of Ysbyty Glan Clwyd, North Wales (UK). At least 12 sections (4 μm each) were cut from each patient tissue block using a microtome, placed on positively charged glass microscope slides and incubated at 60^0 C for at least 30 min before proceeding with IHC. This process enhances adherence of the tissue to the glass slides and ensures stability of the tissue.

Antibodies

Monoclonal anti-CEACAM-1/CD66a (clone: 283324; R&D systems UK), monoclonal anti-CD31 (clone: JC70; cell marque UK), Polyclonal anti-COX-2 (Clone: SP21; cell marque UK), monoclonal anti-HER-2/neu (Clone: 4B5; Roche diagnostics UK), monoclonal anti-S100P (clone: 16/f5; Cell marque UK), monoclonal anti-thrombomodulin (clone: 1009; Cell marque UK) and monoclonal anti-VEGFR-3 (clone: AF349; R&D systems UK) were used in this study. Antibodies were stored and treated according to manufacturer's instructions.

Immunohistochemistry

Tissue slides were dewaxed using 1X EZ prep solution (Ventana Medical Systems, UK), heat and vortex mixing and antigen retrieval was carried out using cell condition 1. VENTANA Antibody Diluent with Casein was used to block endogenous proteins. This was followed by the application of primary antibodies which primarily were mouse and rabbit IgG. The antigens were then visualised using Ventana Ultraview DAB universal detection kit. The slides were then counter stained using Ventana haermatoxylin 1. The slides were washed in warm soapy water to remove residual liquid coverslip (oil) and the then dehydrated in a series of alcohol and DPX mounted on Dako HE autostainer. For each IHC stain, both positive and negative control tissue were used to ensure validity of the results.

Assessing recurrence

In all patients recruited into this research study, follow up data immediately available from follow up clinics was retrieved. This information was obtained from outpatient clinic as well as BCUHB clinical portal.

Investigating the long-term overall survival rates, 5-year and 10-year recurrence and progression data are, however, beyond the scope of this research. However, the short-term information available (up to 2 years post TURBT) will be discussed in relation to the biomarkers measured and may ultimately provide sufficient and accurate clinical data that may help predict or forecast NMIBC recurrence and progression.

Statistical analysis

Statistical analysis was undertaken using SPSS (version 26). With regards to tissue analysis, a chi-square test was performed to determine the difference between antibody staining in bladder tumour cells in comparison with normal urothelium. A Kruskal Wallis test was used to determine the association between clinopathological features (such as cancer grade and stage) and expression. In cases where there was a significant difference, further post-hoc testing was performed using the Mann–Whitney test.

Results

CD31 tissue expression in BC patients

Anti-CD31 primary monoclonal antibody demonstrated cytoplasmic and membranous staining patterns in endothelial cells (Fig. 1). Vascular endothelial cells in BC tissues had significantly higher anti CD31 expression, compared to normal underlying tissues ($X^2(3) = 20.353$, $p < 0.001$), as determined by the Chi-square test. With respect to cancer grading and staging, there was no significant association between patients' cancer grade and CD31 ($X^2(2) = 2.719$, $p = 0.257$), as determined by the Kruskal–Wallis test. However, there was a significant association with cancer stage ($X^2(2) = 12.276$, $p = 0.002$), as determined by the Kruskal–Wallis test.

Thrombomodulin tissue expression in BC patients

The anti-thrombomodulin primary monoclonal antibody used in this study shows membranous staining patterns in BC tissue sections (Fig. 2). Positive membranous staining was reported based on colour intensity and percentage of cells that were expressed. Generally, there was a significantly reduced thrombomodulin in Bladder tumours, compared to normal underlying tissues ($X^2(3) = 11.29$, $p < 0.010$), as determined by the Chi-square test.

With respect cancer grading and staging, there was no significant association between patients' cancer grade and Thrombomodulin ($X^2(2) = 0.380$, $p = 0.83$), as determined by the Kruskal–Wallis test. There was however a significant association between patient's cancer stage and Thrombomodulin ($X^2(2) = 6.50$, $p = 0.039$), as determined by the Kruskal-Wallis test.

HER-2/neu tissue expression in BC patients

The anti-HER-2/neu primary monoclonal antibody used in this study shows membranous staining patterns in BC tissue sections (Fig. 3). Positive membranous staining was reported based on colour intensity and percentage of cells staining positive. Generally, there was a significantly

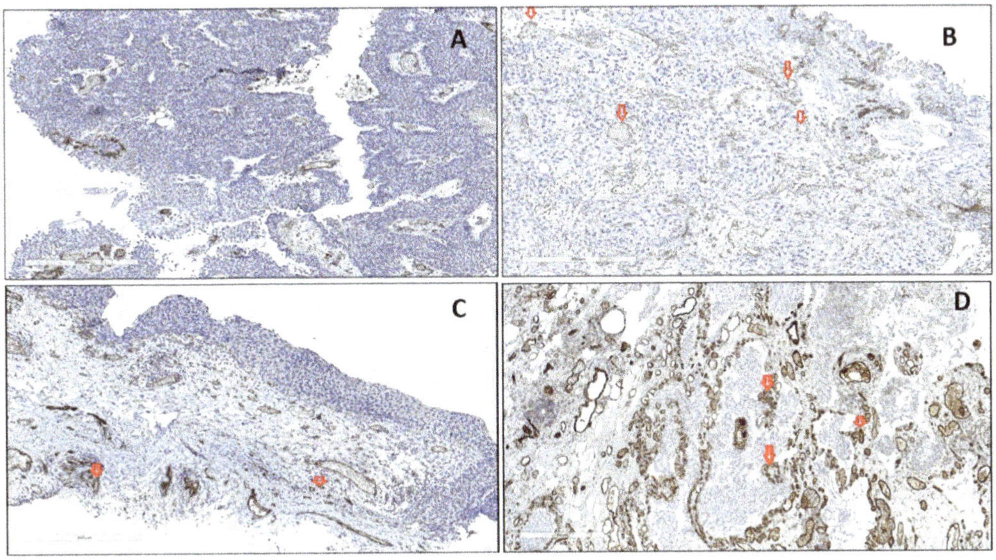

Fig. 1 Anti-CD31 antibody staining in BC tissues. **a** Negative: No staining or positive cytoplasmic/membranous staining in < 5% of VE cells in BC tissues. **b** Positive (+: Weak intensity cytoplasmic/membranous staining in up to 20% of VE cells in BC tissues. **c** Positive (++): Moderate intensity cytoplasmic/membranous staining in 20–50% of VE cells in BC tissues. **d** Positive (+++): Strong cytoplasmic/membranous staining in > 50% of VE cells in BC tissues. DAB detection. ×40 magnification. VE, vascular endothelial

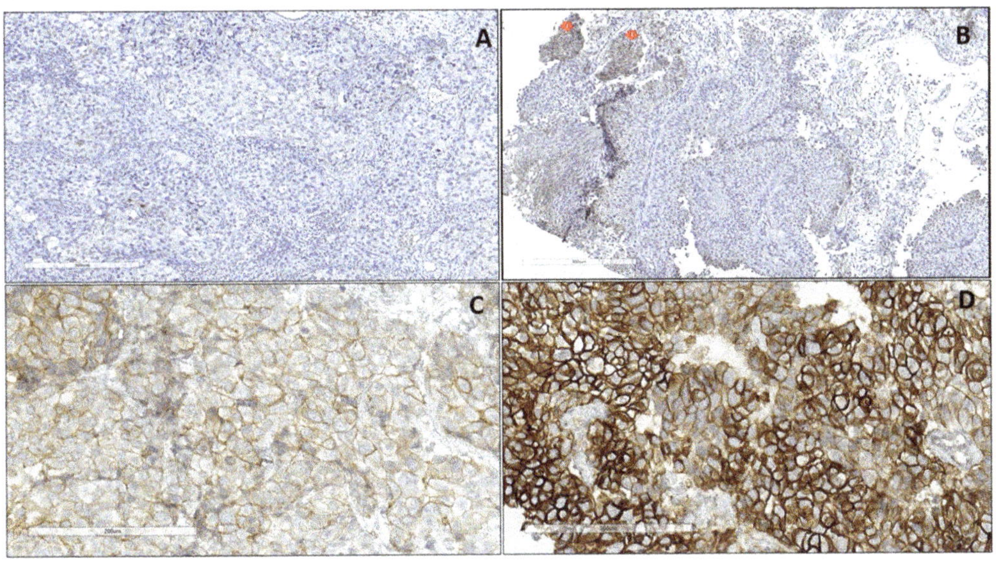

Fig. 2 Anti-thrombomodulin IHC staining in BC tissues. **a** Negative: No membranous staining in < 5% of Bladder tumours **b** Positive (+): Positive membranous staining in up to 20% of Bladder tumours. Note the weak positive membranous staining (red arrows). **c** Positive (++): Positive membranous staining in up to 20–50% of Bladder tumours. Note the Moderate colour intensity. **d** Positive (+++): Positive membranous staining in > 50% of Bladder tumours. Note the high colour intensity. DAB detection. ×40 magnification

higher HER-2/neu expression in Bladder tumours, compared to normal underlying tissues ($X^2(3) = 8.82$, $p < 0.032$), as determined by the Chi-square test.

With respect cancer grading, there was a significant association between patients' cancer grade and HER-2/neu ($X^2(2) = 11.407$, $p = 0.003$), as determined by the Kruskal–Wallis test. Further post-hoc testing using the Mann–Whitney test revealed significant difference between grade 1 and grade 2 ($Z = -3.042$, $p = 0.002$, $r = 0.673$) and a significant difference between grade 1

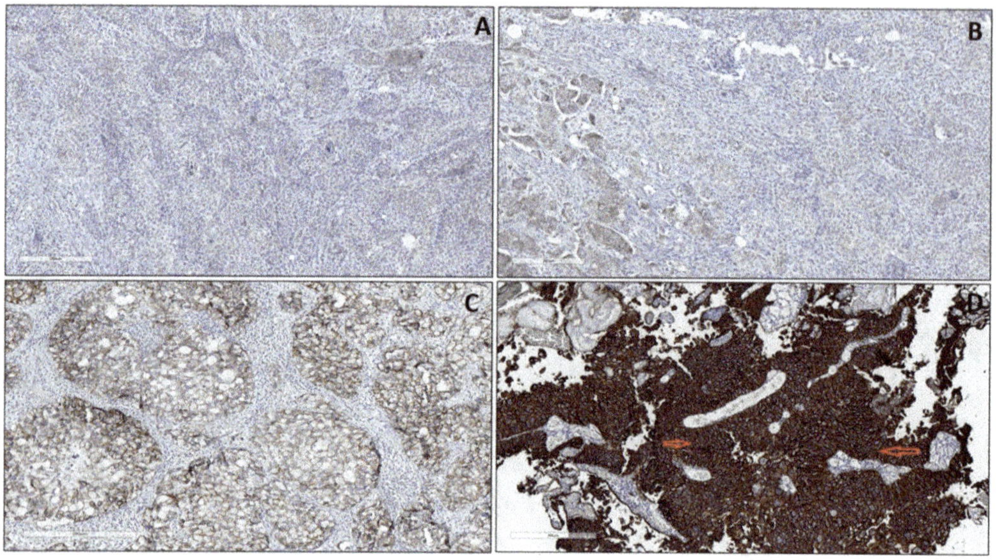

Fig. 3 Anti-HER-2/neu antibody staining in BC tissues. **a** Negative: No staining or weak membranous staining in < 5% of BC tissues. **b** Positive (+): Weak intensity membranous staining in up to 20% BC tumours. **c** Positive (++): Moderate intensity membranous staining in 20–50% of BC tissues. **d** Positive (+++): Strong intensity membranous staining in > 50% of BC tissues (Brown colour, red arrows). DAB detection. ×40 magnification

and grade 3 (Z = -2.843, $p = 0.004$, r = 0.606), both with a high Eta^2 effect size. There was also a significant association between patient's cancer stage and HER-2/neu ($X^2(2) = 16.092$, $p < 0.001$), as determined by the Kruskal–Wallis test.

S100P tissue expression in BC patients

The anti-S100p primary monoclonal antibody used in this study shows cytoplasmic and nuclear staining patterns in BC tissue sections (Fig. 4). Generally, there was a significant increase in S100P expression in Bladder tumours

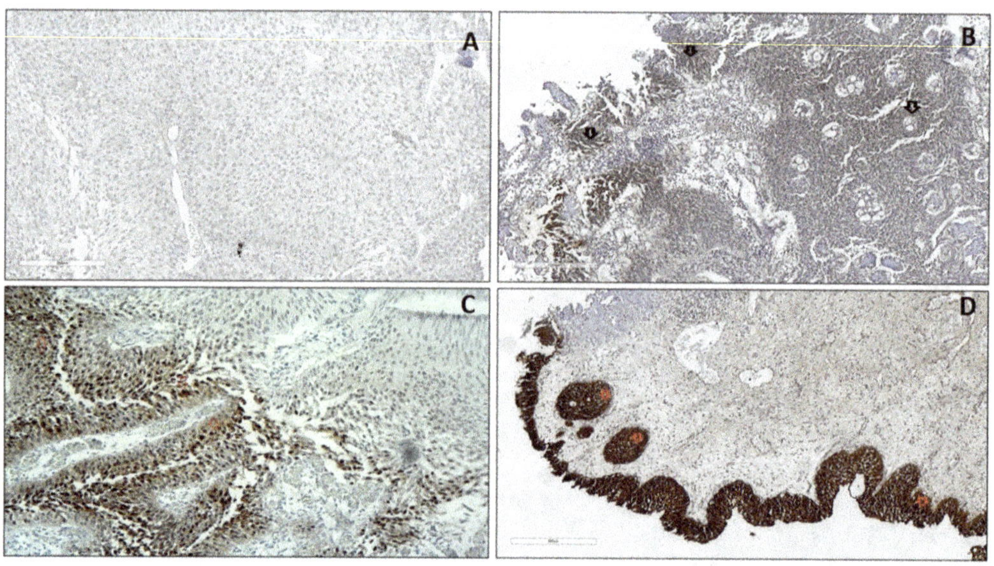

Fig. 4 Anti-S100P antibody staining in BC tissues. **a** Negative: No staining or positive cytoplasmic/nuclear staining in < 5% of Bladder tumours. **b** Positive (+): Weak Nuclear/cytoplasmic staining in up to 20% of Bladder tumours (black arrows). **c** Positive (++): Moderate/strong positive nuclear and cytoplasmic staining 20–50% of Bladder tumours. **d** Positive (+++): Strong positive nuclear and cytoplasmic staining in > 50% of Bladder tumours. DAB detection. X40 magnification

compared to those in normal tissues (X2(3) = 41.686, $p < 0.001$), as determined by the Chi-square test.

With respect to cancer grading, there was no significant association between patients' cancer grade and anti-S100P expression ($X^2(2) = 0.206$, $p = 0.902$), as determined by the Kruskal–Wallis. There was also no significant association between patient's cancer stage and S100P ($X^2(2) = 2.134$, $p = 0.344$), as determined by the Kruskal–Wallis test.

COX-2 tissue expression in BC patients

The anti-COX-2 primary monoclonal antibody used in this study shows cytoplasmic and membranous staining patterns in BC tissue sections (Fig. 5). Generally, there was a significant increase in COX-2 expression in Bladder tumours, compared to those in normal tissues (X2(3) = 19.97, $p < 0.001$), as determined by the Chi-square test. With respect to cancer grading, there was no significant association between patients' cancer grade and anti-COX-2 ($X^2(2) = 0.96$, $p = 0.61$), as determined by the Kruskal–Wallis test. There was also no significant association between patient's cancer stage and S100P ($X^2(2) = 1.65$, $p = 0.45$), as determined by the Kruskal–Wallis test.

Anti-CEACAM-1 tissue expression in BC patients

The anti-CEACAM-1 primary monoclonal antibody used in this study shows cytoplasmic/membranous staining patterns in BC tissue sections (Fig. 6). Generally, there was a significant change (loss of tissue expression) in CEACAM-1 in Bladder tumour, compared to normal tissues (X2(3) = 11.29, $p < 0.001$), as determined by the Chi-square test.

There was a significant association between patients' cancer grade and CEACAM-1 expression ($X^2(2) = 6.19$, $p = 0.045$), as determined by the Kruskal–Wallis. Further post-hoc testing using the Mann–Whitney test revealed significant difference between grade 1 and grade 3 (Z = -2.444, $p = 0.015$, r = 0.509). With respect to cancer staging, there was a significant association between patient's cancer stage and CEACAM-1 expression ($X^2(2) = 10.78$, $p = 0.005$), as determined by the Kruskal–Wallis test.

Anti-VEGFR-3 tissue expression in BC patients

The anti-VEGFR-3 primary monoclonal antibody used in this study shows nuclear and cytoplasmic staining patterns in BC tissue sections (Fig. 7). Generally, there was a significant increase in VEGFR-3 expression in Bladder tumours, compared to normal tissues (X2(3) = 41.71, $p < 0.001$), as determined by the Chi-square test.

With respect to cancer grading, there was a significant association between patients' cancer grade and VEGFR-3 ($X^2(2) = 4.18$, $p = 0.12$), as determined by the Kruskal–Wallis. There was also no significant association between patient's cancer stage and VEGFR-3 ($X^2(2) = 2.94$,

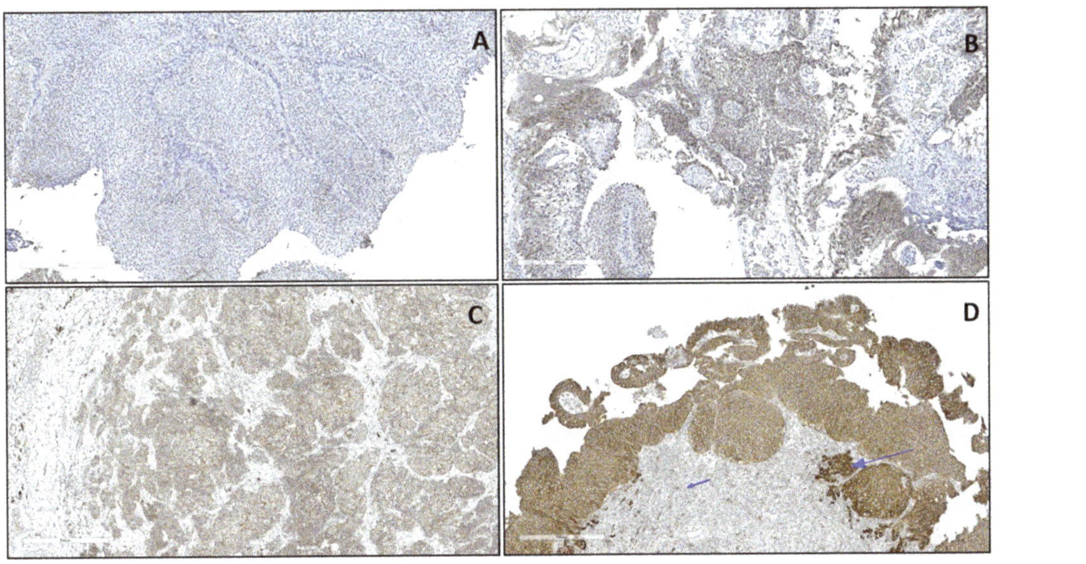

Fig. 5 Anti-COX-2 antibody staining in BC tissues. **a** Negative: No staining/Positive cytoplasmic/membranous staining in < 5% of Bladder tumours. **b** Positive (+): Weak positive cytoplasmic/membranous staining in up to 20% of Bladder tumour cells (Brown colour). **c** Positive (++): Moderate/high positive cytoplasmic/membranous staining (brown colour) in in up to 20–50% of Bladder tumours. **d** Positive (+++): Strong positive cytoplasmic/membranous staining in in up to > 50% of Bladder tumours (bigger arrow). Note the absence of staining in underlying tissue (smaller arrow). DAB. ×40 magnification

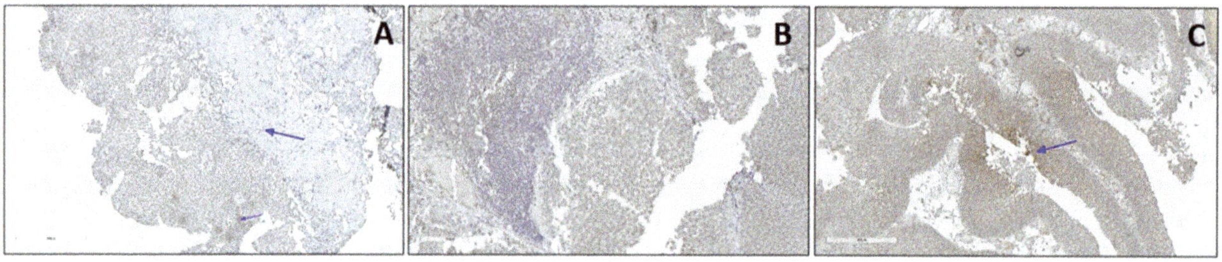

Fig. 6 Anti-CEACAM-1 staining in BC tissues. **a** Negative: No staining/Positive membranous staining in < 5% of Bladder tumours. Small blue arrow shows weakly expressed bladder tumours. Big blue arrow shows underlying connective tissue. **b** Positive (+): Moderate membranous staining in up to 20% of Bladder tumours. **c** Positive (++): Positive membranous staining in 20–50% of Bladder tumour cells (Blue arrows). Ventana ultraview DAB detection. ×40 magnification

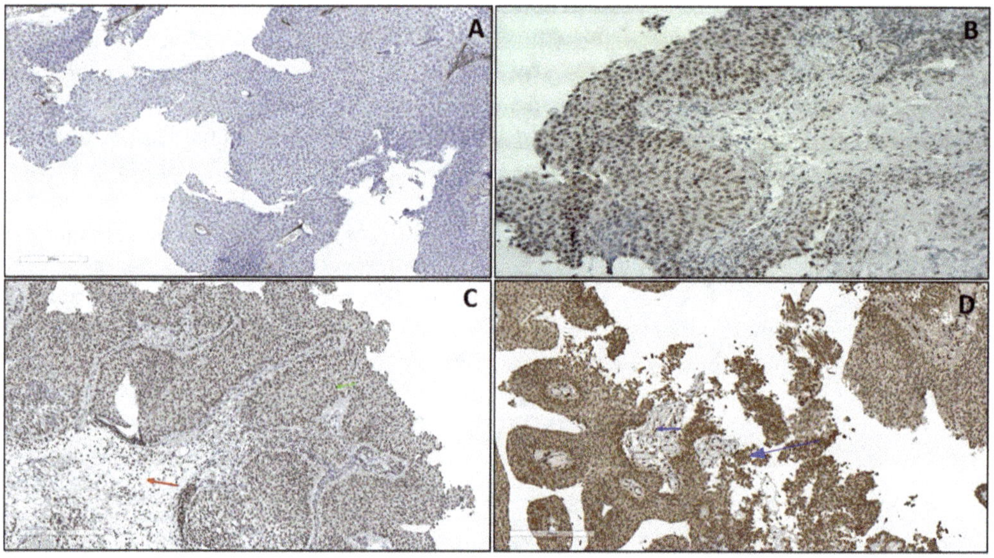

Fig. 7 Anti-VEGFR3 staining in BC tissues. **a** Negative: No Staining or < 5% nuclear/cytoplasmic Staining. **b** Positive (+): Moderate intensity Nuclear/cytoplasmic staining in up to 25% of Bladder tumours **c** Positive (++) Moderate intensity nuclear/cytoplasmic staining in 25–50% of Bladder tumours (Green arrows). Nonspecific staining in underlying stroma cells (red arrows). **d** Positive (+++): Strong intensity nuclear/cytoplasmic staining in > 50% of Bladder tumour (big blue arrows). Smaller arrow shows nonspecific staining in stroma cells. Ventana Ultraview DAB. ×40 magnification

$p = 0.23$), as determined by the Kruskal–Wallis test. Table 2 summarises the results for antibody staining in bladder cancer patients.

Discussion

The main aim of this study was to evaluate the expression of various tissue-based biomarkers in BC patients and their association with cancer recurrence. This was done by assessing IHC staining in patient tissues following TURBT for the treatment of BC.

The results from this study showed a significant increase in anti-CD31 in vascular endothelial cells located in bladder tumour cells with some staining also located close to the tumour cells. As a marker of angiogenesis, these findings potentially show the presence of increased angiogenesis within the Bladder tumours. The scoring system used in this research examines both staining intensity and percentage positivity in tumour cells and has been used by others [27].

Anti-CD31 patterns reported in this study complements results by others [28] although those author's used a different patient cohort. Both studies however show that, CD31 is a good marker for measuring angiogenesis using IHC. Results from this present study disagree with others [29] as no association between CD31 and cancer grade was observed. This could be

Table 2 Summarised statistical results for antibody staining in BC

Antibody	Overall staining pattern in patients' Bladder tumours (Chi square)	Association between antibody expression and cancer grade (Kruskal–Wallis test)	Association between antibody expression and cancer stage (Kruskal–Wallis test)	Association between antibody expression and cancer recurrence (Mann–Whitney test)
CD31	Increased expression in vascular cells ($p < 0.001$)	Not significant ($p = 0.257$)	Significant ($p = 0.002$)	Not significant ($p = 0.69$)
Thrombomodulin	Reduced/loss of expression ($p < 0.010$)	Not significant ($p = 0.827$)	Not significant ($p = 0.039$)	Not significant ($p = 0.89$)
HER-2	Increased expression ($p < 0.032$)	Significant ($p = 0.003$)	Significant ($p < 0.001$)	Not significant ($p = 0.91$)
S100P	Increased expression ($p < 0.001$)	Not significant ($p = 0.902$)	Not significant ($p = 0.344$)	Not significant ($p = 0.23$)
CEACAM-1	Reduced/loss of expression ($p < 0.001$)	Not significant ($p = 0.045$)	Significant ($p = 0.005$)	Not significant ($p = 0.65$)
COX-2	Increased expression ($p < 0.001$)	Not significant ($p = 0.619$)	Not significant ($p = 0.439$)	Not significant ($p = 0.98$)
VEGFR-3	Increased expression ($p < 0.001$)	Not significant ($p = 0.123$)	Not significant ($p = 0.231$)	Not significant ($p = 0.38$)

due to differences in cancer types and grading systems. Patients with cancer stage pTa presented with higher CD31 compared to other BC stages. These findings suggest that increased CD31 in low pTa tumours may have an association with angiogenesis.

In this study, loss of expression or reduced thrombomodulin was observed within bladder tumour cells compared to normal bladder cells. Due to its tumour suppressive properties [30], loss of thrombomodulin observed in this present study, could potentially cause increased tissue differentiation, metastasis and recurrence. Although the exact mechanisms are not fully understood, earlier studies show that, thrombomodulin maintains cell–cell interactions and also inhibits degradation of the ECM; important factors in cancer proliferation [31, 32]. Our findings therefore further complement these earlier studies by highlighting the loss of Thrombomodulin within BC cells. In terms of Bladder specific research however, our research provides new information on Thrombomodulin staining patterns in bladder tumours.

High stage BC was significantly associated with reduced thrombomodulin suggesting that there was reduced cell to cell interaction due to the absence of thrombomodulin. This observation is in agreement with an earlier study which reported that, decreased thrombomodulin was significantly correlated with high cancer stage, differentiation and 5 year survival [33]. In this current study, there was no association between thrombomodulin (at diagnosis) and cancer recurrence. This observation should however be further investigated using larger sample sizes and increasing the length of follow up.

Our results also showed reduced CEACAM-1 in Bladder tumour cells compared to other tissues. Due to its angiogenic properties, an increase in CECAM-1, was expected in BC patients before TURBT. Although increased tissue expression of CEACAM-1 has been reported in human cancers [34], our findings of decreased expression may further explain earlier reports of a dual role of CEACAM-1 in BC [35]. Furthermore, the two IHC reporting systems (traditional scoring system using stain intensity/percentage vrs MVD) produced different results and raises further issues with validation.

Some studies have associated CEACAM-1 with aggressive tumour behaviour (i.e. high grade, advanced stage, metastasis and survival) in different human cancers [36, 37]. In our study, we report a significant association between loss of CEACAM-1 and BC stage and grade. Our study further attempts to evaluate this association with cancer recurrence. In this regard, there was no association between patients' CEACAM-1 (at diagnosis) and BC recurrence.

There was generally a significant increase in COX-2 in Bladder tumour cells, compared to those in normal tissues. These findings are in agreement with a recent study by others in colonic adenocarcinoma tissues [4]. The results suggest that tumour cells of epithelial origin express high levels of COX-2 probably due to chronic inflammation and may potentially be a good biomarker. Furthermore, high stage and high grade patients presented with high staining intensity and percentage of tumour cells [4]. These observations were also present in the current study and suggests that COX-2 in cancer tissues (especially staining intensity) should be further investigated in BC.

With regards to cancer stage, our results are in contrast with others [5] who reported significant associations between COX-2 and cancer stage. Although both endometrial carcinoma (EC) and BC are of epithelial origin, differences in sample size (183 EC vrs 35 BC), duration of follow up (5 yrs. for EC vrs 2 yrs. for BC) and different antibody clones, may explain the differences in results reported by both studies.

The relationship between antibody expression (at diagnosis) vs BC recurrence was not significant. Nonetheless, the expression patterns of COX-2 in BC, reported in this present study, should be investigated further using larger sample sizes and longer follow up periods. COX-2 seems to be epithelial cancer specific and may be a useful marker for monitoring and management of BC patients following TURBT.

Anti-S100P was investigated in this present study because its cellular expression may interact with growth factors and their receptors, leading to several effects such as tumour proliferation [9]. The results from this present study showed that S100P was significantly expressed in BC cells in comparison with normal Bladder tissue and suggests this protein may be a good marker for identification of BC. In a similar study, S100A8 (which belongs to the same family as S100P) was highly expressed in TCC tissues compared to normal cells [38]. In disagreement with that study however, there was no correlation between S100P expression and patients' cancer grade and stage in this present study.

Although it can be appreciated that S100P will be higher in high grade tumours due to increased cell proliferation [39], that observation was not made in this present study and could potentially be due to low sample size. Furthermore, comparing S100P at diagnosis, with S100P at 2–5 years following treatment, may provide confirmatory information with regards to recurrence and long-term outcome measures.

With regards to recurrence however, findings disagree with other researchers [39] who observed that positive S100P expression was strongly associated with early recurrence in HCC patients. Difference in patient cohorts and sample sizes may explain these variations. The results from this study nonetheless provides new information with regards to S100P staining in bladder tumour cells as well as its association with cancer grade, stage and recurrence following treatment via TURBT.

In various human cancers, different HER-2 rates and patterns have been reported [40–42]. HER-2 expression was therefore investigated in this present study due to its links to cancer growth in various human cancers, especially its utility in breast cancer treatment and management.

Our findings suggest that HER-2 was significantly higher in bladder tumour cells, compared to normal tissues. As a protein involved in signal transduction leading to increased cell proliferation, the increased expression observed in this present study potentially implicates HER-2 in BC growth. These observations complement results by others [43] who reported higher HER-2 expression in colorectal cancer cells compared to normal controls and another group [44] who also reported higher HER-2 in breast cancer patients. The differences between the studies however is that, this present study provides detailed information with regards to antibody clone, scoring system and optimises IHC protocol to the Ventana IHC autostainer.

High grade (G3) patients presented with higher HER-2 expression compared with low grade (G1), in agreement with [45], although their observations were made in breast cancer patients. These findings nonetheless suggest that HER-2 results in higher rate of cell differentiation that potentially leads to increased risk of recurrence and metastasis in BC patients.

High stage tumours (pT1/pT2) also presented with high HER-2, which complement findings from a previous study [45] involving breast cancer. It can be appreciated that, increasing HER-2 will lead to increased activation of the so-called MAPK pathway, which explains the association with aggressive tumour behaviour.

There was also a significant increase in VEGFR-3 in bladder tumour cells, compared to those in normal tissues. In a previous study [4], VEGF in colonic adenocarcinoma showed intensely positive staining compared to normal control tissues. However, control tissues were moderately positive for VEGF indicating the potential likelihood of false positive reporting. In this present study, there was also non-specific VEGFR-3 staining within nuclei of some underlying muscle cells, lymphatic endothelial cells and basal tissue cells. This observation in this and other study highlights the unspecific nature of VEGF staining, and raises the issues with standardisation in reporting slides.

A limiting factor for this study is the relatively low sample size. Validation of the findings larger multicentre studies could provide clear evidence of a usable biomarker profile as an adjuvant to BC management.

Future studies may also investigate antibody tissue immunoreaction, serum expression and urine levels simultaneously in all patients. This could provide much clearer data to enhance the search for a usable biomarker profile.

Conclusion

It is proposed that by allowing urological surgeons access to laboratory markers such as HER-2, Thrombomodulin, CEACAM-1 and CD31, potentially, in the future, these biomarkers may be used in addition to, or in combination with, currently used scoring systems to predict cancer recurrence and progression.

Ultimately, our research findings may allow current NHS post-operative care protocols to be revised, improved and implemented within 6–8 years, although larger studies are needed in this area of research in order to make an impact on a national scale, and to promote good practice in the field of urology, pertaining to BC.

Abbreviations

BC: Bladder cancer; COX-2: Cyclooxygenase-2; DAB: Diaminobenzidine; FFPE: Formalin-fixed paraffin-embedded; HER-2: Human epidermal growth factor-2; IHC: Immunohistochemistry; MAPK: Mitogen-activated protein kinase; NMIBC: Non-muscle invasive bladder cancer; TCC: Transitional cell carcinoma; TURBT: Transurethral resection of the bladder tumour.

Acknowledgements

The authors are grateful to the patients who consented to participate in this study. The authors wish to thank all the staff at the Department of Urology, Wrexham Maelor Hospital and Histopathology department, Glan Clwyd Hospital at Betsi Cadwaladr University Health Board (BCUHB), North Wales, UK, for their support regards our continued research activities.

Authors' contributions

Conceived concept, study designed and supervision: SFH and IS. Patient recruitment and laboratory experiments: PET, RML and AM. Analysed and interpreted the data: PET and AM. Wrote the paper: PET, SFH and IS. All authors read and approved the final manuscript.

Author details

[1] North Wales Clinical Research Centre, Betsi Cadwaladr University Health Board (BCUHB), Wrexham Maelor Hospital, Wrexham, Wales, UK. [2] Faculty of Social and Life Sciences, Wrexham Glyndwr University, Wrexham, UK. [3] Department of Histopathology, Ysbyty Glan Clwd, Betsi Cadwaladr University Health Board (BCUHB), Wrexham, UK. [4] Department of Biological Sciences, University of Chester, Chester, UK. [5] Department of Urology, BCUHB Wrexham Maelor Hospital, Wrexham, Wales, UK.

References

1. Bray F, Ferlay J, Soerjomataram I, Siegel RL, Torre LA, Jemal A. Global cancer statistics 2018: GLOBOCAN estimates of incidence and mortality worldwide for 36 cancers in 185 countries. CA Cancer J Clin. 2018;68(6):394–424.
2. Mariappan P, Zachou A, Grigor KM. Detrusor muscle in the first, apparently complete transurethral resection of bladder tumour specimen is a surrogate marker of resection quality, predicts risk of early recurrence, and is dependent on operator experience. Eur Urol. 2010;57(5):843–9.
3. Yu S-M, Kim S-J. Endoplasmic reticulum stress (ER-stress) by 2-deoxy-D-glucose (2DG) reduces cyclooxygenase 2 (COX-2) expression and N-glycosylation and induces a loss of COX-2 activity via a Src kinase-dependent pathway in rabbit articular chondrocytes. Exp Mol Med. 2010;42(11):777–86.
4. Hedaya M, Helmy A, Ezzat H, Hammam O. Cyclo-oxygenase-2 and vascular endothelial growth factor expression in colorectal cancer patients. Egypt J Surg. 2015;34(1):35–40.
5. Cai S, Zhang Y-x, Han K, Ding Y-q. Expressions and clinical significance of COX-2, VEGF-C, and EFGR in endometrial carcinoma. Arch Gynecol Obstetr. 2017;296(1):93–8.
6. Song J, Ma D, Liu X, Chen Y, Fang J, Lui VWY, et al. Thrombomodulin (TM) in tumor cell differentiation and periphery blood immune microenvironment in oral squamous cell carcinoma. Clin Immunol. 2018;191:27–33.
7. Greineder CF, Johnston IH, Villa CH, Gollomp K, Esmon CT, Cines DB, et al. ICAM-1-targeted thrombomodulin mitigates tissue factor-driven inflammatory thrombosis in a human endothelialized microfluidic model. Blood Adv. 2017;1(18):1452–65.
8. Wu C-T, Chang Y-H, Lin P-Y, Chen W-C, Chen M-F. Thrombomodulin expression regulates tumorigenesis in bladder cancer. BMC Cancer. 2014;14(1):375.
9. Jiang H, Hu H, Lin F, Lim YP, Hua Y, Tong X, et al. S100P is Overexpressed in squamous cell and adenosquamous carcinoma subtypes of endometrial cancer and promotes cancer cell proliferation and invasion. Cancer Invest. 2016;34(10):477–88.
10. Gibadulinova A, Tothova V, Pastorek J, Pastorekova S. Transcriptional regulation and functional implication of S100P in cancer. Amino Acids. 2011;41(4):885–92.
11. Liu Y, Wang C, Shan X, Wu J, Liu H, Liu H, et al. S100P is associated with proliferation and migration in nasopharyngeal carcinoma. Oncol Lett. 2017;14(1):525–32.
12. Guo L, Chen S, Jiang H, Huang J, Jin W, Yao S. The expression of S100P increases and promotes cellular proliferation by increasing nuclear translocation of beta-catenin in endometrial cancer. Int J Clin Exp Pathol. 2014;7(5):2102–12.
13. Tabrizi MEA, Lancaster TL, Ismail TM, Georgiadou A, Ganguly A, Mistry JJ, et al. S100P enhances the motility and invasion of human trophoblast cell lines. Sci Rep. 2018;8(1):11488.
14. Wang Z, Wang W, Xu S, Wang S, Tu Y, Xiong Y, et al. The role of MAPK signaling pathway in the Her-2-positive meningiomas. Oncol Rep. 2016;36(2):685–95.
15. Siddiqa A, Long LM, Li L, Marciniak RA, Kazhdan I. Expression of HER-2 in MCF-7 breast cancer cells modulates anti-apoptotic proteins Survivin and Bcl-2 via the extracellular signal-related kinase (ERK) and phosphoinositide-3 kinase (PI3K) signalling pathways. BMC Cancer. 2008;8:129.
16. Blackwell KL, Burstein HJ, Storniolo AM, Rugo HS, Sledge G, Aktan G, et al. Overall survival benefit with lapatinib in combination with trastuzumab for patients with human epidermal growth factor receptor 2–positive metastatic breast cancer: final results from the EGF104900 study. J Clin Oncol. 2012;30(21):2585–92.
17. Gerhardt H, Golding M, Fruttiger M, Ruhrberg C, Lundkvist A, Abramsson A, et al. VEGF guides angiogenic sprouting utilizing endothelial tip cell filopodia. J Cell Biol. 2003;161(6):1163–77.
18. Eroglu A, Ersoz C, Karasoy D, Sak S. Vascular endothelial growth factor (VEGF)-C, VEGF-D, VEGFR-3 and D2–40 expressions in primary breast cancer: association with lymph node metastasis. Adv Clin Exp Med Off Organ Wroclaw Med Univ. 2017;26(2):245–9.
19. Tammela T, Zarkada G, Wallgard E, Murtomäki A, Suchting S, Wirzenius M, et al. Blocking VEGFR-3 suppresses angiogenic sprouting and vascular network formation. Nature. 2008;454(7204):656.
20. Neumaier M, Paululat S, Chan A, Matthaes P, Wagener C. Biliary glycoprotein, a potential human cell adhesion molecule, is down-regulated in colorectal carcinomas. Proc Natl Acad Sci. 1993;90(22):10744–8.
21. Luo W, Tapolsky M, Earley K, Wood CG, Wilson DR, Logothetis CJ, et al. Tumor-suppressive activity of CD66a in prostate cancer. Cancer Gene Ther. 1999;6(4):313.
22. Sha QQ, Wei QZ, Zhu JK, Wang KX, Wang C, Liu HT, et al. Loss of membranous carcinoembryonic antigen-related cell adhesion molecule 1 expression is related to decreased relapse-free survival of hepatocellular carcinoma following liver transplantation. Chin Med J. 2012;125(16):2841–5.
23. O'Brien CD, Lim P, Sun J, Albelda SM. PECAM-1-dependent neutrophil transmigration is independent of monolayer PECAM-1 signaling or localization. Blood. 2003;101(7):2816–25.
24. El Gehani K, Al-Kikhia L, Mansuri N, Syrjanen K, Al-Fituri O, Elzagheid A. Angiogenesis in urinary bladder carcinoma as defined by microvessel density (MVD) after immunohistochemical staining for Factor VIII and CD31. Libyan J Med. 2011;6:24.

25. García-Tello A, Angulo JC, Andrés G, Ramón de Fata F, Sánchez-Chapado M, López JI. Impact of p53, MIB-1 and PECAM-1 expression on the prognosis of urothelial carcinoma of the renal pelvis. Actas Urológicas Españolas (English Ed). 2014;38(8):506–14.
26. Mohamed SY, Mohammed HL, Ibrahim HM, Mohamed EM, Salah M. Role of VEGF, CD105, and CD31 in the prognosis of colorectal cancer cases. J Gastrointest Cancer. 2017;5:1–12.
27. Usuda K, Iwai S, Funasaki A, Sekimura A, Motono N, Ueda Y, et al. Expression and prognostic impact of VEGF, CD31 and alphaSMA in resected primary lung cancers. Anticancer Res. 2018;38(7):4057–63.
28. Qian H, Yang L, Zhao W, Chen H, He S. A comparison of CD105 and CD31 expression in tumor vessels of hepatocellular carcinoma by tissue microarray and flow cytometry. Exp Ther Med. 2018;16(4):2881–8.
29. Kuang BH, Wen XZ, Ding Y, Peng RQ, Cai PQ, Zhang MQ, et al. The prognostic value of platelet endothelial cell adhesion molecule-1 in non-small-cell lung cancer patients. Med Oncol (Northwood, Lond, Engl). 2013;30(2):536.
30. Tanaka K, Salunya T, Motomiya Y, Motomiya Y, Oyama Y, Yamakuchi M, et al. Decreased Expression of Thrombomodulin in Endothelial Cells by Fibroblast Growth Factor-23/alpha-Klotho. Ther Apheresis Dial. 2017;21(4):395–404.
31. Koutsi A, Papapanagiotou A, Papavassiliou AG. Thrombomodulin: from haemostasis to inflammation and tumourigenesis. Int J Biochem Cell Biol. 2008;40(9):1669–73.
32. Weiler H, Lindner V, Kerlin B, Isermann BH, Hendrickson SB, Cooley BC, et al. Characterization of a mouse model for thrombomodulin deficiency. Arterioscler Thromb Vasc Biol. 2001;21(9):1531–7.
33. Hanly A, Redmond M, Winter D, Brophy S, Deasy J, Bouchier-Hayes D, et al. Thrombomodulin expression in colorectal carcinoma is protective and correlates with survival. Br J Cancer. 2006;94(9):1320.
34. Dango S, Sienel W, Schreiber M, Stremmel C, Kirschbaum A, Pantel K, et al. Elevated expression of carcinoembryonic antigen-related cell adhesion molecule 1 (CEACAM-1) is associated with increased angiogenic potential in non-small-cell lung cancer. Lung Cancer. 2008;60(3):426–33.
35. Oliveira-Ferrer L, Tilki D, Ziegeler G, Hauschild J, Loges S, Irmak S, et al. Dual role of carcinoembryonic antigen-related cell adhesion molecule 1 in angiogenesis and invasion of human urinary bladder cancer. Can Res. 2004;64(24):8932–8.
36. Thies A, Moll I, Berger J, Wagener C, Brummer J, Schulze HJ, et al. CEACAM1 expression in cutaneous malignant melanoma predicts the development of metastatic disease. J Clin Oncol. 2002;20(10):2530–6.
37. Thom I, Schult-Kronefeld O, Burkholder I, Schuch G, Andritzky B, Kastendieck H, et al. Expression of CEACAM-1 in pulmonary adenocarcinomas and their metastases. Anticancer Res. 2009;29(1):249–54.
38. Cui Y-y, Shi A-p, Xu N. Expression of S100A8 protein in human bladder cancer and its clinical significance. Chin J Lab Diagn. 2012;2:017.
39. Yuan RH, Chang KT, Chen YL, Hsu HC, Lee PH, Lai PL, et al. S100P expression is a novel prognostic factor in hepatocellular carcinoma and predicts survival in patients with high tumor stage or early recurrent tumors. PLoS ONE. 2013;8(6):e65501.
40. Hammam O, Nour HH, Mosaad M, Akl M, Khalil H, al Ganzory H, et al. The clinical significance of HER2 protein amplification/expression in urinary bladder lesion. Arab J Urol. 2015;13(2):146–52.
41. Slamon DJ, Leyland-Jones B, Shak S, Fuchs H, Paton V, Bajamonde A, et al. Use of chemotherapy plus a monoclonal antibody against HER2 for metastatic breast cancer that overexpresses HER2. N Engl J Med. 2001;344(11):783–92.
42. Smith I, Procter M, Gelber RD, Guillaume S, Feyereislova A, Dowsett M, et al. 2-year follow-up of trastuzumab after adjuvant chemotherapy in HER2-positive breast cancer: a randomised controlled trial. Lancet. 2007;369(9555):29–36.
43. Hasan R, Bhatt D, Khan S, Khan V, Verma AK, Anees A, et al. Association of Her-2 expression and clinicopathological parameters in colorectal carcinoma in Indian population. Open Access Macedonian J Med Sci. 2018;7(1):6–11.
44. Du JW, Xu KY, Fang LY, Qi XL. Clinical significance of Mena and Her-2 expression in breast cancer. Eur J Gynaecol Oncol. 2012;33(5):455–8.
45. Jana D, Mandal S, Mukhopadhyay M, Mitra D, Mukhopadhyay SK, Sarkar DK. Prognostic significance of HER-2/neu and survival of breast cancer patients attending a specialized breast clinic in Kolkata, Eastern India. Asian Pacific J Cancer Prev APJCP. 2012;13(8):3851–5.

5

MicroRNA-219c-5p regulates bladder fibrosis by targeting FN1

Bowen Liu[1,2], Yafei Ding[1], Peng Li[1], Tao Wang[1], Siyuan He[1], Zhankui Jia[1,2] and Jinjian Yang[1,2*]

Abstract

Background: We found that the bladders of multiple sclerosis mice were significantly fibrotic. This study aimed to investigate the relationship between fibronectin 1 (FN1) and bladder fibrosis, as well as the microRNAs involved in FN1 regulation.

Methods: The degree of bladder smooth muscle fibrosis was observed by immunohistochemistry. In addition, we used quantitative real-time polymerase chain reaction (RT-qPCR) and Western blotting to determine FN1 expression in bladders with different grades of fibrosis. Bioinformatics analysis revealed that miR-199a-3p, miR-219c-5p and miR-3572-3p could inhibit FN1 synthesis. Therefore, miR-199a-3p, miR-219c-5p and miR-3572-3p were overexpressed or knocked down in bladder smooth muscle cells (BSMCs), and the respective transfection and FN1 knockdown efficiencies were detected by RT-qPCR. Only miR-219c-5p overexpression and knockdown produced the expected results. A dual luciferase reporter assay was used to determine the targeting relationship between miR-219c-5p and FN1. Flow cytometry and Cell Counting Kit 8 (CCK8) experiments confirmed that miR-219c-5p reduced FN1 expression and affected the biological activity of smooth muscle cells. Agomir and anagomir of miR-219c-5p were transfected in vivo to observe the change of bladder fibrosis in mice.

Results: With increasing bladder fibrosis, FN1 expression increased, while miR-199a-3p, miR-219c-5p, and miR-3572-3p expression levels decreased. The RT-qPCR results after transfection showed that only miR-219c-5p could regulate FN1. Indeed, the dual luciferase reporter assay results indicated that miR-219c-5p targeted FN1 directly. CCK8 and cell cycle assays showed that miR-219c-5p overexpression inhibited BSMC proliferation, while miR-219c-5p knockdown promoted BSMC proliferation. An apoptosis assay showed that miR-219c-5p overexpression promoted apoptosis, while miR-219c-5p knockdown inhibited BSMC apoptosis. The agomir and anagomir transfected with miR-219c-5p in vivo found that the bladder fibrosis of the mice in the agomir group was reduced, and the anagomir group was worse.

Conclusions: Our findings indicate that FN1 up-regulation and miR-219c-5p down-regulation play an important role in the development of bladder fibrosis, and miR-219c-5p participates in bladder fibrosis by regulating FN1 expression. Thus, a novel antifibrotic function of miR-219c-5p is proposed, which may represent a potential target for the diagnosis and treatment of bladder fibrosis.

Keywords: Multiple sclerosis, Experimental autoimmune encephalomyelitis, Bladder fibrosis, Fibronectin-1, MicroRNA-219c-5p

Background

Multiple sclerosis (MS) is a diffuse inflammatory autoimmune disease characterized by multiple symptoms and signs [1, 2]. It is currently believed that MS patients suffer mainly from myelin-specific T cell-mediated

*Correspondence: yangjinjian2011@163.com
[1] Department of Urology, Zhengzhou University First Affiliated Hospital, Zhengzhou 450052, China
Full list of author information is available at the end of the article

autoimmune demyelination diseases. Demyelination of the urinary reflex nerve leads to inconsistent bladder detrusor and sphincter movement. Therefore, MS patients often suffer frequent urination, urgency and urinary retention [3–5]. Although many reports have investigated the possible mechanisms of lower urinary tract symptom development in MS, the mechanism of bladder fibrosis as the ultimate outcome of bladder dysfunction has not been clearly elucidated [6, 7]. The experimental autoimmune encephalomyelitis (EAE) model is currently the most commonly used animal model of MS. The myelin autoantigen specifically activates helper T cells in the brain, causing inflammatory infiltration of the central nervous system and loss of myelin. The biochemical, immunological and pathological features of EAE are very similar to those of MS, so this model is widely used to assess the etiology of MS and to find different treatment options [8–10]. PLP139 sensitized SJL/J mice established a relapsing and relieving MS model, while MOG35-55 immunized C57BL/6J mice established an irreversible chronic progressive MS model, where demyelination and axonal damage were obvious. Considering the long-term chronic progression of bladder fibrosis, the C57BL/6J mouse model was chosen. Bladder fibrosis is the ultimate outcome of bladder dysfunction [11, 12]. Fibrosis is described as the "wrong wound healing process", and while many mechanisms may be involved in its development, they are all based on BSMCs activation and the resulting extracellular matrix (ECM) components [13]. Wang et al. [14] reported for the first time that hypoxia induced microRNA-101b and inhibited the TGF-β signaling pathway, thereby inhibiting fibrosis in BSMC. Altuntas et al. [7] were the first to report that bladder fibrosis and bladder remodeling corresponding to the severity of EAE may be due to increased CTGF expression and increased connective tissue growth. Antifibrotic therapy may be an effective way to control bladder dysfunction, but it has not been well studied [15–17].

Fibronectin is an extracellular macromolecular membrane protein present on the surface of animal cells and is the main noncollagen glycoprotein in the ECM and basement membrane. It is also very abundant in the ECM of various tumors, including osteosarcoma, leiomyosarcoma, and gastric cancer [18]. Fibronectin 1 (FN1), which belongs to the FN family, is involved in a variety of cellular biological processes and plays a role in diseases such as fibrosis [19]. Wei Wang et al. [20] first reported that lncRNA GAS5 can adsorb miR-96-5p, reduce the inhibition of miR-96-5p on fibrosis protein FN1, and then aggravate renal fibrosis. We found that the more severe the bladder fibrosis is, the higher the FN1 levels are. We speculate that by inhibiting FN1 synthesis, the process of fibrosis in bladder smooth muscle cells (BSMCs) can be reduced.

A large number of studies have shown that miRNA is involved in a variety of cell biological processes such as cell proliferation and apoptosis. Therefore, miRNAs may be critical for the diagnosis and treatment of certain diseases [21]. Many miRNAs have been found in the brain and spinal cord tissue of EAE mice as biomarkers for MS. Ilona B. Bruinsma et al. [22] reported that detecting the loss of miR-219 in patient cerebrospinal fluid may be a candidate biomarker for MS diagnosis. MicroRNAs (miRNAs) are short-chain noncoding RNAs of approximately 22 nucleotides in length whose primary function is to participate in biological processes by inducing mRNA degradation. Many miRNAs, including miR-26b-5p and miR-200c, are involved in the development of fibrosis [23, 24]. Notably, regulating the expression of these miRNAs can prevent fibrogenesis in vitro and in vivo, suggesting the importance of miRNAs as potential targets for the treatment of fibrotic diseases [25]. In this study, we used miRDB (http://mirdb.org/) to predict potentially targeted miRNAs for FN1. After comparative analysis, miR-199a-3p, miR-219c-5p and miR-3572-3p were all predicted to target FN1.

The bladder wall is composed mainly of a mucosal layer, a submucosa layer, a muscle layer and perimuscular connective tissue. Bladder fibrosis is caused mainly by the pathological proliferation of BSMCs in the muscular layer of the bladder wall. A considerable amount of matrix deposition in the cytoplasm of BSMCs affects bladder detrusor compliance and leads to bladder remodeling and fibrosis. Therefore, BSMCs were used as an experimental model in our study. To investigate whether microRNAs can inhibit FN1 synthesis and block the progression of BSMC fibrosis, we overexpressed and knocked down microRNAs in BSMCs in vitro. The RT-qPCR results after transfection showed that miR-219c-5p was able to regulate FN1.

In this study, we established an EAE model to simulate bladder fibrosis in MS patients and found that bladder fibrosis was directly proportional to FN1. Through in vitro and vivo experiments, we found that miR-219c-5p could inhibit the progression of bladder smooth muscle fibrosis by targeting FN1. This study aimed to investigate the significance of miR-219c-5p expression in bladder fibrosis in vitro and in vivo. In addition, this study determined that miR-219c-5p may target the FN1 gene directly, and the miR-219c-5p/FN1 signaling pathway may be useful in the diagnosis and treatment of bladder fibrosis.

Methods

Animals

80 female C57BL/6 J mice (4–9 weeks old) were purchased from Charles River. All mice were kept in a specific pathogen-free (SPF) animal room at the Zhengzhou University Animal Experimental Center and exposed to a 12:12 h light–dark cycle (light from 6 am to 6 pm).

EAE model

To induce chronic EAE, 40 animals were injected subcutaneously with an emulsion of MOG 35–55 in complete Freund's adjuvant (CFA) (Sigma, USA). Then, pertussis toxin (Sigma, USA; 0.2 μg per animal) in PBS was administered on days 0, 3, and 7 after immunization [7]. The mice were scored daily according to the following signs of nerve damage: 0, no disease; (1) tail weakness and/or moderately awkward gait and/or poor righting ability; (2) tail weakness and/or moderately awkward gait; (3) hind limb paralysis or mild forelimb weakness (or both); (4) limb paralysis; and (5) quadriplegia with detained urine or death. Another group of animals was injected subcutaneously with CFA emulsion and used as the normal control group. Forty mice were scored daily for signs of neurological impairment according to clinical symptom (CS) score criteria up to 50 days after induction. Animals received standard Purina chow and had free access to water. On the 50th day after immunization, the mice were placed in transparent glassware, and excess isoflurane was added. When the mouse does not have spontaneous breathing and blinking reflexes, the follow-up operation can be performed. The experimental protocol was approved by the Ethics Committee of the First Affiliated Hospital of Zhengzhou University and confirmed with the Guide for the Care and Use of Laboratory Animals.

In order to analyze the effect of miR-219c-5p in mice on bladder fibrosis in EAE mice, another 40 mice were used to establish an EAE mouse model. On the 30th day, randomly selected CS3 mice were divided into EAE-miR-219c-5p agomir group, EAE-miR-219c-5p antagomir group and EAE-NC group, 3 mice in each group. MiR-219c-5p agomir (10 nmol), miR-219c-5p antagomir (10 nmol) and PBS were injected into the tail vein once a week. On the 50th day, the mice were killed by cervical dislocation after anesthesia. The bladder tissues of the mice were taken for HE and Masson`s trichrome staining. The degree of fibrosis and the expression of FN1 were observed by FN1 immunohistochemistry.

Prediction of potentially targeted miRNAs that inhibit FN1

The miRDB (http://mirdb.org/) and miRBase (http://www.mirbase.org) databases were used to predict FN1-targeting microRNAs. After comparing the context score, context score percentile, weighted context score, and conserved branch length, miR-199a-3p, miR-219c-5p and miR-3572-3p were predicted to interact with FN1.

Mouse BSMC primary culture

BSMCs were purchased from Otwo Biotech (HTX3129; Shenzhen, China) and verified by a-SMA immunofluorescence. The BSMCs were cultured in Dulbecco's modified Eagle's medium—high glucose (DMEM-H; Gibco, Thermo Fisher Scientific, Waltham, MA) containing 10% fetal bovine serum (FBS) (Gibco, Thermo Fisher Scientific) and 100 U/ml cyan-streptomycin. Anti-α-SMA (MA1-06110; Thermo Fisher Scientific; 1:200) and goat anti-rabbit IgG H&L (Alexa Fluor488) (ab150077; Abcam, USA; 1:1000) immunofluorescence staining was used to identify BSMCs. Only cells at passage numbers 3 to 10 were used for all experiments.

Overexpression or knockdown of miRNAs in BSMCs

One day before transfection, cells were starved by seeding in medium supplemented with 2% FBS at a density of 5×10^4 cells/ml. On the day of transfection, the medium was changed to 10% FBS medium, and the cells were transfected with miRNA mimic, NC mimic, miRNA inhibitor or NC inhibitor (RiboBio, Guangzhou, China) using a riboFECT™ CP Transfection Kit (RiboBio, Guangzhou, China) according to the manufacturer's instructions. The miRNA mimic and inhibitor used are listed in Table 1.

miR-219c-5p target prediction and luciferase reporter assay

Potential miR-219c-5p binding sites were predicted using online database programs with different algorithms, including miRDB (http://mirdb.org/) and miRBase (http://www.mirbase.org). For the luciferase assay, BSMCs (3×10^3 cells/well) were first seeded in 96-well plates. Then, 1 day later, luciferase reporter plasmids [pmiR-FN1-wild type (WT) or pmiR-FN1-mutant (Mut)

Table 1 List of gene

Gene name	Sequence
miR-199a-3p mimics	5′-AUUGGUUACACGUCUGAUGACA-3′
miR-199a-3 inhibitor	5′-UAACCAAUGUGCAGACUACUGU-3′
miR-219c-5p mimics	5′-GGACGUCCAGACGCAACUCUCG-3′
miR-219c-5p inhibitor	5′-CGAGAGUUGCGUCUGGACGUCC-3′
miR-3572-3p mimics	5′-UACACUUGUCCUUCUUUCCCCAG-3′
miR-3572-3p inhibitor	5′-CUGGGGAAAGAAGGACAAGUGUA-3′
mimics NC	5′-UUUGUACUACACAAAAGUACUG-3′
inhibitor NC	5′-UUUGUACUACACAAAAGUACUG-3′

(RiboBio, Guangzhou, China)] were cotransfected with miR-219c-5p mimic or NC mimic into BSMCs. Luciferase activity was determined 48 h after transfection using a GLOMAX 96 spectrophotometer (Promega Corporation) following the manufacturer's protocol. Firefly luciferase activity was normalized to Renilla luciferase activity.

Quantitative real-time polymerase chain reaction

Total RNA was isolated from bladder tissue or BSMCs using TRIzol (Leagene Biotechnology, Beijing, China) according to the manufacturer's protocol. For miRNA RT-qPCR, reverse transcription was performed using ReverTra Ace qPCR RT Master Mix (FSQ-101; TOYOBO, Japan). For FN1 RT-PCR, reverse transcription was performed using ReverTra Ace qPCR RT Master Mix and gDNA Remover (FSQ-301; TOYOBO, Japan). As described above, cDNA obtained by reverse transcription was used for real-time PCR. qPCR was performed using a SYBR Green Mix (Applied Biosystems; Roche, Inc.) in a 20-μl reaction at 95 °C for 2 s, 60 °C for 20 s, and 70 °C for 10 s (40 cycles). Relative miRNA expression levels and other indicators were calculated in triplicate using the $2^{-\Delta\Delta CT}$ method. Expression levels were normalized to β-actin or U6 levels, and the primers used are listed in Table 2.

Hematoxylin and eosin and Masson's trichrome staining

Mouse bladders were soaked overnight in 4% paraformaldehyde. The tissues were cut into 5-μm paraffin sections for bladder fibrosis analysis. According to the protocol, the paraffin sections were stained with hematoxylin and eosin (H&E) and Masson's trichrome. The amount of collagen, the number of smooth muscle cells, and the ratio of collagen to smooth muscle cells were calculated by using an image analysis system (ImageJ 1.80). The ratio of collagen to smooth muscle cells was used to quantify the degree of fibrosis in the bladder tissue.

Immunohistochemistry

Immunohistochemical (IHC) staining for streptavidin-peroxidase (SP) was used to detect FN1 expression in bladder tissue. After sectioning, conventional dewaxing, gradient ethanol hydration, and antigen retrieval were performed in sequence. Subsequently, the sections were incubated with 3% hydrogen peroxide for 20 min, blocked with serum for 10 min, and incubated with the primary antibody rabbit anti-mouse FN1 (ab45688; Abcam, USA; 1:200) overnight at 4 °C. The sections were then incubated with horseradish peroxidase-labeled goat anti-rabbit secondary antibody (ab205718; Abcam, USA; 1:2000) for 30 min and stained with DAB (Sigma, USA). After counterstaining with hematoxylin, all slides were hydrated, clarified, fixed and observed, and the positive cell index was determined.

Table 2 List of primers

Gene name	Primer sequences
β-actin	F-AAATGTGGCTGAGGACTTTGTAC
	R-GGACTTCCTGTAACCACTTATTTCA
U6	F-GCTCGCTTCGGCAGCACA
	R-GAGGTATTCGCACCAGAGGA
FN1	F-ACCCGTTTTCATCCAACAAGAG
	R-CGGTATCCAGACACCACACTATCA

FN1 Fibronectin 1, *F* forward, *R* reverse

Cell proliferation assay

Cell proliferation was tested using a Cell Counting Kit 8 (CCK8) (CK04; DOJINDO, Japan; 10 μl) assay. The BSMCs to be transfected were inoculated into 96-well plates. Each well was inoculated with approximately 1000 cells, and 6 replicate wells were assayed for each group. After 24, 48, 72 and 96 h of transfection, 10 μl of CCK8 reagent was added to each well and incubated for 1 h. Sample absorbance was read at 450 nm on a microplate reader (SpectraMax-M5, Sunnyvale, CA).

Flow cytometry

After 48 h of transfection, cells were treated with 0.25% trypsin and harvested. Approximately 1×10^5 cells were counted, fixed with 75% cold ethanol (Solarbio Life Sciences, Shanghai, China) for 4 h, and then treated with 0.5% Triton-X100 for 10 min. Triton-X100 was removed by centrifugation, and the cells were stained with 200 μl propidium iodide (PI) (BD, USA) at room temperature for 30 min in the dark. A flow cytometer (ACCURI C6 PLUS, BD, USA) was used to analyze the cell cycle, and the experiments were repeated three times. Similarly, cells were treated with 0.25% trypsin without ethylenediaminetetraacetic acid. Approximately 1×10^5 cells were counted, and 10 μl Annexin V-fluorescein isothiocyanate (FITC) (BD, USA) and PI (BD, USA) each was added and incubated at room temperature for 15 min in the dark. The rate of apoptosis (percentage of apoptotic cells relative to the total number of cells) was estimated by flow cytometry. Representative results of three independent experiments are shown.

Western blot assay

An equal amount of each protein sample (20 μg) was separated using 12% sodium dodecyl sulfate polyacrylamide gel electrophoresis (SDS-PAGE) at 120 V. The proteins were transferred to a polypropylene difluoride (PVDF) membrane at a constant flow of 400 mA for 5 h under ice bath conditions. The PVDF membrane was incubated for 30 min at room temperature in 5% skim milk to block nonspecific banding. Then, the PVDF membrane was incubated with rabbit anti-mouse-FN1 (ab45688; Abcam, USA; 1:10,000) or anti-β-actin (AC026; ABclonal, Wuhan, China; 1:10,000) primary antibody at 4 °C overnight. After washing once with TBS and 3 times with TBST, the PVDF membrane was incubated with horseradish peroxidase-conjugated goat anti-rabbit IgG secondary antibody (AS003; ABclonal, Wuhan, China; 1:10,000) for 1 h at room temperature. The PVDF membrane was washed 5 times with TBST, and the proteins of interest were detected using an enhanced chemiluminescence (ECL) system. Densitometry analysis of the protein bands was performed using ImageJ software (National Institutes of Health, Bethesda, MA, USA) and normalized to the gray value of β-actin. This experiment was replicated three times.

Statistical analysis

All data were obtained from three independent replicates and are shown as the mean ± standard deviation. Comparisons between two sets of samples were performed using Student's t test. One-way ANOVA or two-way ANOVA was used for comparisons between single-factor or two-factor multiple groups. $P < 0.05$ was chosen to represent a statistically significant difference. Statistical analysis was performed using SPSS software (SPSS for Windows 21.0; SPSS Inc., Chicago, IL, USA).

Results

EAE induced bladder wall fibrosis in mice

On the 10th day after immunization, EAE mice were observed to show signs of neurological deficits, while the normal control mice (immunized with CFA alone) were normal. We found that the symptoms of EAE mice were not persistent but rather presented a cycle of sustained remission-relapse. However, mice in the remission phase were not completely normal and still had tail weakness. Figure 1a shows the mean CS score of mice in the EAE model group from day 0 to day 50. The control group (NC) did not show any clinical symptoms throughout the time period. Fifty days after immunization, the mice were scored by CS, including 10 in the NC group, 7 in the CS1 group, 9 in the CS2 group, 12 in the CS3 group, and 2 in the CS4 group. At 50 days postimmunization, the bladder-body weight ratio was significantly higher for the EAE model group (CS1/2/3 group) than for the NC group (Fig. 1b, $P < 0.0001$), whereas the mean body weight was not significantly different between NC mice and EAE mice (Table 3, $P > 0.05$).

To further determine whether prolonged urinary retention of the neurogenic bladder can lead to bladder wall fibrosis, we performed histological and morphological analyses by H&E and Masson's trichrome staining. Only the degree of bladder smooth muscle layer tissue fibrosis was evaluated. H&E and Masson's staining showed that the CS3 group was significantly more fibrous than the NC group (Fig. 1c, $P < 0.01$). Only the degree of bladder smooth muscle layer tissue fibrosis was evaluated. These results suggest that the higher the CS score of EAE mice is, the more severe the bladder fibrosis is.

FN1 expression in EAE-induced fibrotic bladder tissue

We found a potential correlation between bladder fibrosis and FN1 by detecting protein and mRNA expression levels in bladders with varying degrees of fibrosis. As the clinical symptoms of EAE model mice deteriorated, the FN1 expression level increased significantly. We detected an increase in FN1 expression by immunohistochemistry (Fig. 2a, $P < 0.01$), Western blot analysis (Fig. 2b, $P < 0.0001$) and RT-qPCR (Fig. 2c, $P < 0.0001$) as bladder fibrosis was aggravated. These results indicate that the more severe the fibrosis of the bladder tissue is, the higher the FN1 content of the bladder tissue will be. In other words, the degree of bladder tissue fibrosis is positively correlated with the expression of FN1.

Prediction of miRNAs targeting FN1 and detection of miRNA expression in bladders with different degrees of fibrosis

The miRDB (http://mirdb.org/) and miRBase (http://www.mirbase.org) databases were used to predict FN1-targeting microRNAs. After comparing the context score, context score percentile, weighted context score, and conserved branch length, it was found that miR-199a-3p, miR-219c-5p and miR-3572-3p could interact with FN1 (Fig. 3a). Next, the miRNA expression levels in the bladder with different scores were detected by RT-qPCR (Fig. 3b–d). We found that the miR-199a-3p, miR-219c-5p and miR-3572-3p expression levels decreased with increasing bladder fibrosis, which was the opposite of the FN1 expression trend. These results indicate that the high FN1 expression during bladder fibrosis may potentially be related to the reductions in these miRNAs.

Identification of BSMCs and miRNA transfection

Since the main component of the bladder wall is BSMCs, we cultured BSMCs in vitro for experiments. BSMCs were identified by immunofluorescence staining for α-SMA (Fig. 4a). The transfection efficiencies of miR-199a-3p, miR-219c-5p and miR-3572-3p were detected by RT-qPCR (Fig. 4b). Then, the effect of miR-199a-3p, miR-219c-5p and miR-3572-3p on FN1 was detected by RT-qPCR (Fig. 4c). We found that only miR-219c-5p produced the expected results when the transfection efficiencies among miR-199a-3p,

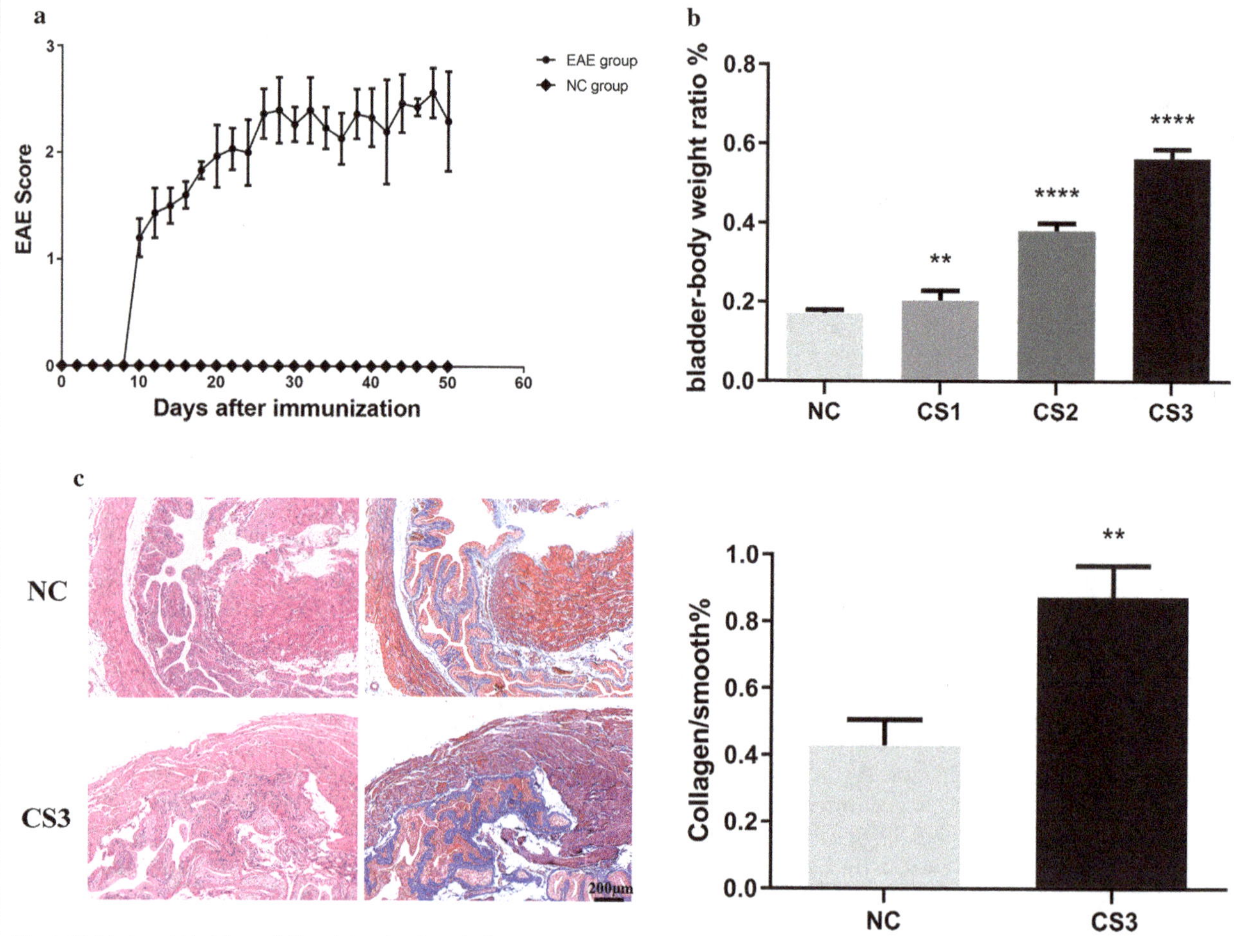

Fig. 1 EAE-induced bladder wall fibrosis in mice. Female C57BL/6 mice were used to establish EAE using MOG 35–55. After immunization, the disease development was scored according to clinical symptoms (CS), and the body weight and neurological deficit of the mice were examined daily and scored on a scale of 0–5, where CS0 = no disease; CS1 = tail weakness and/or moderately awkward gait and/or poor righting ability; CS2 = tail weakness and/or moderately awkward gait; CS3 = hind limb paralysis or mild forelimb weakness (or both); CS4 = limb paralysis; and CS5 = quadriplegia with detained urine or death. **a** EAE progression in mice is indicated by the mean clinical score. The error bars show ± SE. **b** The bladder-to-body weight ratios were significantly greater in EAE mice than in normal control mice (NC) (n = 3 mice/group). **c** Only the degree of bladder smooth muscle layer tissue fibrosis was evaluated. Left: H&E, Right: Masson's trichrome stain. The red areas indicate smooth muscle, and the blue areas indicate connective tissue. The collagen-smooth-muscle ratio was determined by the mean Masson's trichrome staining data in the NC and CS3 groups (n = 3 mice/group). The data are expressed as the mean ± SD. NC, normal control group; CS, clinical symptoms. $^{**}P < 0.01$, $^{****}P < 0.0001$ versus control. Scale bar = 200 μm

Table 3 Bladder weight, FN1 and miR-219c-5p expression in mice with different EAE scores

Variable	EAE score				F Value	*P* Value
	0	1	2	3		
Body weight/g	27.99 ± 0.56	27.91 ± 0.78	25.81 ± 1.05	25.68 ± 0.87	0.5882	0.646
Bladder weight to total body weight (%)	0.17 ± 0.01	0.20 ± 0.02	0.38 ± 0.02	0.56 ± 0.02	1002	< 0.0001
FN1	1.00 ± 0.10	1.23 ± 0.70	1.59 ± 0.14	3.01 ± 0.10	342.7	< 0.0001
miR-199a-3p	3.40 ± 0.53	2.73 ± 0.25	1.93 ± 0.40	1.03 ± 0.15	23.6	< 0.0001
miR-219c-5p	3.10 ± 0.10	1.73 ± 0.08	1.23 ± 0.06	1.00 ± 0.10	376.4	< 0.0001
miR-3572-3p	4.50 ± 0.50	3.53 ± 0.55	2.03 ± 0.25	1.03 ± 0.15	44.6	< 0.0002

Values are means ± SE; n = 3 mice/group. $P < 0.05$ by ANOVA among four groups; expression levels were normalized to β-actin or U6

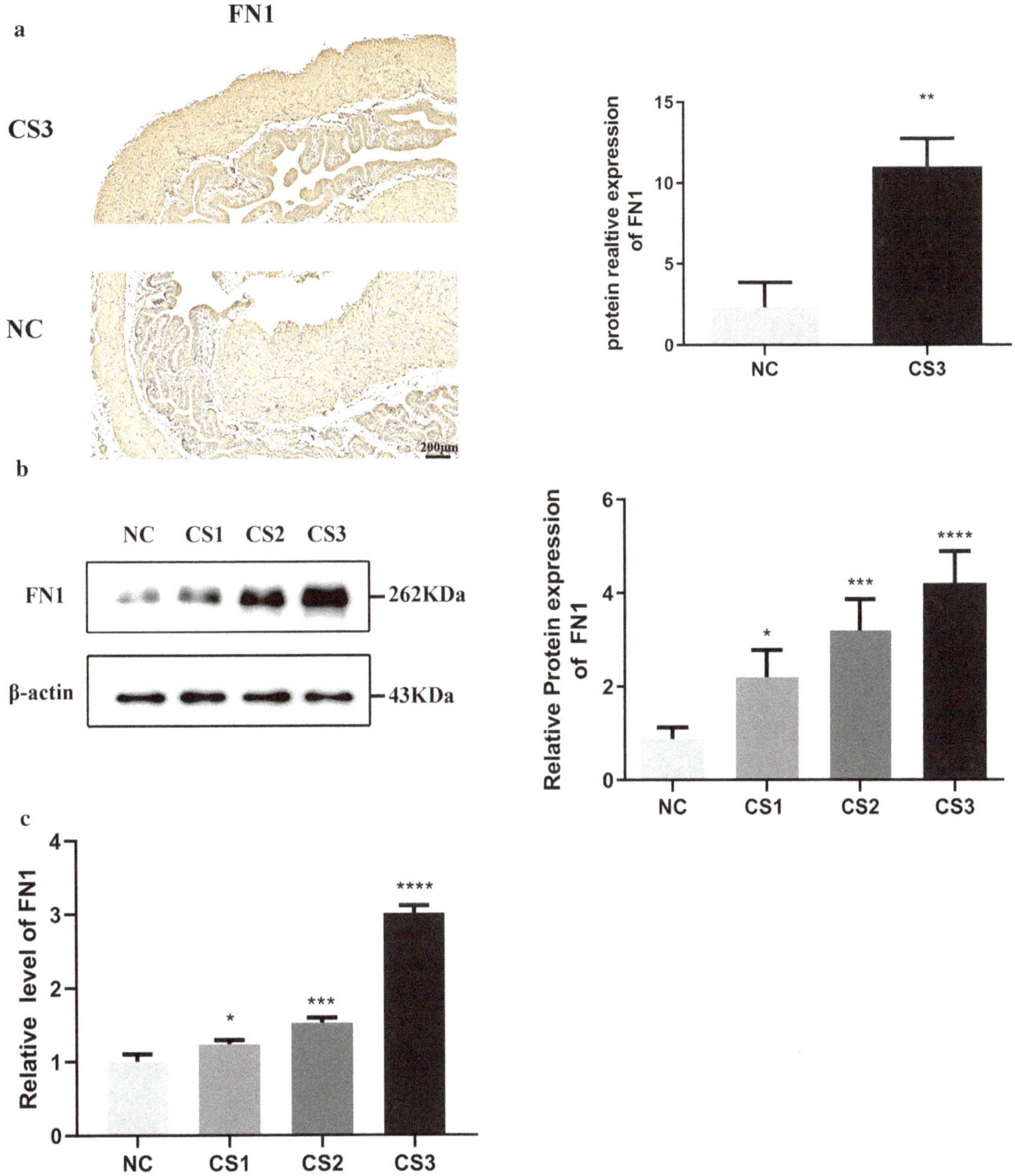

Fig. 2 FN1 expression in EAE-induced fibrotic bladder tissue. **a** The expression of FN1 in bladder fibrosis with different scores was analyzed by immunohistochemistry. **b** The expression of FN1 in bladder fibrosis with different scores was analyzed by Western blotting. **c** The expression of FN1 in bladder fibrosis with different scores was analyzed by RT-qPCR. The findings were from three separate experiments. The data are expressed as the mean ± SD. NC, normal control group; CS, clinical symptoms; FN1, fibronectin 1. $^{ns}P > 0.05$, $^{*}P < 0.05$, $^{**}P < 0.01$, $^{***}P < 0.001$, $^{****}P < 0.0001$ versus control. Scale bar = 200 μm

miR-219c-5p and miR-3572-3p were the same. That is, FN1 was decreased ($P < 0.001$) when miR-219c-5p was overexpressed, and FN1 was increased ($P < 0.0001$) when miR-219c-5p was knocked down. In summary, miR-219c-5p is most likely one of the miRNAs targeting FN1.

miR-219c-5p binding to FN1

Bioinformation prediction websites such as miRDB (http://mirdb.org/) and miRBase (http://www.mirbase.org) were used to infer the potential targeting relationship between miR-219c-5p and FN1. The sequence of the predicted 3′-UTR site where miR-219c-5p binds

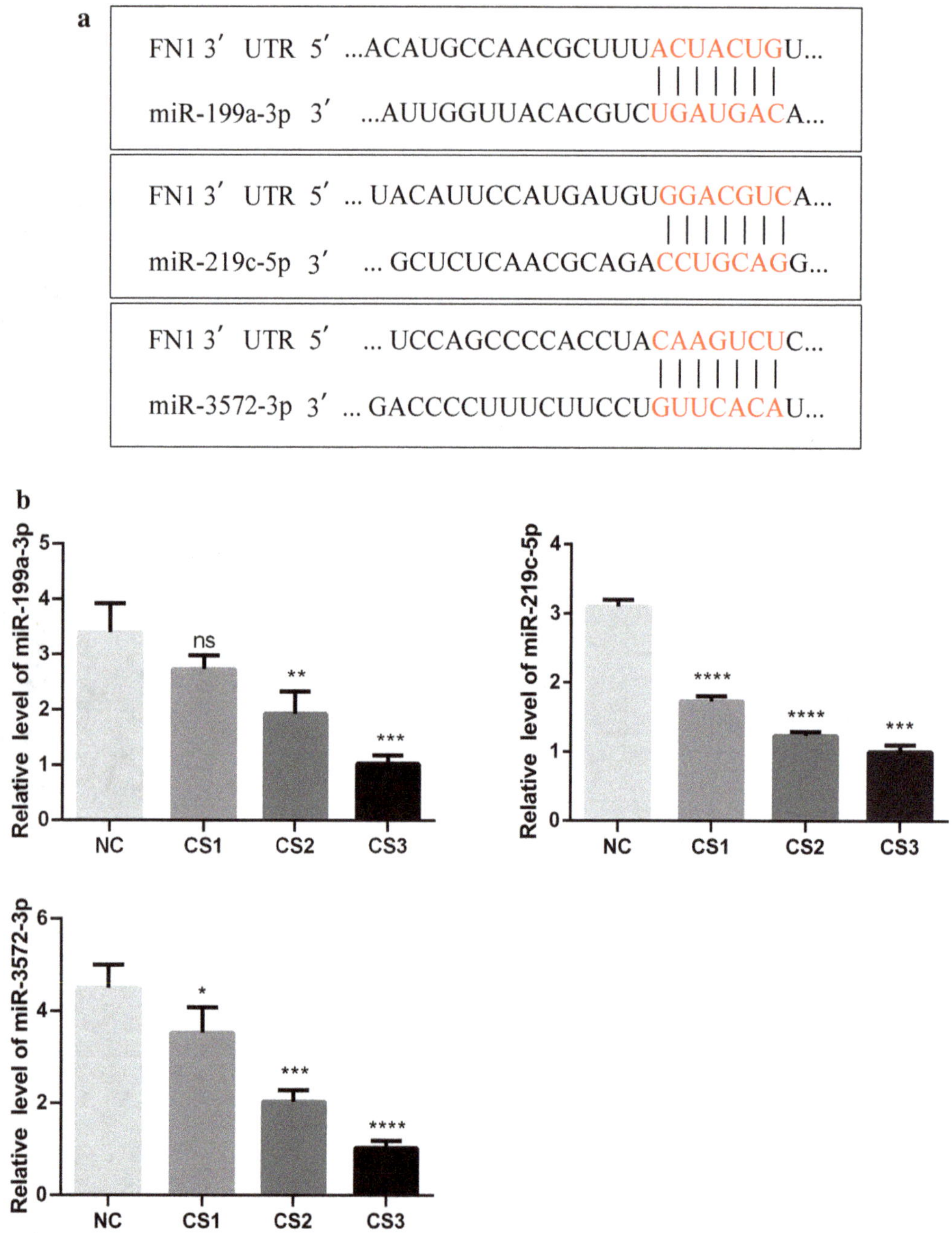

Fig. 3 Prediction of miRNAs targeting FN1 and detection of miRNA expression in bladders with different degrees of fibrosis. **a** Database prediction that miR-199a-3p, miR-219c-5p, and miR-3572-3p target FN1. **b–d** The expression levels of miR-199a-3p, miR-219c-5p, and miR-3572-3p in different fibrotic bladders were detected by RT-qPCR. The findings were from three separate experiments. The data are expressed as the mean ± SD. NC, normal control group; CS, clinical symptoms; FN1, fibronectin 1. $^{ns}P > 0.05$, $^{*}P < 0.05$, $^{**}P < 0.01$, $^{***}P < 0.001$, $^{****}P < 0.0001$ versus control

to FN1 mRNA is shown in Fig. 5a. The dual luciferase reporter assay results showed that miR-219c-5p reduced FN1-WT luciferase activity by 49% ($P < 0.01$) and had no effect on FN1-MUT luciferase activity (Fig. 5a, $P > 0.05$), indicating that miR-219c-5p can target FN1 and affect its synthesis.

miR-219c-5p targeted FN1 to suppress BSMC proliferation

To observe the effect of miR-219c-5p on BSMC proliferation, we overexpressed or knocked down miR-219c-5p in vitro. The effect of miR-219c-5p on proliferation in BSMCs is shown in Fig. 5B. There was no significant difference in the survival rate of BSMCs between the blank

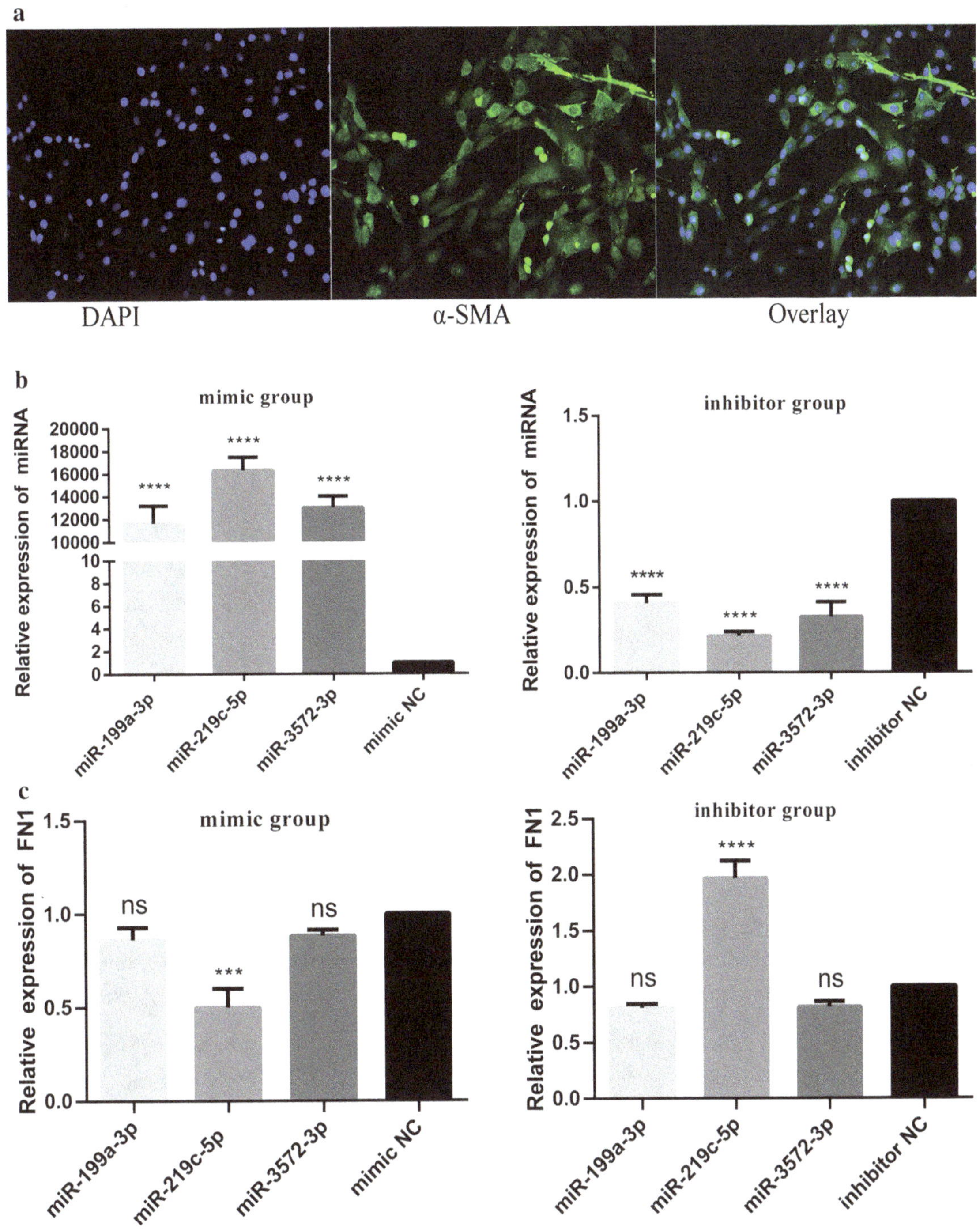

Fig. 4 Identification of BSMCs and miRNA transfection. **a** Under a fluorescence microscope, almost all cells were stained green, indicating the cytoskeleton, and blue, indicating the nucleus (magnification: × 200). **b** The transfection efficiencies of miR-199a-3p, miR-219c-5p and miR-3572-3p were detected by RT-qPCR. **b** The effect of miR-199a-3p, miR-219c-5p and miR-3572-3p on FN1 was detected by RT-qPCR. The findings were from three separate experiments. The data are expressed as the means ± SD. CS, clinical symptoms; FN1, fibronectin 1. $^{ns}P > 0.05$, $^{*}P < 0.05$, $^{**}P < 0.01$, $^{***}P < 0.001$, $^{****}P < 0.0001$ versus control

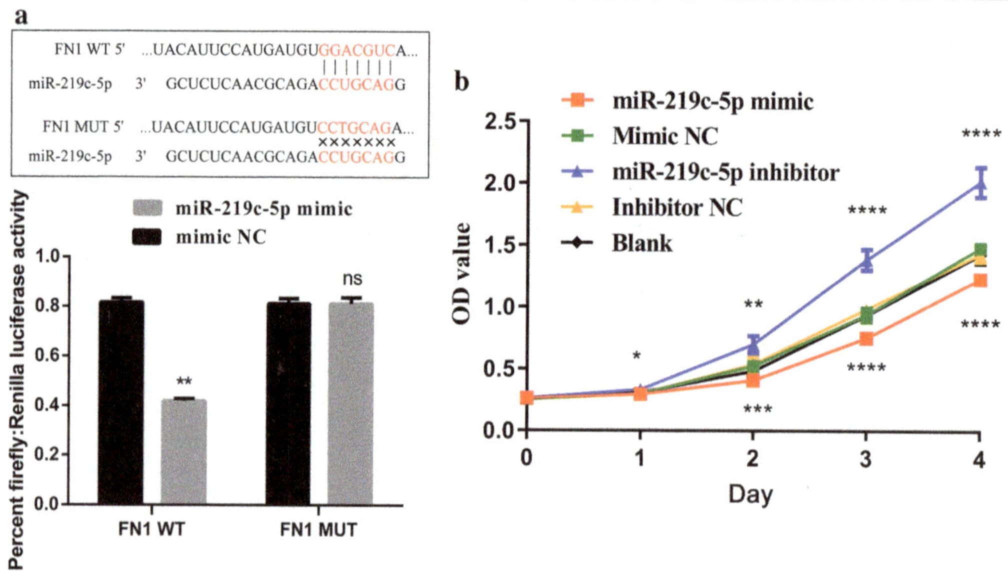

Fig. 5 miR-219c-5p targets FN1 and affects BSMC proliferation. **a** miR-219c-5p and FN1 3′-UTR binding and luciferase activity detection in BSMCs (n = 3). **b** The OD_{450} values of the cells were measured via CCK8 assay. The findings were from three separate experiments. The data are expressed as the mean ± SD. WT, wild type; MUT, mutant; FN1, fibronectin 1; 3′-UTR, three prime untranslated region. $^{ns}P > 0.05$, $^{*}P < 0.05$, $^{**}P < 0.01$, $^{***}P < 0.001$, $^{****}P < 0.0001$ versus mimic NC or inhibitor NC

and NC groups (all $P > 0.05$). Compared with that of the blank and NC groups, the viability of BSMCs in the miR-219c-5p group decreased ($P < 0.05$), whereas cell viability in the miR-219c-5p inhibitor group increased ($P < 0.05$). These results indicate that miR-219c-5p can participate in BSMC proliferation by regulating the expression of FN1.

Effect of miR-219c-5p on the BSMC cycle

Compared with that in the blank and NC groups, the number of BSMCs in the miR-219c-5p group increased in the G1 phase but decreased in the S/G2 phase, while the number of cells in the miR-219c-5p inhibition group decreased in the G1 phase but increased in the S/G2 phase (Fig. 6a, $P < 0.05$ in all cases). These data indicate that miR-219c-5p can inhibit the cell cycle by regulating FN1 gene expression and thereby arresting BSMCs in the G1 phase.

Effect of miR-219c-5p on apoptosis in BSMCs

The apoptosis rate of the miR-219c-5p mock group increased significantly compared with that of the blank and NC groups ($P < 0.05$). However, the apoptosis rate of the miR-219c-5p inhibition group was significantly reduced compared with that of the blank and NC groups (Fig. 6b, $P < 0.05$). These results indicate that miR-219c-5p can promote BSMC apoptosis.

Effects of miR-219c-5p agomir and antagomir on bladder fibrosis in EAE mice

In order to observe the effect of miR-219c-5p on bladder fibrosis in mice EAE model, we overexpressed or knocked down miR-219c-5p in vivo, that is, injection of agomir and antagomir through the tail vein. Compared with the EAE-NC group, bladder fibrosis was significantly reduced in the EAE-miR-219c-5p agomir group (Fig. 7, $P < 0.05$), and the expression of FN1 content was reduced (Fig. 7, $P < 0.05$). The EAE-miR-219c-5p antagomir group had significantly increased bladder fibrosis (Fig. 7, $P < 0.05$), and the expression of FN1 increased (Fig. 7, $P < 0.05$). The above results suggest that miR-219c-5p can participate in the occurrence and development of bladder fibrosis through targeted inhibition of FN1 expression.

Discussion

In this study, we found that bladder fibrosis in EAE mice was aggravated by clinical symptoms. Moreover, we found that bladder fibrosis severity positively correlated with FN1. Therefore, we speculated that FN1 synthesis could be inhibited by a targeting miRNA, thereby blocking the progression of bladder fibrosis. Two databases, including miRDB (http://mirdb.org/), were used to predict microRNAs that interact with FN1. After comparative analysis, miR-199a-3p, miR-219c-5p and miR-3572-3p were predicted to target FN1. By overexpressing or knocking down miR-199a-3p, miR-219c-5p

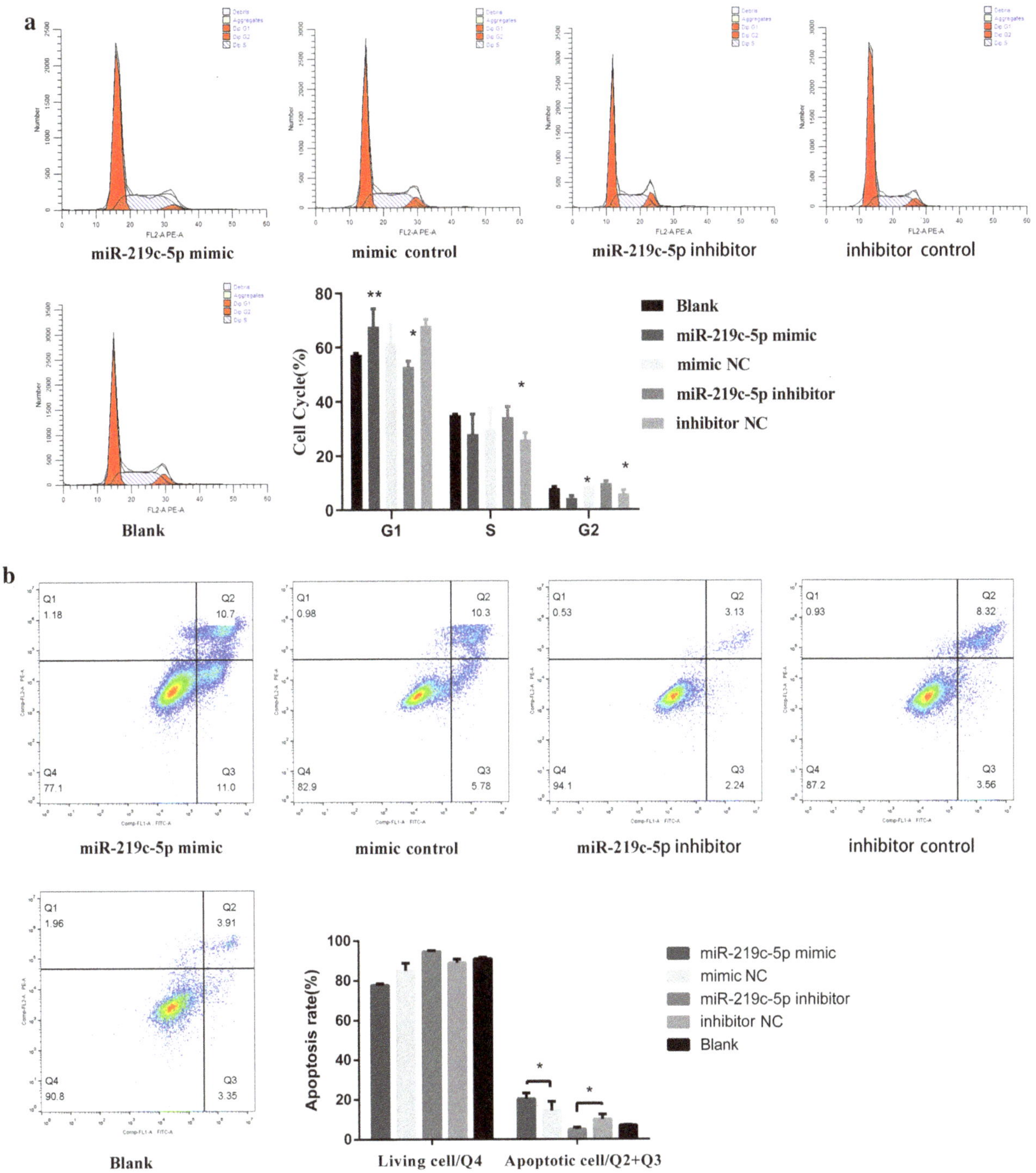

Fig. 6 Effect of miR-219c-5p on the cell cycle and apoptosis in BSMCs. **a** Compared with that in the blank and NC groups, the number of BSMCs in the miR-219c-5p group increased in the G1 phase but decreased in the S/G2 phase, while the number of cells in the miR-219c-5p inhibition group decreased in the G1 phase but increased in the S/G2 phase ($P < 0.05$ in all cases). **b** The apoptosis rate of the miR-219c-5p group increased significantly compared with that of the blank and NC groups ($P < 0.05$). However, the apoptosis rate of the miR-219c-5p inhibition group was significantly reduced compared with that of the blank and NC groups ($P < 0.05$). The findings were from three independent experiments. The data are expressed as the means ± SD. *$P < 0.05$, **$P < 0.01$ versus mimic NC or inhibitor NC

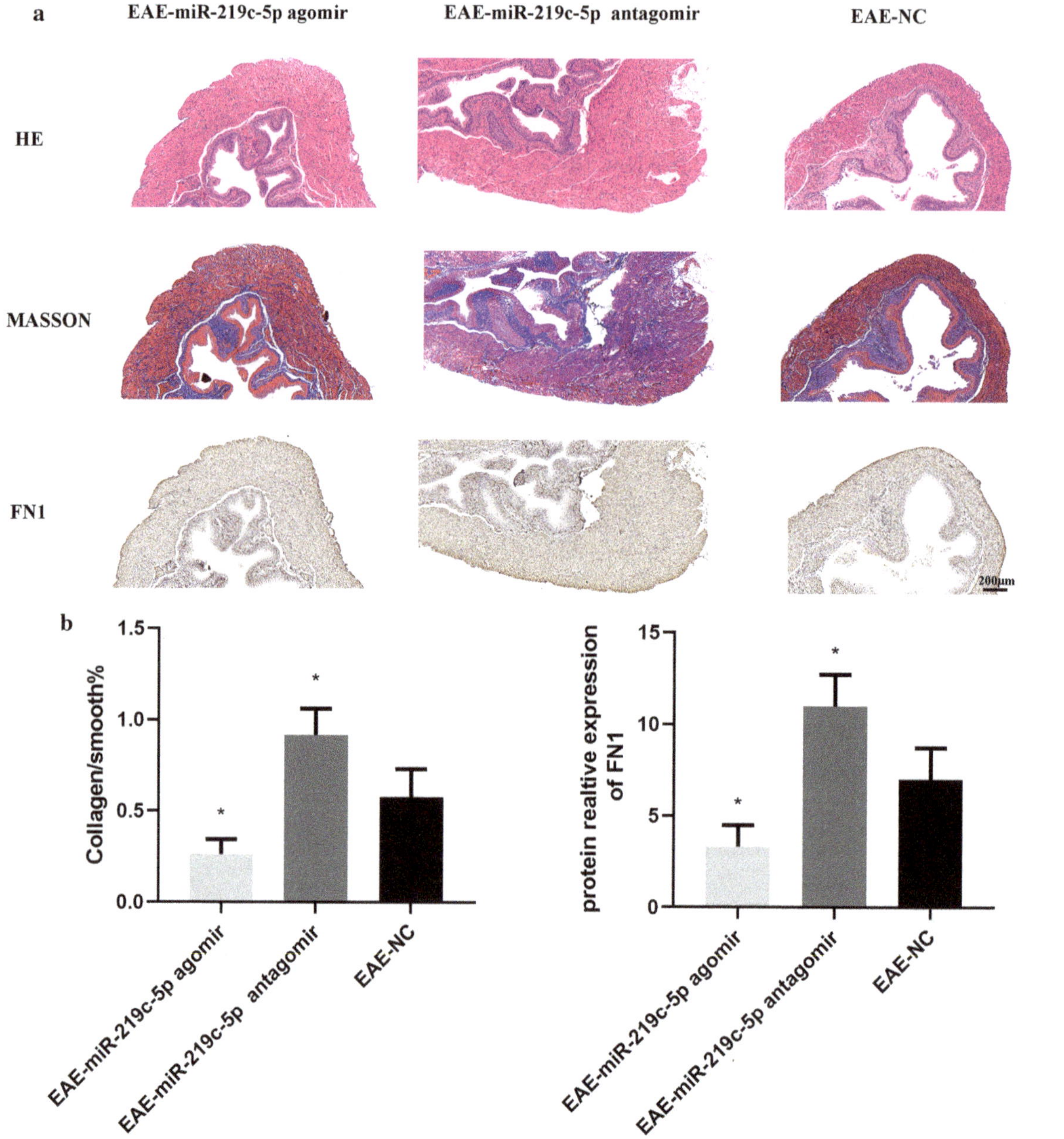

Fig. 7 Effects of miR-219c-5p agomir and antagomir on bladder fibrosis in EAE mice. **a** Only the degree of fibrosis and FN1 expression of bladder smooth muscle layer tissue were evaluated. **b** Compared with the EAE-NC group, bladder fibrosis was significantly reduced in the EAE-miR-219c-5p agomir group ($P < 0.05$), and the expression of FN1 content was reduced ($P < 0.05$). The EAE-miR-219c-5p antagomir group had significantly increased bladder fibrosis ($P < 0.05$), and the expression of FN1 increased ($P < 0.05$). The data are expressed as the means ± SD. *$P < 0.05$ versus EAE-NC

and miR-3572-3p in bladder smooth muscle in vitro, we found that only miR-219c-5p targeted FN1. A luciferase reporter assay confirmed that miR-219c-5p could inhibit FN1 synthesis. Moreover, CCK8 and flow functional assays confirmed that miR-219c-5p could regulate the function of BSMCs by regulating FN1 synthesis.

Urinary dysfunction, such as frequent urination, urgency, and urinary retention, is a common problem in patients with MS. Treating MS patients with bladder dysfunction remains clinically difficult because there is currently no effective treatment. Altuntas et al. [8] were the first to suggest that the EAE model induced by

PEP139-151 is similar to urinary dysfunction in patients with neurogenic bladders. Previous studies have shown that the neurological damage symptoms in EAE mice are associated with prostaglandin E2 E-prostaglandin receptor 3/4 (PGE2 EP3/EP4), providing a new target for neurogenic bladder targeted therapy [26]. Wang et al. [27] reported that human BSMCs proliferation is regulated mainly by extracellular signal-regulated kinase 1/2 activity and by exchange factors directly activated by the cAMP pathway. These findings not only provide new ideas for the treatment of neurogenic bladder but also support our findings.

Fibrosis is described as "wrong body repair", and while its development may involve many mechanisms, myofibroblast activation and the subsequent production of excess extracellular components are essential for fibrosis. Similarly, bladder fibrosis is thought to be involved in BSMC activation and excess extracellular matrix accumulation. Some studies have shown that miRNAs are involved in smooth muscle cell function, including cell proliferation, the cell cycle, and apoptosis [23, 28, 29]. There is growing evidence that many miRNAs play key regulatory roles in bladder fibrosis. Duan et al. [30] demonstrated a novel miR-133 regulatory factor that targets the TGF-β-Smad3 signaling pathway to modulate TGF-β1-induced changes in the BSMC phenotype. A novel antifibrotic function of miR-133 was proposed, which represents a potential target for diagnosis and treatment strategies for bladder fibrosis.

FN1 is a high molecular weight glycoprotein in the extracellular matrix with complex biological functions as a core component. Fibroblasts, vascular endothelial cells, hepatocytes, vascular smooth muscle cells, and other cell types secrete this functional protein, which regulates cell adhesion, proliferation, differentiation, cell morphology maintenance, cell migration promotion, ion exchange, signal transduction, and other functions. Properly increase the expression of FN1 in vitro, the growth of BSMCs increases, but due to the influence of microenvironment (space, nutrition, etc.) in the vivo, when FN1 protein is overexpressed, excessive FN1 protein is deposited in the cytoplasm of the cell, affecting the normal functional activity of the cell causing fibrosis. Numerous studies have reported the regulation of FN1-mediated fibrosis by miRNAs. Gunadi et al. [31] reported that miRNA-206 targeting FN1 is abnormally expressed in multifactorial Hirschsprung's disease and can be used as a potential targeting molecule. Moreover, an interesting phenomenon was found in this study: BSMCs undergo apoptosis after miR-219c-5p is overexpressed. We speculate that BSMC apoptosis may be related to the increase in Bax/Bcl-2 ratio-induced apoptosis after FN1 downregulation [32].

Numerous studies have shown that miRNAs are involved in the tissue fibrosis process. Jing Wu et al. [33] reported that miR-27a can target the AMP-activated protein kinase alpha2 catalytic subunit and activate the TGF-β1 and Smad3 signaling pathways, thereby reducing detrusor fibrosis in streptozotocin-induced diabetic rats. Su-Jin Moon et al. [34] reported that FN1 is an important functional protein in the development of skin fibers. Therefore, we explored whether FN1 is involved in the development of bladder fibrosis and whether miRNAs can target FN1 to regulate bladder fibrosis progression. According to miRBase (http://www.mirbase.org) and miRDB (http://mirdb.org/) predictions, miR-199a-3p, miR-219c-5p and miR-3572-3p may interact with FN1. We overexpressed miR-219c-5p, miR-199a-3p, and miR-3572-3p in vitro and found that FN1 was significantly downregulated when miR-219c-5p was overexpressed. What role might miR-199a-3p and miR-3572-3P play in the development of bladder fibrosis? Ying Tao [35] et al. reported that miR-199a-3p promotes cardiomyocyte proliferation by inhibiting Cd151 expression. We speculated through miRDB (http://mirdb.org/) that miR-3572-3P may inhibit cell proliferation by targeting cyclin-dependent kinase 6. Combining the results of in vivo and in vitro experiments, only miR-219c-5p can better regulate FN1 and participate in bladder fibrosis.

Conclusions

Overall, this study reported that miR-219c-5p is better at targeting FN1 than miR-199a-3p and miR-3572-3p. This study demonstrated that miR-219c-5p blocks bladder fibrosis by inhibiting FN1 expression.

In conclusion, this study confirmed that FN1 and miR-219c-5p are associated with bladder fibrosis in MS mice. We also show that miR-219c-5p can regulate bladder fibrosis by targeting FN1. A novel antifibrotic function of miR-219c-5p is proposed, which may represent a potential target for the diagnosis and treatment of bladder fibrosis.

Abbreviations

MS: Multiple sclerosis; EAE: Experimental autoimmune encephalomyelitis; BSMCs: Bladder smooth muscle cells; ECM: Extracellular matrix; FBS: Fetal bovine serum fetal bovine serum; FN1: Fibronectin 1; qPCR: Quantitative real-time PCR; α-SMA: α-Smooth muscle actin; CS: Clinical score.

Acknowledgements

This work was supported by the National Natural Science Foundation of China (No. 81570685). We acknowledge and appreciate our colleagues for their valuable efforts and comments on this paper.

Authors' contributions

JY and ZJ have made significant contributions to the concept and design. TW collected data. The data was analyzed and interpreted by YD and PL. BL participated in the drafting of the manuscript. JY and SH participated in critical revisions of important knowledge content. All authors have finally approved the version to be released and agree to be responsible for all aspects of the work. All authors read and approved the final manuscript.

Author details

[1] Department of Urology, Zhengzhou University First Affiliated Hospital, Zhengzhou 450052, China. [2] Zhengzhou Institute of Urology, Zhengzhou University First Affiliated Hospital, Zhengzhou 450052, China.

References

1. Hafler DA, Slavik JM, Anderson DE, O'Connor KC, De Jager P, Baecher-Allan C. Multiple sclerosis. Immunol Rev. 2005;204:208–31.
2. Steinman L. Multiple sclerosis: a two-stage disease. Nat Immunol. 2001;2(9):762–4.
3. Fernandez O. Mechanisms and current treatments of urogenital dysfunction in multiple sclerosis. J Neurol. 2002;249(1):1–8.
4. Kalsi V, Fowler CJ. Therapy Insight: bladder dysfunction associated with multiple sclerosis. Nat Clin Pract Urol. 2005;2(10):492–501.
5. Litwiller SE, Frohman EM, Zimmern PE. Multiple sclerosis and the urologist. J Urol. 1999;161(3):743–57.
6. Al-Izki S, Pryce G, Giovannoni G, Baker D. Evaluating potential therapies for bladder dysfunction in a mouse model of multiple sclerosis with high-resolution ultrasonography. Mult Scler. 2009;15(7):795–801.
7. Altuntas CZ, Daneshgari F, Izgi K, Bicer F, Ozer A, Sakalar C, Grimberg KO, Sayin I, Tuohy VK. Connective tissue and its growth factor CTGF distinguish the morphometric and molecular remodeling of the bladder in a model of neurogenic bladder. Am J Physiol Renal Physiol. 2012;303(9):F1363-1369.
8. Steinman L, Zamvil SS. Virtues and pitfalls of EAE for the development of therapies for multiple sclerosis. Trends Immunol. 2005;26(11):565–71.
9. Petry KG, Boullerne AI, Pousset F, Brochet B, Caille JM, Dousset V. Experimental allergic encephalomyelitis animal models for analyzing features of multiple sclerosis. Pathol Biol (Paris). 2000;48(1):47–53.
10. Altuntas CZ, Daneshgari F, Liu G, Fabiyi A, Kavran M, Johnson JM, Gulen MF, Jaini R, Li X, Frenkl TL, et al. Bladder dysfunction in mice with experimental autoimmune encephalomyelitis. J Neuroimmunol. 2008;203(1):58–63.
11. Anumanthan G, Tanaka ST, Adams CM, Thomas JC, Wills ML, Adams MC, Hayward SW, Matusik RJ, Bhowmick NA, Brock JW 3rd, et al. Bladder stromal loss of transforming growth factor receptor II decreases fibrosis after bladder obstruction. J Urol. 2009;182(4 Suppl):1775–80.
12. Taylor JA, Zhu Q, Irwin B, Maghaydah Y, Tsimikas J, Pilbeam C, Leng L, Bucala R, Kuchel GA. Null mutation in macrophage migration inhibitory factor prevents muscle cell loss and fibrosis in partial bladder outlet obstruction. Am J Physiol Renal Physiol. 2006;291(6):F1343-1353.
13. Slama A, Khouni H, Sriha B, Brini K, Ben Sorba N, Taher Mosbah A. Bladder fibrosis caused by eosinophilic cystitis. Ann Urol (Paris). 2003;37(5):272–4.
14. Wang N, Duan L, Ding J, Cao Q, Qian S, Shen H, Qi J. MicroRNA-101 protects bladder of BOO from hypoxia-induced fibrosis by attenuating TGF-beta-smad2/3 signaling. IUBMB Life. 2019;71(2):235–43.
15. Siddiqui NY, Helfand BT, Andreev VP, Kowalski JT, Bradley MS, Lai HH, Berger MB, Mueller MG, Bickhaus JA, Packiam VT, et al. Biomarkers implicated in lower urinary tract symptoms: systematic review and pathway analyses. J Urol. 2019;2019:101097JU0000000000000257.
16. Andersson KE, Fry C, Panicker J, Rademakers K. Which molecular targets do we need to focus on to improve lower urinary tract dysfunction? ICI-RS 2017. Neurourol Urodyn. 2018;37(S4):S117-s126.
17. Peyronnet B, Mironska E, Chapple C, Cardozo L, Oelke M, Dmochowski R, Amarenco G, Game X, Kirby R, Van Der Aa F, et al. A comprehensive review of overactive bladder pathophysiology: on the way to tailored treatment. Eur Urol. 2019;2019:1.
18. Sobolewski P, Murthy NS, Kohn J, El Fray M. Adsorption of fibrinogen and fibronectin on elastomeric poly(butylene succinate) copolyesters. Langmuir. 2019;2019:1.
19. Stribos EGD, Seelen MA, van Goor H, Olinga P, Mutsaers HAM. Murine precision-cut kidney slices as an model to evaluate the role of transforming growth factor-β1 signaling in the onset of renal fibrosis. Front Physiol. 2017;8:1026.
20. Wang W, Jia Y-J, Yang Y-L, Xue M, Zheng Z-J, Wang L, Xue Y-M. LncRNA GAS5 exacerbates renal tubular epithelial fibrosis by acting as a competing endogenous RNA of miR-96-5p. Biomed Pharmacother. 2020;121:109411.
21. Rupaimoole R, Slack FJ. MicroRNA therapeutics: towards a new era for the management of cancer and other diseases. Nat Rev Drug Discov. 2017;16(3):203–22.
22. Bruinsma IB, van Dijk M, Bridel C, van de Lisdonk T, Haverkort SQ, Runia TF, Steinman L, Hintzen RQ, Killestein J, Verbeek MM, et al. Regulator of oligodendrocyte maturation, miR-219, a potential biomarker for MS. Journal of neuroinflammation. 2017;14(1):235.
23. Yang L, Dong C, Yang J, Yang L, Chang N, Qi C, Li L. MicroRNA-26b-5p inhibits mouse liver fibrogenesis and angiogenesis by targeting PDGF receptor-beta. Mol Ther Nucl Acids. 2019;16:206–17.
24. Zhang H, Sun Z, Li Y, Fan D, Jiang H. MicroRNA-200c binding to FN1 suppresses the proliferation, migration and invasion of gastric cancer cells. Biomed Pharmacother. 2017;88:285–92.
25. Si M, Wang Q, Li Y, Lin H, Luo D, Zhao W, Dou X, Liu J, Zhang H, Huang Y, et al. Inhibition of hyperglycolysis in mesothelial cells prevents peritoneal fibrosis. Sci Transl Med. 2019;11:495.
26. Xue R, Jia Z, Kong X, Pi G, Ma S, Yang J. Effects of PGE2 EP3/EP4 receptors on bladder dysfunction in mice with experimental autoimmune encephalomyelitis. Am J Physiol Renal Physiol. 2013;305(12):F1656-1662.
27. Lai J, Ai J, Luo D, Jin T, Liao B, Zhou L, Feng S, Jin X, Li H, Wang K. Beta-Adrenoceptor signaling regulates proliferation and contraction of human bladder smooth muscle cells under pathological hydrostatic pressure. J Cell Biochem. 2019;2019:1.
28. Guo JH, Su C, Jiang SY, Wang F, Feng X, Wang JT. MicroRNA-1 regulates fibronectin expression in human trabecular meshwork cells under oxidative stress. Zhonghua Yan Ke Za Zhi. 2019;55(5):355–60.
29. Ma L, Ma J, Ou HL. MicroRNA219 overexpression serves a protective role during liver fibrosis by targeting tumor growth factor beta receptor 2. Mol Med Rep. 2019;19(3):1543–50.
30. Duan LJ, Qi J, Kong XJ, Huang T, Qian XQ, Xu D, Liang JH, Kang J. MiR-133 modulates TGF-β1-induced bladder smooth muscle cell hypertrophic and fibrotic response: implication for a role of microRNA in bladder wall remodeling caused by bladder outlet obstruction. Cell Signal. 2015;27(2):215–27.
31. Gunadi BNYP, Kalim AS, Santiko W, Musthofa FD, Iskandar K, Makhmudi A. Aberrant expressions of miRNA-206 target, FN1, in multifactorial Hirschsprung disease. Orphanet J Rare Dis. 2019;14(1):5.
32. Li B, Shen W, Peng H, Li Y, Chen F, Zheng L, Xu J, Jia L. Fibronectin 1 promotes melanoma proliferation and metastasis by inhibiting apoptosis and regulating EMT. OncoTargets and therapy. 2019;12:3207–21.
33. Wu J, Liu S, Yuan ZW, Liu JH, Li JM, Chen T, Fang KW. MicroRNA-27a suppresses detrusor fibrosis in streptozotocin-induced diabetic rats by targeting PRKAA2 through the TGF-beta1/Smad3 signaling pathway. Cell Physiol Biochem. 2018;45(4):1333–49.
34. Moon SJ, Bae JM, Park KS, Tagkopoulos I, Kim KJ. Compendium of skin molecular signatures identifies key pathological features associated with fibrosis in systemic sclerosis. Ann Rheum Dis. 2019;78(6):817–25.
35. Tao Y, Zhang H, Huang S, Pei L, Feng M, Zhao X, Ouyang Z, Yao S, Jiang R, Wei K. miR-199a-3p promotes cardiomyocyte proliferation by inhibiting Cd151 expression. Biochem Biophys Res Commun. 2019;516(1):28–36.

6

Survival rate of patients with bladder cancer and its related factors in Kurdistan Province (2013–2018): A population-based study

Mozhdeh Amiri[1], Sofimajidpour Heshmatollah[2], Nader Esmaeilnasab[3], Jamshid Khoubi[4], Ebrahim Ghaderi[3] and Daem Roshani[3*]

Abstract

Background: Bladder cancer is one of the most common urinary tract cancers. This study aims to estimate the survival rate of patients with bladder cancer according to the Cox proportional hazards model based on some key relevant variables.

Methods: In this retrospective population-based cohort study that explores the survival of patients with bladder cancer and its related factors, we first collected demographic information and medical records of 321 patients with bladder cancer through in-person and telephone interviews. Then, in the analysis phase, Kaplan–Meier method and log-rank test were used to draw the survival curve, compare the groups, and explore the effect of risk factors on the patient survival rate using Cox proportional hazards model.

Results: The median survival rate of patients was 63.2 (54.7–72) months and one, three and five-year survival rates were 87%, 68% and 54%, respectively. The results of multiple analyses using Cox's proportional hazards model revealed that variables of sex (male gender) (HR = 11.8, 95% CI: 0.4–100.7), more than 65 year of age (HR = 4.1, 95% CI: 0.4–11), occupation, income level, (HR = 0.4, 95% CI: 0.2–0.8), well differentiated tumor grade (HR = 3.2, 95% CI: 1.7–6) and disease stage influenced the survival rate of patients ($p < 0.05$).

Conclusion: The survival rate of patients with bladder cancer in Kurdistan province is relatively low. Given the impact of the disease stage on the survival rate, adequate access to appropriate diagnostic and treatment services as well as planning for screening and early diagnosis, especially in men, can increase the survival rate of patients.

Keywords: Survival rate, Bladder cancer, Population based, Cox proportional hazards model

Background

Bladder cancer is the most common urinary tract cancer and the ninth most prevalent cancer in both sexes worldwide [1, 2], accounting for 7% and 2% of new cases of cancers in men and women, respectively [3]. According to statistical center of Iran, the ratio of bladder cancer mortality in men was 3.26 times higher than that of women between 2006 and 2010. The incidence of bladder cancer mortality was 1.12 and 1.09 per 100,000 people in 2006 and 2010, respectively, indicating that the trend was relatively stable. According to a 2015 study by Mahdavi et al., the death rate of bladder cancer increases with age, so that people above 70 years of age are more vulnerable to this disease [4]. Currently, bladder cancer mortality in Europe and the United States is declining due to the lower prevalence of smoking [5]. In 2016, 76,960 new

*Correspondence: d.roshani@muk.ac.ir
[3] Social Determinants of Health Research Center, Research Institute for Health Development, Kurdistan University of Medical Sciences, Sanandaj, Iran
Full list of author information is available at the end of the article

cases and 16,390 deaths related to bladder cancer were reported in the United States, of which 76% of new cases were reported in men [6]. Women accounted for fewer cases, but factors like late diagnosis and advanced stages of the disease decreased their survival rate [7–11]. Bladder cancer is the second and the third most common cancer among men in Markazi and Kurdistan province, respectively [12, 13]. Studies on bladder cancer have linked several factors, including occupation, smoking, and sex to the higher prevalence of the disease [11, 14, 15].

The survival rate index is defined as the proportion of cancer patients who survive over a given period of time after diagnosis. Several variables, such as cancer histology and stage, as well as the availability of treatment, affect the survival of the disease [18]. According to the results of our study, despite the rising disease incidence in Iran, there is a paucity of population-based research on the survival rate of patients with bladder cancer in Iran, and most of studies in this field have focused on the cancer trend and epidemiological analysis [12, 16–18].

Hence, the aim of the present study is to estimate the survival rate of bladder cancer patients based on Cox's proportional hazards model and to explore the variables affecting survival rates based on population-based information derived from Kurdistan province. The findings can significant contribute to the health system planning, timely treatment, patient survival and quality of life.

Methods

The present study is a retrospective population-based cohort study conducted in Kurdistan Province from 2013 to 2018. In the first stage, the information on patients diagnosed with bladder cancer was collected by reviewing all cases recorded in cancer registry at the Provincial Health Department, the Cancer Registration Center and the Provincial Mortality Registration Center. In the next step, demographic information (including: gender, age at diagnosis, marital status, place of residence, occupation, level of education, social status, smoking, family history and exposure to toxins and pesticides) and medical and pathological information (including stage of disease, tumor differentiation grade, treatment method, histology, diagnosis method and comorbidity) were collected through interviews, questionnaires and the review of medical records.

Patient information was recorded based on the ICDL10 International Classification (codes C67.0-C67.9). Given that all diagnosed patients in the study were chosen over a 6-year period from 2013 to 2018, the research was undertaken as a population census in Kurdistan province. In this study, of 341 patients diagnosed with bladder cancer, 12 (3.5%) refused to participate in the study, and 8 (2.3%) could not be reached. Hence, finally, 321 subjects were including in the study and their information was recorded. The cause and date of patients' deaths were recorded based on inquiries from the family and death certificates. Patients who were lost to the follow-up or died of bladder cancer were excluded from the study.

Statistical analysis

To determine the relationship between study variables and bladder cancer survival, STATA V.14 statistical software, Kaplan–Meier nonparametric method, and the log-rank test were used. For all variables, the survival curve was drawn and the variables with p values <0.2 in the log-rank test were included in Cox proportional hazards model to estimate the effect of multiple variables on the survival rate by calculating the hazard ratio (HR) at a significant level of less than 0.05. To calculate the total survival rate and one, three and five-year survival rates, the life table (monthly) was used over 1 to 5- year period. Three methods of scaled Schoenfeld residuals, the hazard log cumulative and goodness of fit were used to assess the appropriateness of the hazards.

Results

In this study, the survival rate analysis was conducted for 321 patients with bladder cancer, of which 82.2% were male and 17.7% were female. Also, 77% of patients lived in urban areas, 87.8% were married and 53.9% were above 65 years of age. During the study period, 96 out of 321 participants passed away, 86 due to bladder cancer and 10 due to other causes. According to the results, the overall median survival of patients was 63.2(54.7–72) months and the mean survival (47.1–53.7) was 50.4 ± 1.7 months. Also, the one to five-year survival rates were 87%, 76%, 68%, 61% and 54%, respectively (Fig. 1).

Table 1 shows one-year, two-year, three-year and five-year survival rates for each variable using the life table, as well as p values obtained from the log-rank test.

According to Table 1, the survival rate was higher in women than in men, and according to the log-rank test, the survival curve was not significantly different between the subgroups ($p < 0.05$). Moreover, survival rates were lower in single patients, patients above 65 years of age, and patients living in rural areas. Survival rates in retired and unemployed patients were higher than other groups. The literate and high-income patients also had higher survival rates. In this study, smoking, supplementary insurance, and family history were not statistically significant.

As shown in Table 1, patients at early disease stage who did not have an underlying disease, had a poorly differentiated tumor grade, and their histology was urothelial carcinoma had a higher survival rate. However, the

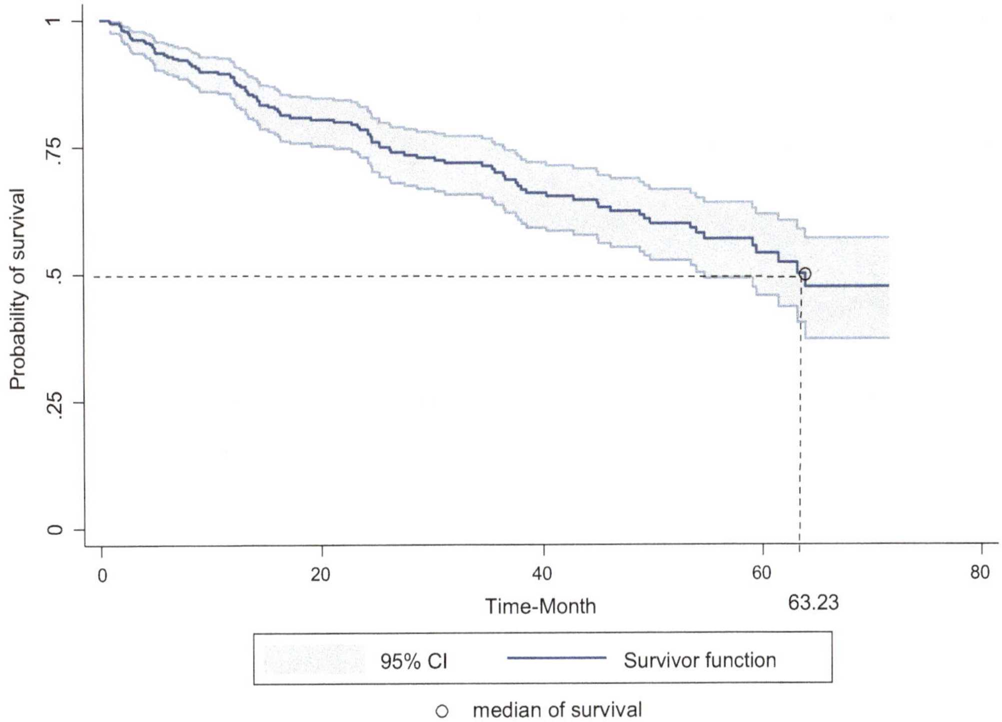

Fig. 1 Survival rate of patients treated with bladder cancer in Kurdistan province (2013–2018) (Kaplan–Meier). CI = confidence interval, BC = bladder cancer

survival rate was not significantly different with regard to the method of diagnosis, type of treatment and exposure to poisons and pesticides. According to the results, group curves, gender ($p = 0.044$), age at diagnosis ($p < 0.001$), residence ($p < 0.001$), marital status ($p < 0.001$), level of education ($p = 0.002$), occupation ($p = 0.008$), socioeconomic status ($p < 0.001$), disease stage ($p < 0.001$), histology ($p = 0.04$) and tumor grade differentiation ($p < 0.001$) were significantly different. Moreover, the curves of the supplementary insurance, smoking, method of diagnosis, family history and underlying disease were not significantly different patients ($p < 0.05$) (Table 1).

In the multivariate analysis, using Cox's proportional hazards, variables of gender, age groups, residence, marital status, level of education, occupation, disease stage, histology, treatment method, differentiation grade, and socioeconomic status were incorporated in the final model of Cox's proportional hazards model ($p < 0.2$). The results of the final model revealed that the hazard ratio was significantly higher in men than in women (HR = 11.8, 95% CI: 0.4–100.7). Moreover, the hazard ratio increased with age (HR = 4.1, 95% CI: 1.5–11.1) and patients from a high socioeconomic background had a lower hazard ratio than those from a poor socioeconomic background (HR = 0.4, 95% CI: 0.2–0.8). The hazard ratio of patients at Stage II (HR = 1.5, 95% CI: 0.7–2.9), Stage III (HR = 2.8, 95% CI: 1.34–5.8) and Stage IV (HR = 6.4, 95% CI: 2.1–19.2) was higher than Stage V. Also, the hazard ratio growth at Stages III and IV was significantly different than Stage I, but it was not the case for Stages I and II ($p < 0.05$).

Moreover, the hazard ratio at well differentiated grade was greater than the poorly differentiated tumor grade (HR = 3.25, 95% CI: 1.7–6). Patients with an office job (HR = 4.9, 95% CI: 1.7–13.9) and workers (HR = 2.6, 95% CI: 1.1–6.2) had a higher hazard ratio than retired and unemployed patients. Meanwhile, the variables of residence, marital status, level of education, type of histology and treatment method were not significantly related to the survival rate of patients ($p < 0.05$) (Table 2).

Figure 1 shows that the median survival of patients with bladder cancer in Kurdistan province was 63.2(54.7–72) months.

The survival rate of patients with bladder cancer versus sex in study participants shows that the five-year survival is higher in women than in men (Fig. 2). Also, the survival rate of patients with bladder cancer versus age at diagnosis shows that the five-year survival in participants with ≥ 65 year is less than the others (Fig. 3).

Figure 4 shows that the five-year survival rate in patients from rich (74%), moderate (61%), and poor (34%)

Table 1 Demographic and clinical characteristics of patients diagnosed with bladder cancer in terms of mean survival rate using Kaplan–Meier method

Characteristic	Category	Frequency (%)	Mean survival per month (95% CI)	p*
Sex	Female	57 (17.7)	57.4 (50–64.8)	0.04
	male	264 (82.2)	48.9 (45.2–52.6)	
Age at diagnosis	≤50 y	43 (13.4)	60.3 (53.1–67.5)	<0.001
	51–64 y	105 (32.7)	55.8 (50.5–61)	
	≥65 y	173 (53.9)	44.3 (39.7–48.9)	
Marital status	Single (unmarried, divorced, widow/widower)	39 (12.1)	32.7 (23.8–41.5)	<0.001
	Married	282 (87.8)	52.9 (49.5–56.4)	
Residence	Rural	74 (23.5)	41.7 (35.3–47.9)	<0.001
	Urban	247 (76.9)	53.9 (50.2–57.7)	
Occupation	Unemployed/Retired	67 (20.8)	58.9 (52.5–65.3)	0.008
	Housewife	47 (14.6)	56.2 (47.9–64.5)	
	Worker	53 (16.5)	48.8 (39.6–57.9)	
	Self-employed	66 (20.5)	48.1 (40.5–55.7)	
	Office job	27 (8.4)	47.7 (39.3–55.9)	
	Agriculturist	61 (19.0)	41.6 (34.9–48.2)	
Education	Illiterate	158 (49.2)	45.3 (40.5–50.1)	0.001
	Literate	163 (50.7)	55.8 (51.4–60.2)	
Socioeconomic status	Poor	106 (33.1)	42.4 (36.9–47.8)	<0.001
	Moderate	107 (33.4)	52.3 (46.5–57.9)	
	Rich	107 (33.4)	58.5 (53.2–63.8)	
Smoking	No	172 (53.5)	51.7 (46.6–56.7)	0.5
	Yes	149 (46.4)	49.4 (45–53.7)	
Family history of BC	No	301 (93.7)	50.0 (46.5–53.4)	0.5
	Yes	20 (6.2)	54.6 (43.3–65.9)	
Comorbidity	No	205 (63.8)	50.8 (46.7–54.8)	0.5
	Yes	116 (34.1)	49.3 (43.6–54.9)	
TNM stage	I	210 (65.4)	58.5 (55–62)	<0.001
	II	74 (23)	44.5 (37.2–51.7)	
	III	29 (9)	21.7 (12.9–30.4)	
	IV	8 (2.5)	21.3 (8.9–33.6)	
Grade	Poorly differentiated	217 (67.6)	59.7 (56.3–62.9)	<0.001
	Well differentiated	104 (32.4)	31.6 (25.8–37.3)	
Treatment	Radiation therapy	13 (4)	48.2 (34.5–61.7)	0.05
	Surgery	207 (64.5)	53.6 (49.6–57.5)	
	Chemotherapy	10 (3.1)	31.9 (20.3–43.5)	
	Combinational treatment (Surgery, Radiotherapy, Chemotherapy or Immunotherapy)	85 (26.4)	44.5 (38–50.8)	
Histology	Adenocarcinoma	10 (3.1)	34.7 (24.8–44.5)	0.03
	Squamous cell carcinoma	7 (2.1)	24.9 (3.7–46)	
	Urothelial carcinoma	304 (94.7)	51.3 (47.9–54.7)	
Method of diagnosis	Urinalysis and ultrasound	55 (17.1)	52.9 (46.5–59.3)	0.5
	Cystoscopy and biopsy	55 (17.1)	45.4 (37.7–53)	
	Biopsy and ultrasound	35 (10.9)	50.0 (40.6–59.3)	
	Combinational method of diagnosis	176 (54.8)	50.8 (46.1–55.6)	
Poison and pesticides exposure	Yes	64 (19.9)	49.9 (43.5–56.4)	0.9
	No	257 (80)	50.5 (46.7–54.3)	

BC bladder cancer

*Log-rank test-*p* value

socioeconomic backgrounds, according to the log-rank test, is significantly different ($p < 0.001$).

Figure 5 shows the five-year survival rate in patients at Stage I (67%), Stage II (45%) and Stage III (15%), according to the log-rank test, is not significantly different ($p < 0.001$).

Discussion

The one-year, three-year and five-year survival rates of patients with bladder cancer in Kurdistan province resembled the survival rates of patients in Shiraz province, as reported by Mohammad Beigi et al. The one-year, three-year, five-year, and ten-year survival rates of patients in their study were 0.9, 0.7, 0.6, and 0.2, respectively [19].

According to the American Cancer Society (ACS) in 2016, the five-year, ten-year, and fifteen-year survival rates at all stages of bladder cancer are 77%, 70%, and 65%, respectively [20]. This suggests that the five-year survival rate of bladder cancer patients in Kurdistan province (54%) in this study is lower than in developed countries. However, the median survival of patients was estimated to be 63.23 months, which is higher than the value reported by Benjamin WF et al. (Median OS = 14, 95% CI: 13.5–14.5) [21]. It is probably due to early diagnosis of the disease because 65.4% of patients were identified at Stage I and 23.05% at Stage II.

In this study, the history of smoking was not significantly related to the survival rate of patients. Most patients had a history of smoking at young age but had abandoned smoking after a while or due to the bladder cancer. This could be attributed to the effect of smoking cessation followed by the reduced devastating effect of the disease. Our findings are consistent with those reported by Mohammad Beigi et al., who did not report a significant relationship between smoking and survival rates [19]. This results illustrated that just as reduced smoking decreased the incidence of bladder cancer, smoking cessation also increased the survival of patients with bladder cancer [22].

In the present study, age and income level influenced the survival rate of patients with bladder cancer ($p < 0.05$), which is aligned with the study of Joshua Lara et al. In their study, the risk of death in adolescents and youths was lower than older people (HR = 0.4, 95% CI: 0.3–0.5). In adolescents and young people from poor socioeconomic background, the specific survival rate (HR = 7.1, $p < 0.001$) and the overall survival rate (HR = 5, $p < 0.001$) were statistically significant [23].

According to the results, the survival rate was higher in women than in men, which is in conflict with the findings reported by Stephen B.W. et al. This could be assigned to

Table 2 Univariate and multivariate Cox proportional hazards model for the overall survival of patients with bladder cancer

	Univariate model		Multivariate model	
	HR (95%)	*p* value	HR (95%)	*p* value
Sex				
Female	1	–	1	–
Male	1.9 (1–3.7)	0.04	11.8 (1.3–100.7)	0.02
Age				
≤ 50	1	–	1	
51–64	1.6 (0.6–4)	0.27	1.1 (0.4–3.1)	0.8
≥ 65	3.3 (1.4–7.5)	0.005	4.1 (1.5–11)	0.004
Marital status				
Single*	1	–	1	–
Married	0.36 (0.2–0.6)	< 0.001	0.7 (0.3–1.3)	0.3
Residence				
Rural	1	–	1	–
Urban	0.5 (0.3–0.7)	0.001	0.8 (0.4–1.6)	0.5
Occupation				
Unemployed/Retired	1	–	1	–
Housewife	1.2 (0.5–26.8)	0.6	11.3 (1.1–116.8)	0.04
Worker	2.2 (1–4.7)	0.04	2.6 (1.1–6.2)	0.03
Self-employed	2.2 (1.1–4.4)	0.03	3.3 (1.5–7.1)	0.002
Office job	1.8 (0.7–4.4)	0.19	4.9 (1.7–13.9)	0.003
Agriculturist	3.1 (1.6–6.1)	0.001	1.8 (0.7–4.4)	0.2
Education				
Illiterate	1	–	1	–
Literate	0.5 (0.3–0.8)	0.003	1.1 (0.6–2)	0.8
Socioeconomic status				
Poor	1	–	1	–
Moderate	0.6 (0.3–0.9)	0.02	0.5 (0.3–1)	0.06
Rich	0.35 (0.2–0.6)	< 0.001	0.4 (0.2–0.8)	0.01
TNM stage				
I	1	–	1	–
II	2.4 (1.5–4)	< 0.001	1.5 (0.7–2.9)	0.2
III	7.9 (4.7–13.4)	< 0.001	2.8 (1.3–5.8)	0.006
IV	7.3 (3.2–16.6)	< 0.001	6.4 (2.1–19.3)	0.001
Grade				
Poorly differentiated	1	–	1	–
Well differentiated	5.2 (3.4–7.9)	< 0.001	3.2 (1.7–6)	< 0.001
Treatment				
Radiation therapy	1	–	1	–
Surgery	0.8 (0.3–2.1)	0.6	0.9 (0.3–2.6)	0.8
Chemotherapy	1.7 (0.4–6.6)	0.4	1.5 (0.3–6.2)	0.6
Combinational treatment	1.3 (0.4–3.7)	0.6	0.9 (0.5–5)	0.4
Histologic type				
Adenocarcinoma	1	–	1	–
Squamous cell carcinoma	1.3 (0.3–5.1)	0.7	4.7 (0.8–26.8)	0.08
Urothelial carcinoma	0.46 (0.19–1)	0.06	1.6 (0.5–4.5)	0.4

HR hazard ratio, *CI* confidence interval

*Unmarried, divorced, widow/widower

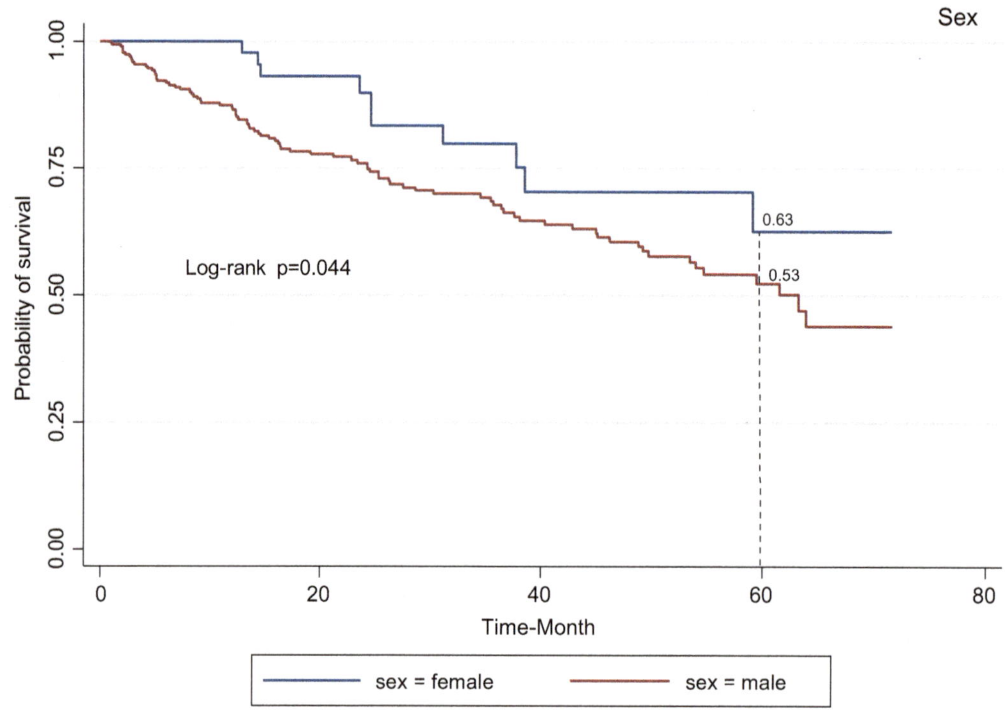

Fig. 2 Kaplan–Meier curves of survival in patients with bladder cancer versus sex

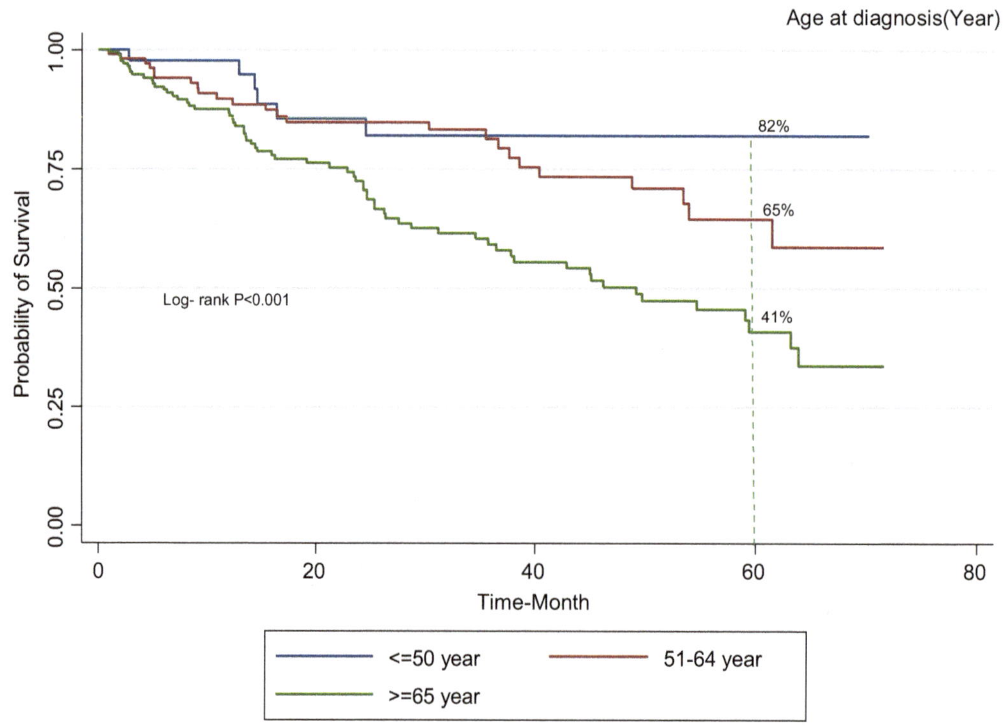

Fig. 3 Kaplan–Meier curves of the survival of patients with bladder cancer versus age at diagnosis

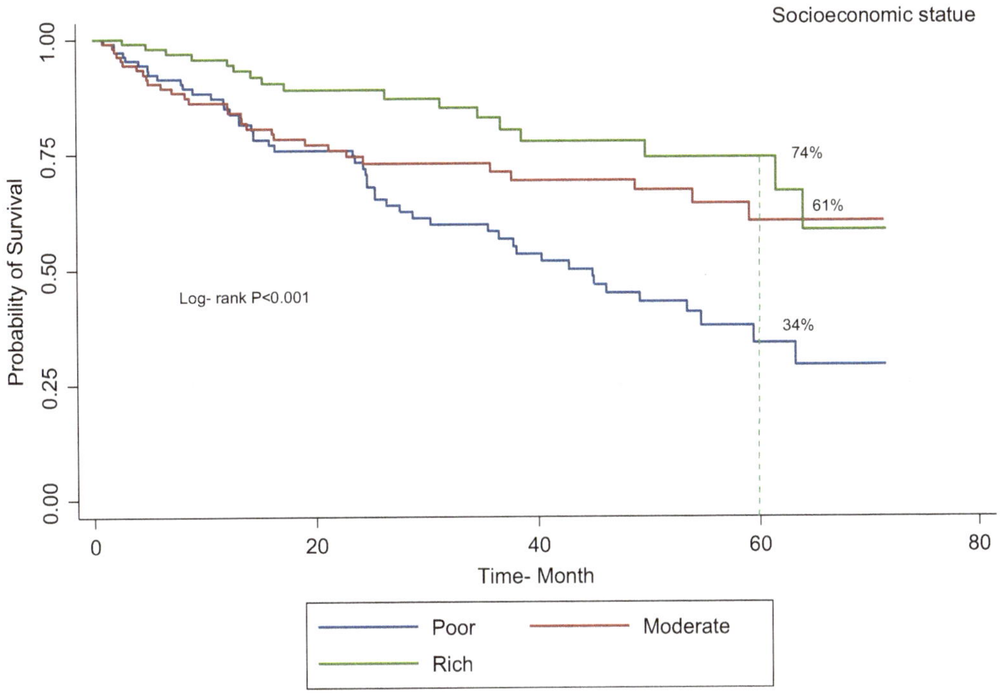

Fig. 4 Kaplan–Meier curves of the survival of patients with bladder cancer versus socioeconomic status

the early detection of the disease and the higher commitment of women with bladder cancer to follow-ups. However, in both studies, the incidence was higher in men. Furthermore, old age, tumor stage and single marital status were found to be significantly related to the lower survival rate ($p < 0.05$). In this study, we observed that the diagnosis of the disease at lower stage was associated with the higher survival of patients, which is consistent with the study of Stephen B.W. [24].

Survival rates were also higher in urban residents than in rural areas, which can be attributed to the greater access to healthcare services and follow-ups. For many cancers, survival is considerably lower in rural areas than in urban areas ($p < 0.05$) [25].

Khoubi et al. introduced exposure to poisons and pesticides as a risk factor for bladder cancer, but in the present study, the history of exposure to pesticides was not significantly correlated with the survival rate of patients with bladder cancer ($p > 0.05$) [26]. We found that most farmers had attended Agricultural Jihad's training classes and put on personal protective gears during spraying. There was a statistically significant association between housework and increased risk of bladder cancer in women, which is in agreement with the findings of Khoubi et al. (ISCO 5152, OR = 5.9, 95% CI = 1.04–34.3) [26]. This is due to the fact that women are more likely to use detergents, cleaners and bleaches, and inhale oil fumes during frying and less likely to engage in physical activities. Our study also showed that an office job and self-employment were significantly correlated with the survival rate ($p < 0.05$).

The univariate and multivariate Cox regression analysis did not reveal a significant relationship between treatment method and survival rate, but in the study of Mark C. et al., the overall survival rate improved in chemotherapy patients (HR = 0.7, 95% CI: 0.6–0.9, $p < 0.001$) [27]. In this study, 64.9% of patients with bladder cancer underwent surgery and 3.1% started chemotherapy, but the surgical procedure was not significantly correlated with the patient survival ($p < 0.05$). This aligns well with the study of Stephen BW et al. who did not report any associations between the survival of the elderly with radical cystectomy and sex at all stages (HR = 1.07, 95% CI: 1.01–1.1, $p = 0.02$) [24].

Literacy was also linked to survival. Literate participants had a higher survival rate than the illiterate ones. This suggests that raising awareness and promoting health literacy can influence the survival rate of patients ($p < 0.05$). The survival rate was higher in married subjects than in the single subjects (never married, widower

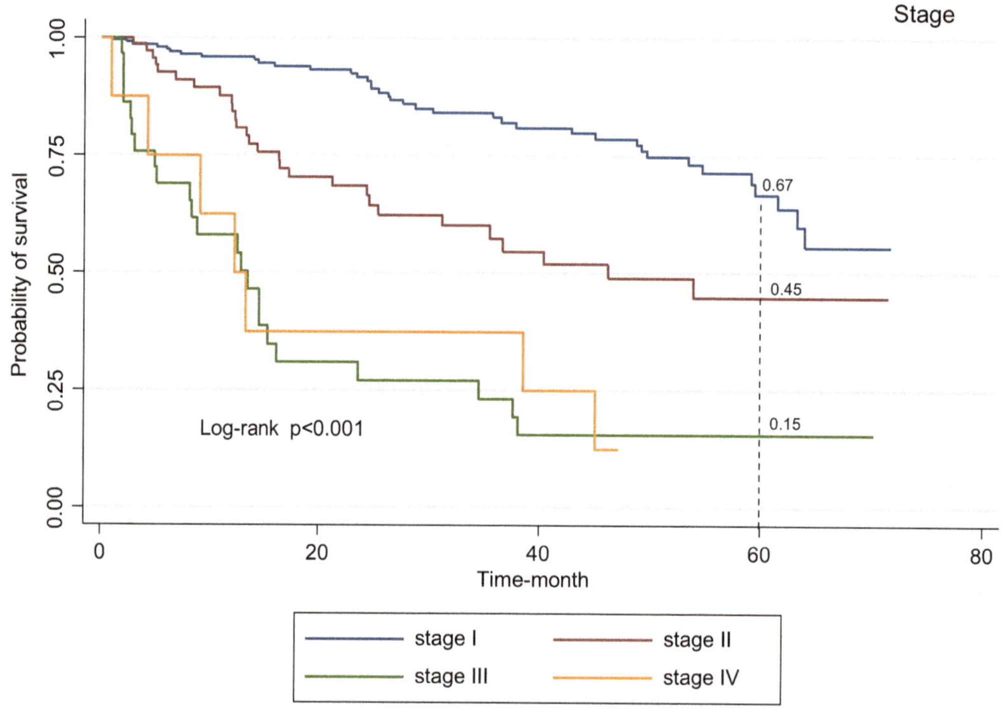

Fig. 5 Kaplan–Meier curves of the survival of patients with bladder cancer versus diagnosis stage

or divorced), which is in agreement with the study of Klapheke et al. [28].

Our study had a number of limitations including incompleteness of patients' medical records. The distinguishing point of this study is its population-based nature, which eliminates the problem of accessing hospital records and biases.

Conclusion

The results of this study demonstrated that the survival rate of patients with bladder cancer in Kurdistan province is relatively low due to lack of access to appropriate diagnostic and treatment services, lack of screening and early diagnosis and sloppy follow-ups, especially amongst men. Variables of gender, over 65 years of age, occupation, socioeconomic background, tumor differentiation grade, and disease stage affected patient survival rates. This suggests the importance of further planning for these factors to increase the survival of patients with bladder cancer.

Acknowledgements

This study was a research project in Kurdistan University of Medical Sciences. We would like to thank the National Cancer Registry in Kurdistan for providing data, as well as all those who were involved in the project and helped us collect data from across the country.

Authors' contributions

Data curtain: DR, MA, HS, NE, JK, EG. Formal analysis: DR, MA. Investigation: DR, MA, HS. Project administration: DR, MA. Writing – original draft: DR, MA. Writing – review & editing: DR, MA, HS, NE, JK, EG. All authors read and approved the final manuscript.

Author details

[1] Department of Epidemiology and Biostatistics, Faculty of Medicine, Kurdistan University of Medical Sciences, Sanandaj, Iran. [2] Department of Urology, Faculty of Medicine, Kurdistan University of Medical Sciences, Sanandaj, Iran. [3] Social Determinants of Health Research Center, Research Institute for Health Development, Kurdistan University of Medical Sciences, Sanandaj, Iran. [4] Environmental Health Research Center, Research Institute for Health Development, Kurdistan University of Medical Sciences, Sanandaj, Iran.

References

1. Koosha A, Farahbakhsh M, Hakimi S, Abdolahi L, Golzari M, Farshad MS. Epidemiologic assessment of cancer disease in East Azerbaijan 2007. Med J Tabriz Univ Med Sci Health Serv. 2010;32(4):74–9.
2. Ploeg M, Aben KK, Kiemeney LA. The present and future burden of urinary bladder cancer in the world. World J Urol. 2009;27(3):289–93.
3. Salehi A, Khezri AA, Malekmakan L, Aminsharifi A. Epidemiologic status of bladder cancer in Shiraz, southern Iran. Asian Pac J Cancer Prev. 2011;12(5):1323–7.
4. Mahdavi S, Amoori N, Salehiniya H, Almasi Z, Enayatrad M. Trend of bladder cancer mortality in Iran (2006 to 2010). Int J Epidemiol Res. 2015;2(4):184–9.
5. Jemal A, Bray F, Center MM, Ferlay J, Ward E, Forman D. Global cancer statistics. CA: Cancer J Clin. 2011;61(2):69–90.
6. Miller KD, Siegel RL, Lin CC, Mariotto AB, Kramer JL, Rowland JH, Stein KD, Alteri R, Jemal A. Cancer treatment and survivorship statistics, 2016. CA: Cancer J Clin. 2016;66(4):271–89.

7. Fajkovic H, Halpern JA, Cha EK, Bahadori A, Chromecki TF, Karakiewicz PI, Breinl E, Merseburger AS, Shariat SF. Impact of gender on bladder cancer incidence, staging, and prognosis. World J Urol. 2011;29(4):457–63.
8. Mungan NA, Aben KK, Schoenberg MP, Visser O, Coebergh JW, Witjes JA, Kiemeney LA. Gender differences in stage-adjusted bladder cancer survival. Urology. 2000;55(6):876–80.
9. Kiemeney L, Mungan N, Aben K, Schoenberg M, Visser O, Coebergh J, et al. Gender differences in stage-adjusted bladder cancer survival. 2000;151(11):S68.
10. Najari BB, Rink M, Li PS, Karakiewicz PI, Scherr DS, Shabsigh R, Meryn S, Schlegel PN, Shariat SF. Sex disparities in cancer mortality: the risks of being a man in the United States. J Urol. 2013;189(4):1470–4.
11. Scosyrev E, Noyes K, Feng C, Messing E. Sex and racial differences in bladder cancer presentation and mortality in the US. Cancer. 2009;115(1):68–74.
12. Mohaghegh F, Hamta A. The study of cancer incidence and cancer registration in Markazi province between 2001–2006 and comparison with national statistics. Iran. J Arak Univ Med Sci. 2008;11(2):84–93.
13. Ahmad E, Ghasem KO, Dastoori P. Recurrence rate and prognostic factors of superficial bladder cancer in shiraz shahid faghihi hospital during the years 1998–2001.
14. Whelan P. Survival from bladder cancer in England and Wales up to 2001. British J Cancer. 2008;99(Suppl 1):S90.
15. Brookfield KF, Cheung MC, Gomez C, Yang R, Nieder AM, Lee DJ, Koniaris LG. Survival disparities among African American women with invasive bladder cancer in Florida. Cancer: Interdiscip Int J Am Cancer Soc. 2009;115(18):4196–209.
16. Nourafkan Z, Yavari P, Roshandel GH, Khalili D, Zayeri F. Estimation of survival rate of esophageal cancer and some of its determinants in Golestan province, north of Iran. Iran J Epidemiol. 2013;9(1):11–8.
17. Farahmand M, Khadem AF, Medhati M, Shokrpour N, Joulaei H, Mehrbani D. Trend of bladder cancer in Fars province, southern Iran, 2002–2006.
18. Toutounchi M, Mazdak H, Najafipour S, Soleymani B. Bladder cancer risk factors among Isfahan population: a case-control study.
19. Mohammadbeigi A, Rezaeian Zadeh A. Application of life table in survival analysis of patients with bladder cancer. Zahedan J Res Med Sci. 2011;13(3).
20. http://www.cancer-org 2016 [bladder cancer].
21. Fischer-Valuck BW, Rao YJ, Rudra S, Przybysz D, Germino E, Samson P, Baumann BC, Gay H, Michalski J. Treatment patterns and overall survival outcomes of octogenarians with muscle invasive cancer of the bladder: an analysis of the national cancer database. J Urol. 2018;199(2):416–23.
22. Cumberbatch MG, Jubber I, Black PC, Esperto F, Figueroa JD, Kamat AM, Kiemeney L, Lotan Y, Pang K, Silverman DT, Znaor A. Epidemiology of bladder cancer: a systematic review and contemporary update of risk factors in 2018. Eur Urol. 2018;74(6):784–95.
23. Lara J, Brunson A, Keegan TH, Malogolowkin M, Pan CX, Yap S, deVere White R. Determinants of survival for adolescents and young adults with urothelial bladder cancer: results from the california cancer registry. J Urol. 2016;196(5):1378–82.
24. Williams SB, Huo J, Dafashy TJ, Ghaffary CK, Baillargeon JG, Morales EE, Kim SP, Kuo YF, Orihuela E, Tyler DS, Freedland SJ. Survival differences among patients with bladder cancer according to sex: critical evaluation of radical cystectomy use and delay to treatment. In: Urologic oncology: seminars and original investigations, vol. 35, no. 10. Elsevier; 2017.
25. Chen W, Zheng R, Baade PD, Zhang S, Zeng H, Bray F, Jemal A, Yu XQ, He J. Cancer statistics in China, 2015. CA: Cancer J Clin. 2016;66(2):115–32.
26. Khoubi J, Pourabdian S, Mohebbi I, Tajvidi M, Zaroorian O, Giahi O. Association between the high risk occupations and bladder cancer in Iran: a case-control study. Int J Occup Med Environ Health. 2013;26(2):205–13.
27. Korpics MC, Block AM, Martin B, Hentz C, Gaynor ER, Henry E, Harkenrider MM, Solanki AA. Concurrent chemotherapy is associated with improved survival in elderly patients with bladder cancer undergoing radiotherapy. Cancer. 2017;123(18):3524–31.
28. Klapheke A, Yap SA, Pan K, Cress RD. Sociodemographic disparities in chemotherapy treatment and impact on survival among patients with metastatic bladder cancer. In: Urologic oncology: seminars and original investigations, vol. 36, no. 6. Elsevier; 2018.

7

Bladder squamous cell carcinoma in a pregnant woman: Case report and review of the literature

Pablo A. Rojas[1], Cristián González[2], Gonzalo P. Mendez[3], Alejandro Majerson[1] and Ignacio F. San Francisco[1*]

Abstract

Background: Bladder tumors in pregnancy are extremely rare. No more than 50 cases have been published to date, including all histologic variants, and only three cases of bladder squamous cell carcinoma have been described.

Case presentation: We present a clinical case of a 31-year-old woman with bladder squamous cell carcinoma in the second trimester of pregnancy. After a C-section at 30 weeks, we performed radical cystectomy with extended bilateral lymphadenectomy, hysterectomy and right oophorectomy. The Studer neobladder technique was performed for urinary tract reconstruction. Definitive pathology showed invasive bladder squamous cell carcinoma, Grade 2, with microscopic infiltration of the perivesical fat, negative margins, and 3/28 lymph nodes with carcinoma (pT3aN2M0). The patient underwent 18 months of surveillance after radical cystectomy, without recurrence by PET-CT.

Conclusions: Bladder cancer in pregnant women is extremely rare but must be considered in those with recurrent gross hematuria and/or recurrent urinary tract infection. To our knowledge, this case involves the longest recurrence-free survival of a pregnant woman with squamous cell bladder cancer published thus far.

Keywords: Bladder cancer, Pregnancy, Radical cystectomy, Case report

Background

Bladder tumors inpregnancy are an extremely rare diagnosis. Currently, no more than 50 cases have been published, including all histologic variants [1].

Case presentation

We present the case of a healthy 31-year-old woman with an obstetric history of 1 pregnancy, 1 live birth, no abortions (G1P1A0), and a urinary tract infection in the first and second trimesters, without complications. At 21 weeks of gestation, the patient had gross hematuria. We performed cystoscopy and observed a lesion of 3–4 cm in the right wall not identifying the right ureteral orifice (Fig. 1). Pelvic magnetic resonance imaging (MRI) without contrast was performed and showed a bladder tumor along the right wall that was $6.3 \times 3.5 \times 6$ cm lateral to the right ureter and lymph nodes, 13×9 mm in the right external iliac vessels and 10×7 mm in the right internal iliac vessels (Fig. 2). The patient had no predisposing factors for bladder cancer.

From an obstetric perspective, the pregnancy was normal without complications.

At 26 weeks of gestation, we performed transurethral resection (TUR) of the bladder lesion. The biopsy showed well-differentiated, invasive bladder squamous cell carcinoma (pT2). Abdominal MRI and chest computed tomography (CT) did not reveal metastatic disease. A staging study was performed after TUR to evaluate possible tumor dissemination and the need for systemic therapy.

*Correspondence: isanfrancisco@med.puc.cl
[1] Departamento de Urología, Escuela de Medicina, Pontificia Universidad Católica de Chile, Diagonal Paraguay 362, Santiago, Chile
Full list of author information is available at the end of the article

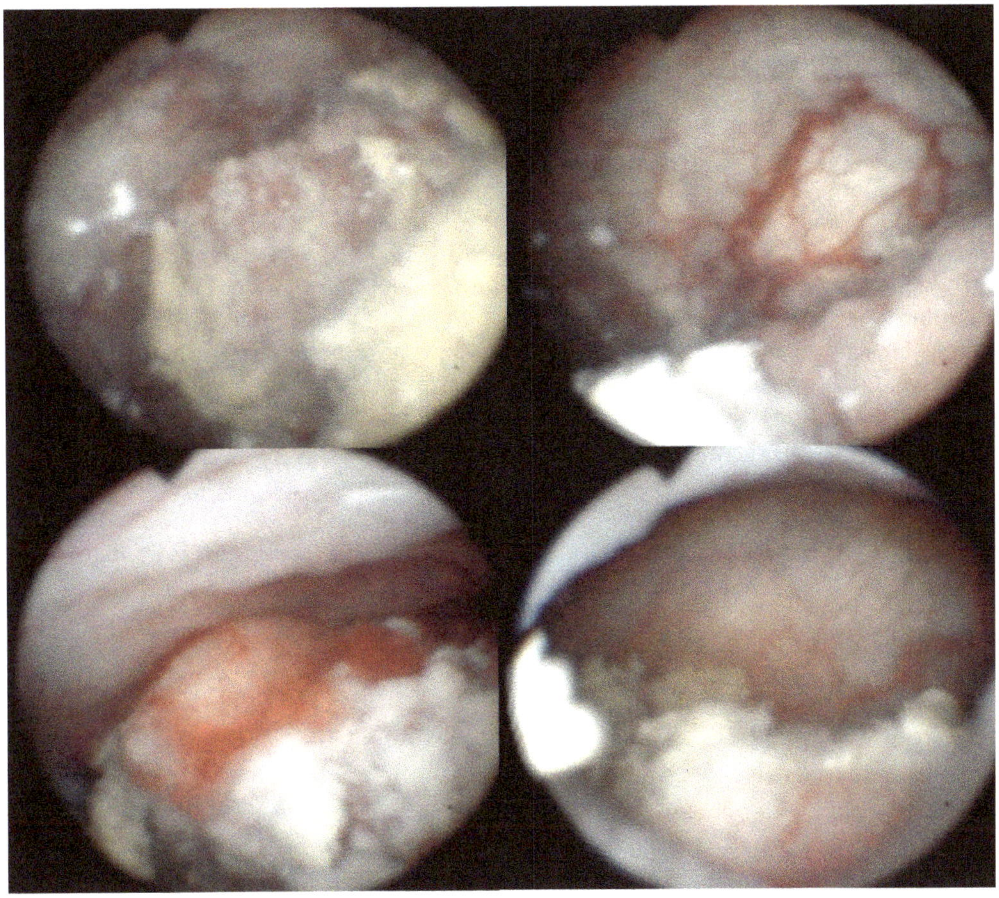

Fig. 1 Cystoscopy at 21 weeks of gestation

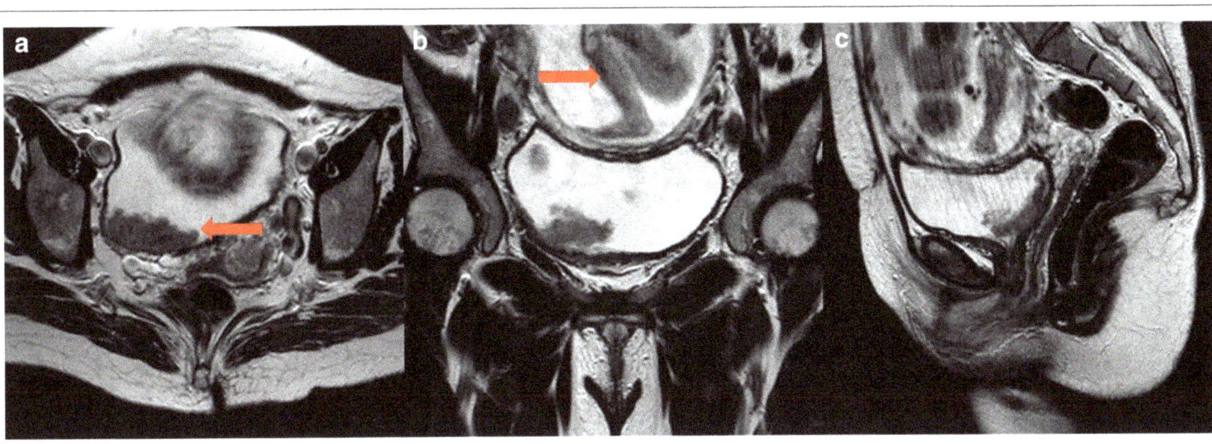

Fig. 2 MRI without gadolinium at 23 weeks of gestation. **a** Axial view of the bladder tumor (arrow). **b** Coronal view of the bladder tumor and fetus (arrow). **c** Sagittal view

The case was presented to a uro-oncology committee meeting and a maternal fetal medicine unit: the patient was offered the alternative of immediately terminating the pregnancy or waiting until 30 weeks for delivery and subsequently performing the surgery. The patient opted for the latter.

The patient underwent C-section at 30 weeks. The newborn was healthy, with no complications.

As recommended by the multidisciplinary committee, the patient did not receive neoadjuvant chemotherapy based on the histology of pure squamous cell carcinoma. One month after delivery, we performed open radical cystectomy with extended bilateral lymphadenectomy through the common iliac vessels and presacrum, a hysterectomy and a right oophorectomy. Blood loss was 1100 cc. There were no other complications from the surgery. The Studer neobladder technique with 60 cm of terminal ileum was performed for urinary tract reconstruction. Cystostomy was carried out, and a urethral catheter was placed for anastomosis.

The patient recovered satisfactorily and was discharged 5 days postoperatively. The ureteral stents and cystostomy were removed two weeks after surgery.

Definitive pathology revealed invasive bladder squamous cell carcinoma, Grade 2, with microscopic infiltration of the perivesical fat, negative margins, and 3/28 lymph nodes with carcinoma (pT3aN2M0, Fig. 3). Again, evaluation by a multidisciplinary committee decided not to apply adjuvant chemotherapy/immunotherapy or radiation based on the histology and the lack of residual macroscopic disease.

Twenty days after the surgery, the patient presented with abdominal pain and fever. CT with contrast revealed uroperitoneum with neobladder filtration. The patient underwent exploratory laparotomy, which revealed 1200 cc of uroperitoneum, leakage through the cystostomy site, suture line of the ileum and ureterovesical anastomosis. The filtration sites were closed with PDS sutures, and a urethral catheter and drainage were again installed. Five days after the surgery, the patient developed abdominal pain, and an increase in drainage output was observed. Cystography showed new filtration

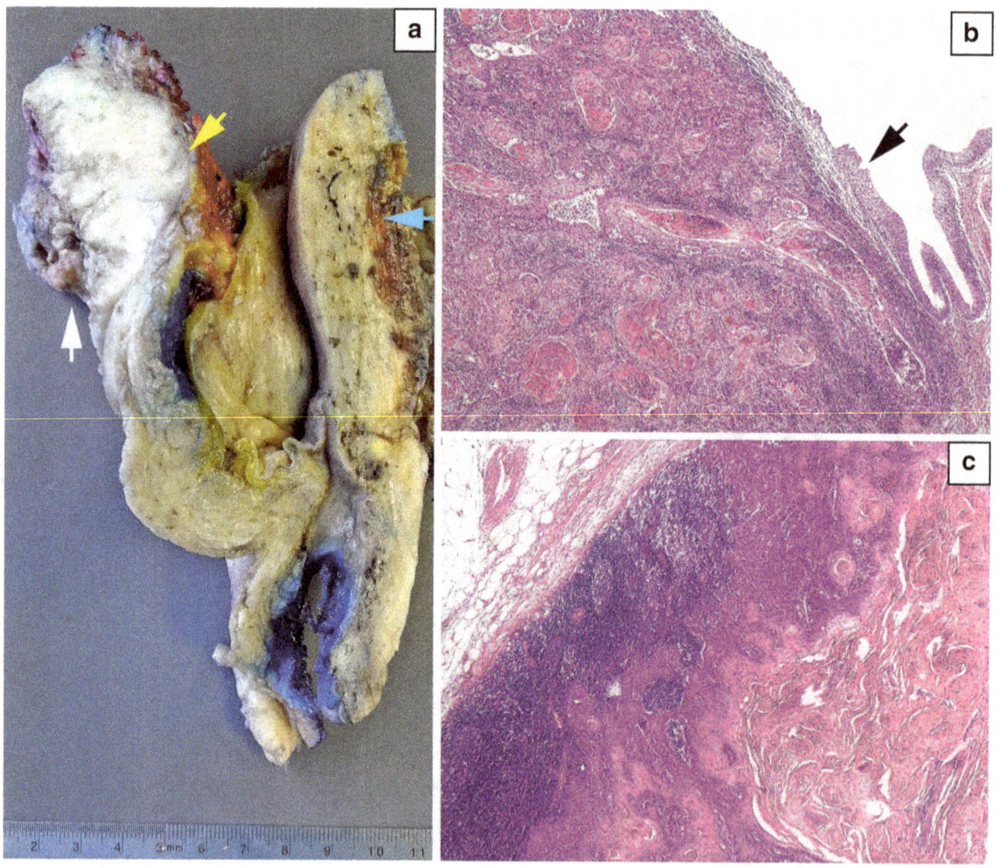

Fig. 3 **a** Longitudinal section of the formalin-fixed bladder and uterus. On the left, the bladder mucosa shows a bulky and exophytic, withe-gray tumor (white arrow) that invades through the complete bladder wall, reaching the perivesical adipose tissue (yellow arrow). On the right, the uterine wall and endometrium are thickened (blue arrow), with no evidence of tumor invasion. In between both walls, the vesico-uterine pouch can be recognized. **b** Microphotograph of the bladder mucosa showing a well-differentiated squamous cell carcinoma with multiple keratinizing epithelial groups (pink nests) invading the subepithelial connective tissue. The mucosa has epithelial denudation, and the residual urothelial lining is hyperplastic (arrow). (Hematoxylin and eosin stain, original magnification × 40). **c** Image of one of the iliac lymph nodes with metastatic squamous cell carcinoma (hematoxylin and eosin stain, original magnification × 40)

in the anterior wall of the neobladder. The patient again underwent exploratory laparotomy, revealing leakage in two points of the suture line. The filtration sites were closed with PDS sutures. No drainage output or abdominal pain occurred but spontaneous diuresis was present. The patient was discharged at 3 weeks after the first reintervention.

At present, the patient has undergone 18 months of surveillance after radical cystectomy, without recurrence by follow-up PET-CT (Fig. 4), with complete continence, day and night, and no metabolic complications. Her baby is currently 19 months old and perfectly healthy.

Discussion and conclusions

Urological tumors in pregnant women are exceedingly rare, with an estimated incidence of 0.0013%. The most frequent tumors are kidney tumors, followed by bladder tumors and finally pheochromocytomas [2].

Bladder tumors during pregnancy have been described since 1927, with transitional cell carcinoma being the most common (70%) [3–7]. To our knowledge, only three cases of squamous cell bladder tumors have been reported in pregnant women (Table 1). Risk factors for squamous cell bladder tumors are a history of catheter use (clean intermittent self-catheterization or an indwelling catheter), smoking and recurrent urinary tract infections [8].

Among reported cases of squamous cell tumors, the women were in the third decade of life with pregnancies in the second trimester, similar to our patient. However, due to the aggressiveness of the disease, patients died within the first year of follow-up after cystectomy [7]. Therefore, to our knowledge, the patient we present in this report has the longest recurrence-free survival described in the literature.

Gross hematuria is frequent in pregnant women (up to 80% can present it), and the most common cause is cystitis [3, 5]; considering the severity of the cases described above, cystoscopy is recommended for pregnant women with recurrent hematuria [7]. MRI can be used as a support tool for diagnosis and staging, and gadolinium can be used from the 23rd week of gestation [2]. An abdomen and pelvis CT scan is not recommended in pregnant women because the fetus will be

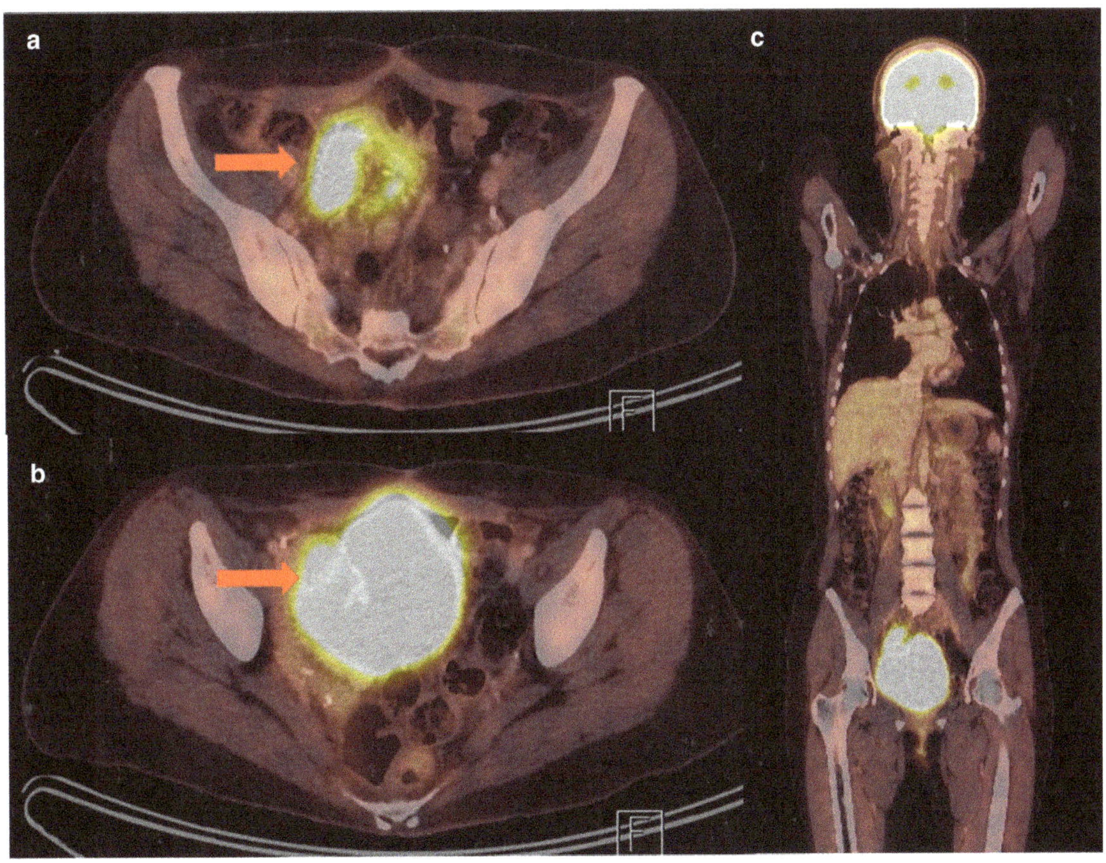

Fig. 4 PET-CT with F18-FDG. There was no evidence of locoregional recurrence or distant metastasis after 18 months of surveillance. **a** Axial view of chimney (arrow). **b** axial view of neobladder (arrow). **c** Coronal view

Table 1 Bladder tumor in pregnant women. Prior studies

Author	Publication's year	Number of patients	Histology
Church [1]	2013	1 patient, 27 years old	Squamous cell carcinoma
Tyagi [3]	2019	1 patient, 30 years old	Transitional cell carcinoma
Mitra [4]	2003	1 patient, 37 years old	Transitional cell carcinoma
Spahn [6]	2005	3 patients	2 transitional cell carcinoma, 1 squamous cell carcinoma
Alleemudder [7]	2016	1 patient, 39 years old	Squamous cell carcinoma
Shrotri [11]	2008	1 patient, 36 years old	Transitional cell carcinoma

exposed to radiation above 50 mGy, though a chest CT scan is an alternative to staging because the radiation exposure of the fetus is minimal [9].

Once the diagnosis of the bladder tumor is established, it is essential to perform TUR, which is considered a low-risk procedure at any stage of pregnancy and only carries the usual risks associated with anesthesia [3]. Bipolar TUR may be safer [7]. Using histology, it is possible to categorize patients into risk groups to define management. Low-risk patients should be monitored with cystoscopy. In high-risk patients, a restaging TUR should be performed, and management should be decided according to the histology [2]. The safety of BCG instillations is currently unclear; however, there are reports of their use during the second trimester in a patient with carcinoma in situ [2]. Mitomycin is contraindicated as intravesical therapy during pregnancy due to its teratogenic effects [4].

When establishing that the tumor is infiltrating (pT2), the case must be staged. In addition, the gestation trimester must be considered. In the first and second trimesters, the pregnancy should be terminated, followed by cystectomy [4]; in the third trimester, the recommendation is to wait until 28–30 weeks of gestation and then perform cystectomy (after 3–4 weeks). These recommendations are based on the predicted percentage survival of the fetus, which is only 3% at 22 weeks of gestation but increases to 84% at 28 weeks [4].

Performing both surgeries at once is not recommended, as it would increase the risk of bleeding, considering pelvic congestion and the difficulty of performing a hysterectomy of a pregnant uterus [2]. Regarding urinary diversion, continent and noncontinent diversions have been described, without specific recommendations for the most appropriate surgical technique.

Currently, there is no evidence regarding adjuvant therapy with chemotherapy or systemic immunotherapy in pure squamous cell bladder tumors. Postoperative radiation therapy is an alternative to local control or in cases of positive margins [10].

In conclusion, bladder cancer in pregnant women is extremely rare and must be considered in women with recurrent gross hematuria and/or recurrent urinary tract infection. The management of these cases should be performed by a multidisciplinary team. The best time to perform radical cystectomy seems to be at least 4 weeks after C-section and not at the same time. To our knowledge, this case constitutes the longest recurrence-free survival of a pregnant woman with squamous cell bladder cancer published in the literature.

Abbreviations

MRI: Magnetic resonance imaging; TUTR: Transurethral resection; CT: Computed tomography; PNLMP: Papillary neoplasms of low malignant potential.

Authors' contributions

PAR drafted and designed the article. CG reviewed the clinical case and current literature. GPM drafted and designed the article and contributed to the pathology analyses and images. AM performed the TURBT and reviewed the clinical case and current literature. IFS designed and reviewed the article, revising it critically for important intellectual content, performed radical cystectomy surgery and continued the patient's follow-ups. All authors have read and approved the manuscript.

Author details

[1] Departamento de Urología, Escuela de Medicina, Pontificia Universidad Católica de Chile, Diagonal Paraguay 362, Santiago, Chile. [2] División de Ginecología y Obstetricia, Escuela de Medicina, Pontificia Universidad Católica de Chile, Santiago, Chile. [3] Departamento de Anatomía-Patológica, Escuela de Medicina, Pontificia Universidad Católica de Chile, Santiago, Chile.

References

1. Church E, Dieh A. A rare case of aggressive squamous cell carcinoma of the bladder in pregnancy. Obstet Med. 2013;6:182–3.
2. Khochikar MV. Management of urological cancers during pregnancy. Nat Rev Urol. 2010;7:195–205.
3. Tyagi S, Nelivigi G, Bhagat S. Management of bladder cancer in the second trimester of pregnancy. J Obstet Gynaecol India. 2019;69:20–3.
4. Mitra S, Williamson JG, Bullock KN, Arends M. Bladder cancer in pregnancy. J Obstet Gynaecol. 2003;23:440–2.
5. Muezzinoglu T, Inceboz U, Baytur Y, Nese N. Bladder carcinoma in pregnancy: unusual cause for frequent urinary tract infection-case report. Arch Gynecol Obstet. 2013;287:833–4.
6. Spahn M, Bader P, Westermann D, Echtle D, Frohneberg D. Bladder carcinoma during pregnancy. Urol Int. 2005;74:153–9.

7. Alleemudder DI, Alleemudder AI, Harry D, Fountain S. Bladder squamous cell carcinoma in pregnancy. J Obstet Gynaecol. 2016;36:388–9.
8. Manley KV, Hubbard R, Swallow D, Finch W, Wood SJ, Biers SM. Risk factors for development of primary bladder squamous cell carcinoma. Ann R Coll Surg Engl. 2017;99:155–60.
9. Yoon I, Slesinger TL. Radiation exposure in pregnancy. https://www.ncbi.nlm.nih.gov/books/NBK551690/. Accessed 2 Oct 2020.
10. Flaig TW, Spiess PE, Agarwal N, Bangs R, Boorjian SA, Buyyounouski MK, et al. Bladder Cancer, Version 3.2020, NCCN Clinical Practice Guidelines in Oncology. J Natl Compr Canc Netw. 2020;18:329–54.
11. Shrotri KN, Ross GC. Bladder carcinoma presenting during twin pregnancy. J Obstet Gynaecol. 2008;28:750–1.

8

Role of microRNA-381 in bladder cancer growth and metastasis with the involvement of BMI1 and the Rho/ROCK axis

Dayin Chen†, Liang Cheng†, Huifeng Cao* and Wensi Liu

Abstract

Background: Emerging evidence has noted the important participation of microRNAs (miRNAs) in several human diseases including cancer. This research was launched to probe the function of miR-381 in bladder cancer (BCa) progression.

Methods: Twenty-eight patients with primary BCa were included in this study. Cancer tissues and the adjacent normal tissues were obtained. Aberrantly expressed miRNAs in BCa tissues were analyzed using miRNA microarrays. miR-381 expression in the bladder and paired tumor tissues, and in BCa and normal cell lines was determined. The target relationship between miR-381 and BMI1 was predicted online and validated through a luciferase assay. Gain-of-functions of miR-381 and BMI1 were performed to identify their functions on BCa cell behaviors as well as tumor growth in vivo. The involvement of the Rho/ROCK signaling was identified.

Results: miR-381 was poor regulated in BCa tissues and cells (all $p < 0.05$). A higher miR-381 level indicated a better prognosis of patients with BCa. Artificial up-regulation of miR-381 inhibited proliferation, invasion, migration, resistance to apoptosis, and tumor formation ability of BCa T24 and RT4 cells (all $p < 0.05$). miR-381 was found to directly bind to BMI1 and was negatively correlated with BMI1 expression. Overexpression of BMI1 partially blocked the tumor suppressing roles of miR-381 in cell malignancy and tumor growth (all $p < 0.05$). In addition, miR-381 led to decreased RhoA phosphorylation and ROCK2 activation, which were also reversed by BMI1 (all $p < 0.05$). Artificial inhibition of the Rho/ROCK signaling blocked the functions of BMI1 in cell growth and metastasis (all $p < 0.05$).

Conclusion: The study evidenced that miR-381 may act as a beneficiary biomarker in BCa patients. Up-regulation of miR-381 suppresses BCa development both in vivo and in vitro through BMI1 down-regulation and the Rho/ROCK inactivation.

Keywords: miR-381, BMI1, Rho/rock signaling pathway, Bladder cancer, Microarray analysis

Background

Cancer is a major public health concern across the globe, and the urinary bladder cancer (BCa) is the most common neoplastic diseases in the urinary system with 81,400 estimated cases in 2020 in the United States alone according to the up-to-date Cancer Statistics [1]. Nearly 165,000 cases die from this malignancy around the world every year, and males have a threefold predominance in morbidity against females, possibly because of the long-term smoking prevalence and exposure to occupational carcinogens [2]. BCa is allocated to two important branches according to the disease states, which are non-muscle invasive BCa (NMIBC, < T2 stage) and the more risky and metastatic type, muscle invasive BCa (MIBC,

*Correspondence: huifengG010601@163.com
†Dayin Chen and Liang Cheng contributed equally to this work
Department of Urology, The First Affiliated Hospital of Jiamusi University, No. 348, Dexiang Street, Jiamusi 154002, Heilongjiang, People's Republic of China

T2-T4 stage) with the current or future distant invasion potential [3]. However, tumor recurrence is a major challenge in BCa treatment with a rate of 61% in the first year, and approximately 3–15% recurrent NMIBC may progress to the invasive type MIBC when obtaining additional genetic mutations [4]. The current treatment for BCa is far below expectations, with the survival rate of patients seeing little improvement during the last decades [2]. Identifying more molecular mechanisms may help develop novel effective treatments for this disease.

MicroRNAs (miRNAs), a large family of non-coding RNAs with 22 nucleotides in length, regulate multiple biological processes and are aberrantly expressed in human diseases including cancers [5]. miRNAs are well-known to exert key functions by inducing complementary target mRNA repression post-transcriptionally through the 3′ untranslated region (3′ UTR) [6]. Here in the paper, the miRNA microarray analysis was performed with miR-381 found as a major down-regulated miRNA in the BCa tissues. miR-381 has been noted as a tumor inhibitor in many human cancers [7, 8]. In addition, it is noteworthy that miR-381-3p may inhibit CDK6 and MET-mediated epithelial-mesenchymal transition (EMT) and cell cycle progression of BCa cells [9]. But the roles of miR-381 in BCa progression are far away from being fully researched. Here, our study identified BMI1 as a putative mRNA target of miR-381. BMI1 is a key protein of polycomb repressive complex 1 that functions in integrity maintenance, and it has been increasingly known as a factor in the development of multiple human cancers [10]. Considering the potential downregulation of miR-381 in BCa and its anti-tumor effects reported in other malignancies, we hypothesized that miR-381 inhibits its malignant behaviors of BCa through the down-regulation of BMI1. To identify this hypothesis, the expression profiles of miR-381 and BMI1 in BCa tissues and cells was determined. The binding relationship between miR-381 and BMI1 was validated through a luciferase assay. Altered expression of miR-381 and BMI1 was induced to explore their roles in BCa development in both cell and animal experiments, and the potential downstream signaling pathway was identified.

Methods

Clinical sample collection

BCa tissues and the paired adjacent tissues were obtained by tumor resection surgery from 28 BCa patients (22 males and 6 females) who were admitted into the First Affiliated Hospital of Jiamusi University from January 2013 to January 2015 with a median age of 63 years. A 4-year follow-up study was performed to record the prognosis of patients at a 3-month interval. The patients were divided into T1 to T4 stages according to the Tumor-Node-Metastasis (TNM) staging, with 7 in T1, 13 in T2, 5 in T3, and 3 in T4. All included patients had neither pre-surgery treatment history nor chemoradiotherapy history, and they were pathologically diagnosed as primary BCa free of other diseases. The tumor tissues and the adjacent tissues (at least 3 cm away from the tumor tissues) were resected during surgery and preserved in liquid nitrogen. The demographic characteristics of the respondents are exhibited in Table 1.

miRNA microarray analysis

Four patients in T1, T2, T3 or T4 stage (one in each stage) were enrolled for miRNA microarray analysis. The tumor and the paired adjacent tissues from patients were collected for total RNA extraction using TRIzol Reagent (Invitrogen, Carlsbad, CA, USA). Total RNA was concentrated in isopropanol, and then the RNA purity was detected using NanoDrop 2000C (Thermo Fisher Scientific Inc., Waltham, MA, USA) and the RNA quality was determined by formaldehyde denatured agarose gel electrophoresis. Then, 50 μg total RNA was purified using a Taqman miRNA ABC purification kit (Thermo Fisher) and hybridized with the beads. The beads were then washed with magnet, and the miRNAs were eluted 3 times to collect the miRNAs. Thereafter, the collected miRNAs were labeled using a miRNA Complete Labeling and Hyb Kit (Agilent, USA). In brief, 100 μg total RNA was incubated in 10 μg Labeling Spike-In at 37 °C for 30 min, treated with DMSO at 16 °C for 2 h, dried in a vacuum concentrator at 45 °C for 3 h, and then treated with Hybridization Mixture and Hyb labeling at 55 °C for 20 h of hybridization. Then, the miRNAs were further hybridized with Human miRNA Microarray Release

Table 1 Clinical feature of included patients

Item	Group	n
Gender	Male	22
	Female	6
Age	≤60	5
	>60	23
TNM stage	T1	7
	T2	13
	T3	5
	T4	3
Tumor number	Multiple	10
	Single	18
Tumor size (cm)	≤3	18
	>3	10
Lymph nodes metastasis	yes	8
	no	20

TNM Tumor Node Metastasis

14.0,8 (Agilent, USA) and scanned using a SureScan Dx Microarray Scanner (Agilent, USA). The obtained data were subjected to Quality Center analysis and normalization to produce the heatmap for differentially expressed miRNAs.

Reverse transcription quantitative polymerase chain reaction (RT-qPCR)

Total RNA from cells or tissues was extracted using the TRIzol Reagent and reversely transcribed into cDNA using a PromeScript™RT Master Mix Kit (Takara Bio, Jan). Relative gene expression was quantitated using a SYBR®Premix Ex Taq™II Kit (Takara Bio, Jan). The qPCR was performed on a Mx3005P System (Stratagene, USA). Quantification of each sample was repeated by three times. Relative expression was evaluated using the $2^{-\Delta\Delta Ct}$ method with U6 and GAPDH as internal references. Table 2 exhibits the primer sequences.

Cell culture and transfection

Human bladder cell lines T24 and RT4, normal bladder epithelial cell line SV-HUC-1, and HEK-293T cells were acquired from ATCC (Manassas, USA). Cells were cultivated in Dulbecco's modified Eagle's medium with 10% fetal bovine serum (FBS, all from Gibco Company, Grand Island, NY, USA) at 37 °C with 5% CO_2. The miR-381 mimic and BMI1-overexpressing vectors (BMI1-OE) were synthesized by GenePharma Co., Ltd. (Shanghai, China). To minimize the off-target effects, 3 RNA fragments were loaded into the vectors and transfected into cells. Then cells were plated into 24-well plates once the cell confluence reaching 70%. miR-381 mimic and BMI1-OE vectors were transfected into T24 and RT4 cells in line with the protocols of the Lipofectamine 2000 (Invitrogen). After 6 h, the fluorescence expression in cells was observed under a fluorescence microscope (Olympus Optical Co., Ltd, Tokyo, Japan). In addition, 50 μmol/L Rho/Rock-specific antagonist, Y-27632 (MedChemExpress, Monmouth Junction, NJ, USA) [11], was further administrated into cells overexpressing BMI1. Cells transfected with an equal volume of DMSO were set as control. The cells were used for following experiments 48 h later.

Table 2 Primer sequences for RT-qPCR

Gene	Primer sequence (5′–3′)
miR-381	F: TATACAAGGGCAAGCTCUCTGT
	R: TGCGGGTGCTCGCTTCGGCAGC3
BMI1	F: TGGATCGGAAAGTAAACAAAGAC
	R: TGCATCACAGTCATTGCTGCT
GAPDH	F: GGGAGCCAAAAGGGTCATCA
	R: TGATGGCATGGACTGTGGTC
U6	F: CTCGCTTCGGCAGCACA
	R: AACGCTTCACGAATTTGCGT

RT-qPCR reverse transcription quantitative polymerase chain reaction, *miR-381* microRNA-381, *GAPDH* glyceraldehyde-3-phosphate dehydrogenase, *F* forward, *R* reverse

Cell proliferation by the cell counting kit-8 (CCK-8) method

A total of 100 μL cell suspension was loaded on 96-well plates and pre-incubated for 24 h. Next, each well was loaded with 10 μL CCK-8 reagent, and then the plates with cells were further incubated for 12, 24, 48 and 72 h. Then the optical density at 450 nm was evaluated using a microplate reader (SoectraMax iD5, Molecular Devices, USA). The CCK-8 kit was from Dojindo Laboratories (Kumamoto, Japan).

Cell migration by scratch test

Guide lines were produced on the back side of 6-well plates at a 1-cm interval, and 5×10^5 cells were added into the plates. On the second day, a pipette was used to produce a scratch perpendicular to the back side guide lines, and the scratched cells were washed away by phosphate buffer saline (PBS). Then the plates were loaded with serum-free medium and cultured at 37 °C with 5% CO_2. Twenty-four hours later, the cells were observed and photographed under a microscope (CX22, Olympus). The scratch area was analyzed using the Image J software (version 1.48, NIH, USA). Relative migration distance (%) = (0 h scratch area—24 h scratch area)/0 h scratch area [12].

Cell invasion by transwell assay

Matrigel was diluted in serum-free DMEM, and then 100 μL Matrigel was loaded onto each apical chamber at 37 °C for 4 h. Then, cells were resuspended in 10% FBS to 5×10^5 cells/mL, and each apical chamber was loaded with 200 μL cell suspension, while each basolateral chamber was loaded with 600 μL cell medium (containing 5 μg/mL fibronectin). Then the transwells were incubated at 37 °C for 20 h, and the non-invaded cells in the apical chambers were removed, while the invaded cells in each well were stained with 500 μL 0.1% crystal violet at 37 °C for 30 min. Then the number of invaded cells were observed and counted under the microscope with 5 random fields included.

Cell apoptosis by flow cytometry

In short, 27 mL ddH_2O was used to dilute 3 mL binding buffer (10 ×). Cells in each group were resuspended in 1 mL 1 × binding buffer, centrifuged at 300 g for 10 min to discard the supernatant, and resuspended in 1 mL 1 × binding buffer again till a density of 1×10^6 cells/mL.

Next, each tube was loaded with 100 μL cells and then 5 μL Annexin V-fluorescein isothiocyanate (FITC) for 10 min of reaction, and then with 5 μL propidium iodide (PI) in the dark for 5 min. The apoptosis was determined using an Annexin V-FITC/PI Apoptosis Kit (Solarbio Science & Technology Co., Ltd., Beijing, China) and run on a flow cytometer (Attune Nxt, Thermo Fisher) within an hour.

Xenograft tumors in nude mice

A total of 48 specific-pathogen-free nude mice (4–6 weeks old, 20 ± 2 g) purchased from Vital River Laboratory Animal Technology Co., Ltd. (Beijing, China) were randomly allocated into 6 groups, 8 in each. Then, each mouse was subcutaneously injected with 4×10^6 T24 or RT4 cells with stable transfection of miR-381 mimic or mimic control, or cells with transfection of BMI1-OE and vector control. The volume (V) of xenograft tumors was calculated as the following formula every 7 days: $V = (L \times W^2)/2$, where 'L' indicates the length while 'W' indicates the width [13]. On the 28th day after cell implantation, mice were euthanized by overdose of pentobarbital sodium (150 mg/kg), and the tumors were taken out and weighed.

Dual-luciferase reporter gene assay

The binding relationship between miRNA and mRNA was predicted on StarBase (http://starbase.sysu.edu.cn/). The 3′UTR sequence of BMI2 and miR-381 was inserted into pMIR-REPORT™ luciferase reporter vector (Thermo Fisher) using Lipofectamine 3000 (Invitrogen) and then transfected into HEK293T cells. Cells were lysed 24 h later, and the luciferase activity was determined using a Dual-Luciferase Reporter Assay System (Promega Corporation, WI, USA) [14]. Three independent experiments were performed.

Western blot analysis

Radio-Immunoprecipitation assay cell lysis buffer (Amresco Inc., Texus, USA) was used to collect total protein. In brief, single cell suspension was centrifuged at 800 g at 4 °C for 5 min with the supernatant discarded. Then the cells were ice-bated in a fivefold volume of lysis buffer for 10 min, and then centrifuged at 12,000 g at 4 °C for 10 min to collect the supernatant. The collected protein was run on SDS-PAGE and transferred to polyvinylidene fluoride membranes (EMD Millipore). Subsequently, the membranes were blocked with 5% skimmed milk and then incubated with the primary antibodies against RhoA (1:5000, ab187027), p-RhoA (1:1000, ab41435), ROCK2 (1:5000, ab71598) and β-actin (1:1000, ab8227) (Abcam Inc., Cambridge, MA, USA) at 4 °C for 16 h, and then with the secondary antibody (1:3000, ab205718) at room temperature for 2 h. The immunoblotting image were visualized using the Image J software (Version 1.8.0, National Institute of Health, USA). Three independent experiments were performed.

Statistical analysis

SPSS 22.0 (IBM Corp. Armonk, NY, USA) was used for data analysis. Data were in normal distribution according to Kolmogorov–SmiRnov test and are exhibited as mean ± standard deviation (mean ± SD). Differences in multiple groups were analyzed using one-way or two-way analysis of variance (ANOVA). Tukey's multiple comparisons test was used for the post-hoc test after ANOVA analysis. Survival curve was drawn using the Kalpan-Meier method and analyzed using the log rank test. p was obtained by two-tailed tests and $p < 0.05$ was regarded statistically significant.

Results

Poor miR-381 expression in BCa patients indicates unfavorable prognosis

The tumor tissues and paired adjacent tissues from 4 BCa patients (T1 to T4) were used for miRNA microarray analysis. It was found that miR-381 was the greatest down-regulated one in tumor tissues as compared to the paired normal ones (Fig. 1a). Then, the RT-qPCR results validated that miR-381 was significantly poorly expressed in the tumor tissues in all the included BCa patients (Fig. 1b). According to the average miR-381 expression (0.46), the patients were allocated into high-expression group (n = 16) and low-expression group (n = 12). The follow-up study data suggested that patients with higher miR-381 had relatively higher survival rates and longer lifetime (Fig. 1c). In addition, we also determined miR-381 expression in cell levels, and it is noteworthy that miR-381 expression was much lower in BCa cell lines T24 and RT4 than that in normal bladder epithelial cells (Fig. 1d).

miR-381 inhibits malignant behaviors of BCa cells

To further figure out the roles of miR-381 in BCa development, up-regulation of miR-381 was introduced in both T24 and RT4 cell lines by administrating miR-381 mimic or mimic control (Fig. 2a). Then, we found that miR-381 mimic treatment led to a significant decline in proliferation in both cells (Fig. 2b). Accordingly, cells with increased miR-381 expression presented decreased migration distance (Fig. 2c) and reduced number of invaded cells (Fig. 2d). In addition, it was found that miR-381 mimic led to increased cell apoptosis (Fig. 2e). As for in vivo experiments, the implantation of cells with miR-381 mimic led to a significant decline in tumor growth

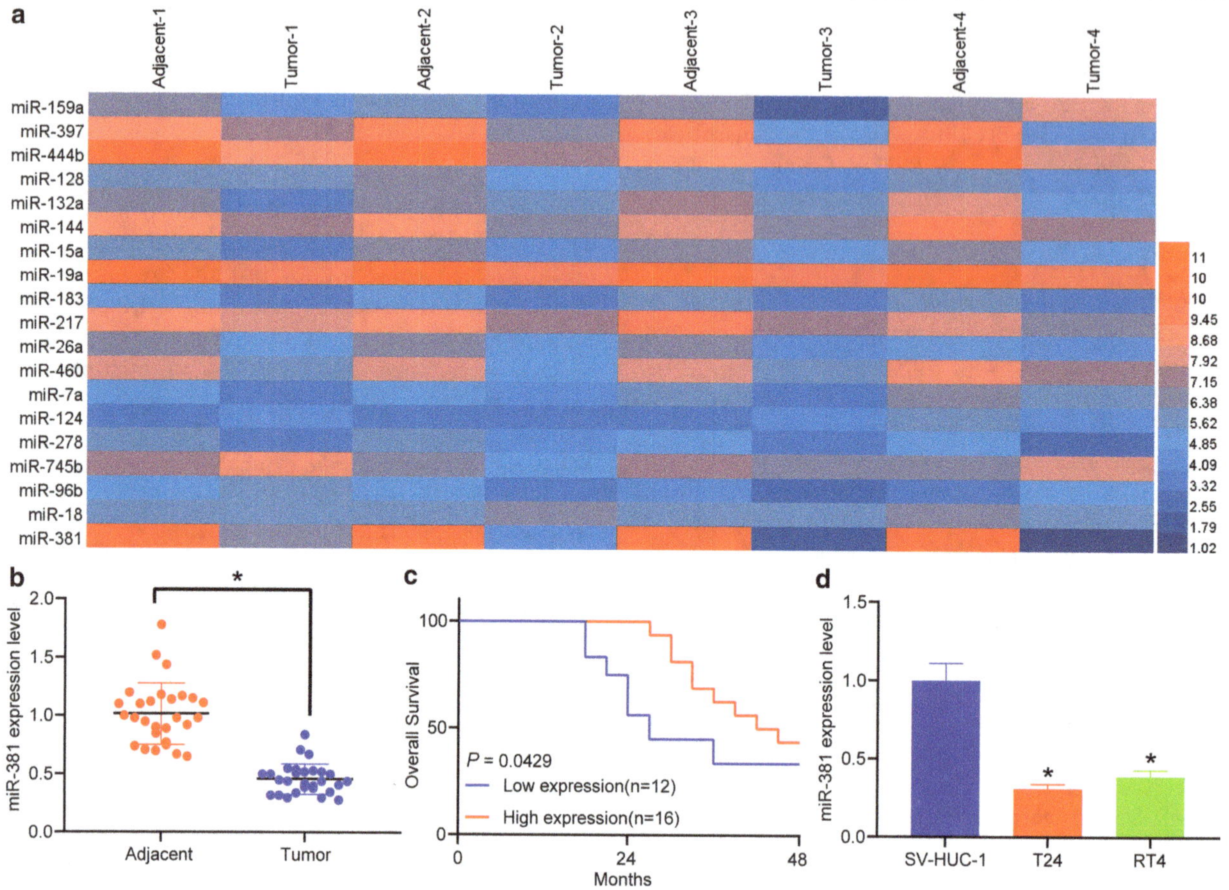

Fig. 1 Poor miR-381 expression in BCa patients indicates unfavorable prognosis. **a** differentially expressed miRNAs between BCa tissues and the paired adjacent tissues determined by microarray analysis ($p < 0.05$, $|\log FC| \geq 1.5$); **b** miR-381 expression in the BCa and paired adjacent tissues determined by RT-qPCR (*$p < 0.05$, two-way ANOVA); **c** survival analysis of BCa patients with different level of miR-381; **d** miR-381 expression in BCa cells (T24 and RT4) and in normal bladder epithelial cell line SV-HUC-1 determined by RT-qPCR (*$p < 0.05$, one-way ANOVA); Repetition = 3

in mice, and the tumor weight was decreased on the 28th day (n = 8) (Fig. 2f).

miR-381 targets BMI1 to inactivate the Rho/Rock pathway

We next explored the potential downstream molecules involved. We first predicted BMI1 as a target of miR-381 on a computer-based bioinformation system, and then had the binding relationship between miR-381 and BMI1 validated through a luciferase assay (Fig. 3a). Then, it was found that BMI1 expression was increased in tumor tissues as compared to the adjacent tissues (Fig. 3b), and similarly, the BMI1 expression was also higher in BCa cell lines than that in bladder epithelial cells (Fig. 3c). The BMI1 expression in the tumor tissues of BCa patients was negatively correlated with miR-381 expression (Fig. 3d). Importantly, BMI1 expression in BCa cells was decreased upon miR-381 upregulation (Fig. 3e). BMI1-OE vectors were administrated into T24 cells and RT4 cells, and BMI1-OE#2 presented a best overexpressing efficiency (Fig. 3f). Intriguingly, the Rho/ROCK signaling pathway has been noted to be significantly associated with the aggressiveness of BCa [15]. After miR-381 control, miR-381 mimic, BMI1-NC or BMI1-OE vector transfection, the protein levels of RhoA and ROCK2 were detected. It was found that miR-381 mimic inhibited the ROCK2 expression and RhoA phosphorylation while BMI1-OE led to increased activation of the Rho/ROCK signaling pathway (Fig. 3g). The above results indicated that miR-381 could target BMI1 to inactivate the Rho/Rock pathway.

Overexpression of BMI1 promotes BCa progression

To further identify the exact roles of BMI1 in BCa pathogenesis, overexpression of BMI1 was artificially upregulated in T24 and RT4 cells. BMI1-OE vector led to an increase in cell proliferation (Fig. 4a). Likewise, the migration rate (Fig. 4b) and invasion rate (Fig. 4c) of cells was notably increased following BMI1 overexpression.

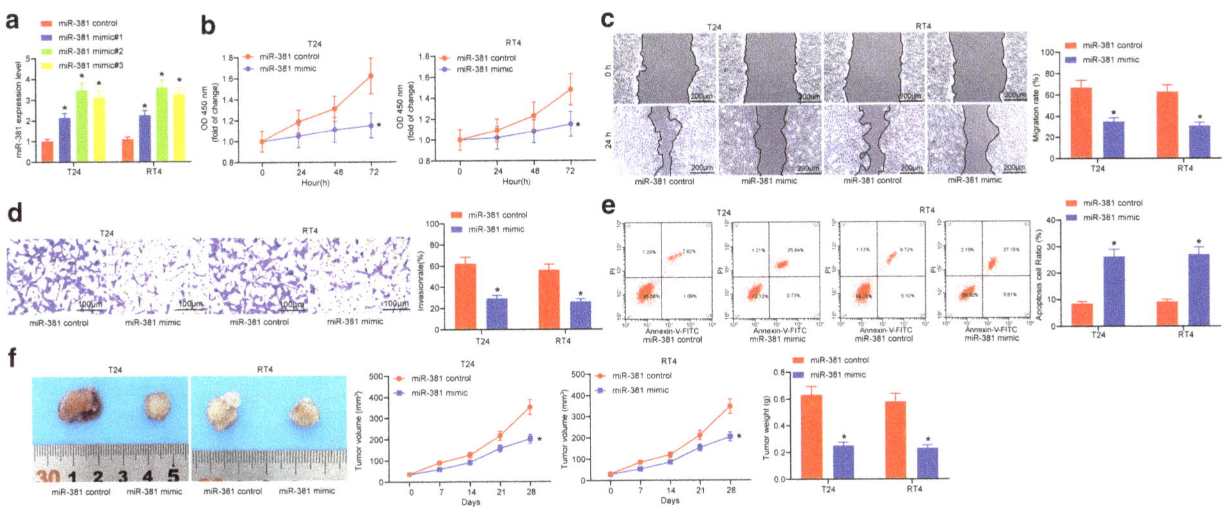

Fig. 2 miR-381 inhibits malignant behaviors of BCa cells. **a** miR-381 expression in cells after miR-381 mimic transfection detected by RT-qPCR, and it was found that miR-381 mimic#2 showed the best efficacy (*$p<0.05$, two-way ANOVA); **b** optical density at 450 nm measured by two-way ANOVA (*$p<0.05$, two-way ANOVA); **c** migration rate of each group of cells at the 24th h (*$p<0.05$, two-way ANOVA); **d** invasion rate of each group of cells measured by transwell assay (*$p<0.05$, two-way ANOVA); **e** apoptosis rate of cells determined by flow cytometry (*$p<0.05$, two-way ANOVA); **f** tumor volume change and weight on the 28th day after implantation of cells transfected miR-381 mimic (*$p<0.05$, two-way ANOVA); Repetition = 3

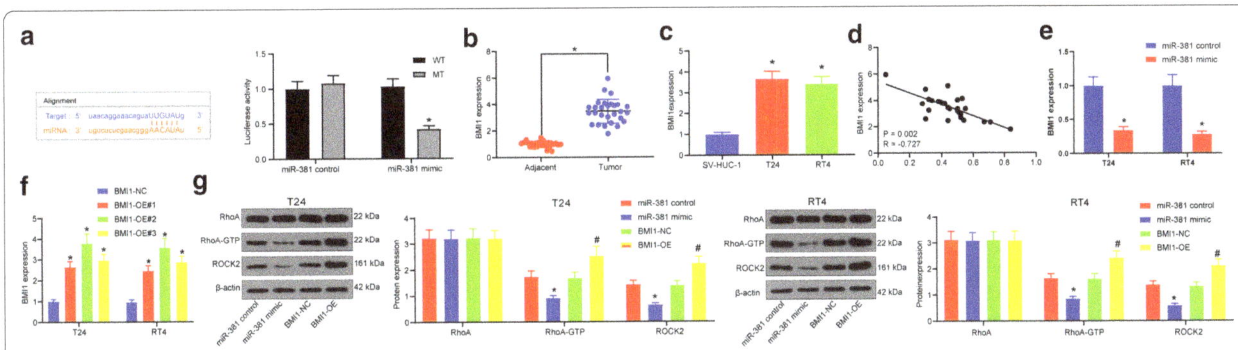

Fig. 3 miR-381 targets BMI1 to inactivate the Rho/Rock pathway. **a** target relationship between miR-381 and BMI1 predicted on StarBase (http://starbase.sysu.edu.cn/) and validated through a dual luciferase reporter assay (*$p<0.05$, two-way ANOVA); **b** BMI1 expression in BCa tissues determined by RT-qPCR (*$p<0.05$, two-way test); **c** BMI expression in BCa cell lines (T24 and RT4) and in normal bladder epithelial cells determined by RT-qPCR (*$p<0.05$, one-way ANOVA); **d** correlation analysis between miR-381 and BMI1 expression in BCa tumor tissues; **e** BMI1 expression in T24 and RT4 cells after miR-381 mimic transfection measured by RT-qPCR (*$p<0.05$, two-way ANOVA); **f** BMI1 expression in BCa tumor tissues after BMI1-OE vector transfection detected by RT-qPCR (*$p<0.05$, two-way ANOVA). **g** protein levels of ROCK2, RhoA and RhoA-GFP (phosphorylated RhoA) in each group of cells measured by western blot analysis (*$p<0.05$, two-way ANOVA); Repetition = 3

In addition, overexpression of BMI1 reduced the apoptosis rate in both cell lines (Fig. 4d). As for in vivo, we found cells transfected with BMI1-OE led to significantly increased tumor growth rate and weight in nude mice (n = 8) (Fig. 4e). These results identified BMI1 presented a reverse regulating role in BCa cells as relative to miR-381.

BMI1 partially blocks the role of miR-381

To further confirm the involvement of BMI1 in the miR-381-mediated events. Overexpression of BMI1 was introduced in cells pre-transfected with miR-381 mimic (Fig. 5a). It was found that further overexpression of BMI1 partially recovered cell proliferation (Fig. 5b), cell migration (Fig. 5c) and cell invasion (Fig. 5d) that were suppressed by miR-381 mimic. In addition, the miR-381-triggerred cell apoptosis was inhibited when BMI1 was further overexpressed (Fig. 5e). Accordingly, cells transfected miR-381 mimic and BMI-OE vector led to an increased tumor growth rate in nude mice compared to cells with miR-381 mimic alone (Fig. 5f). These

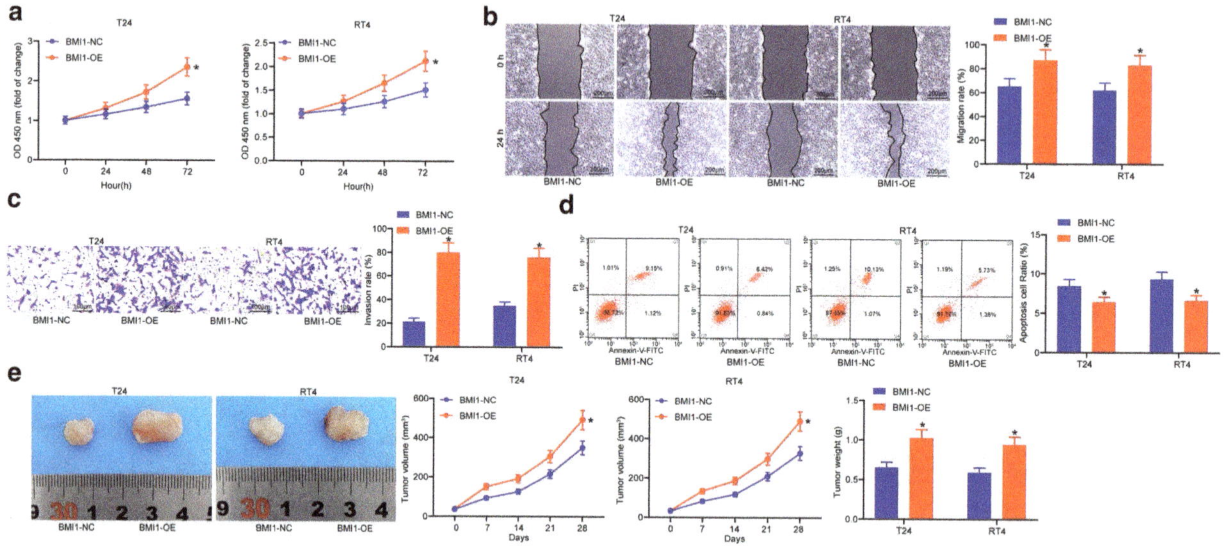

Fig. 4 Overexpression of BMI1 promotes BCa progression. **a** optical density at 450 nm of each group of cells according the CCK-8 method (*$p < 0.05$, two-way ANOVA); **b** migration distance at the 24th hour measured by the scratch test (*$p < 0.05$, two-way ANOVA); **c** number of invaded cells at the 24th hour determined by the transwell assay (*$p < 0.05$, two-way ANOVA); **d** number of PI-Annexin V-double positive cells detected by flow cytometry (*$p < 0.05$, two-way ANOVA); **e** tumor growth rate change and weight on the 28th day in nude mice (n = 8) (*$p < 0.05$, two-way ANOVA); Repetition = 3

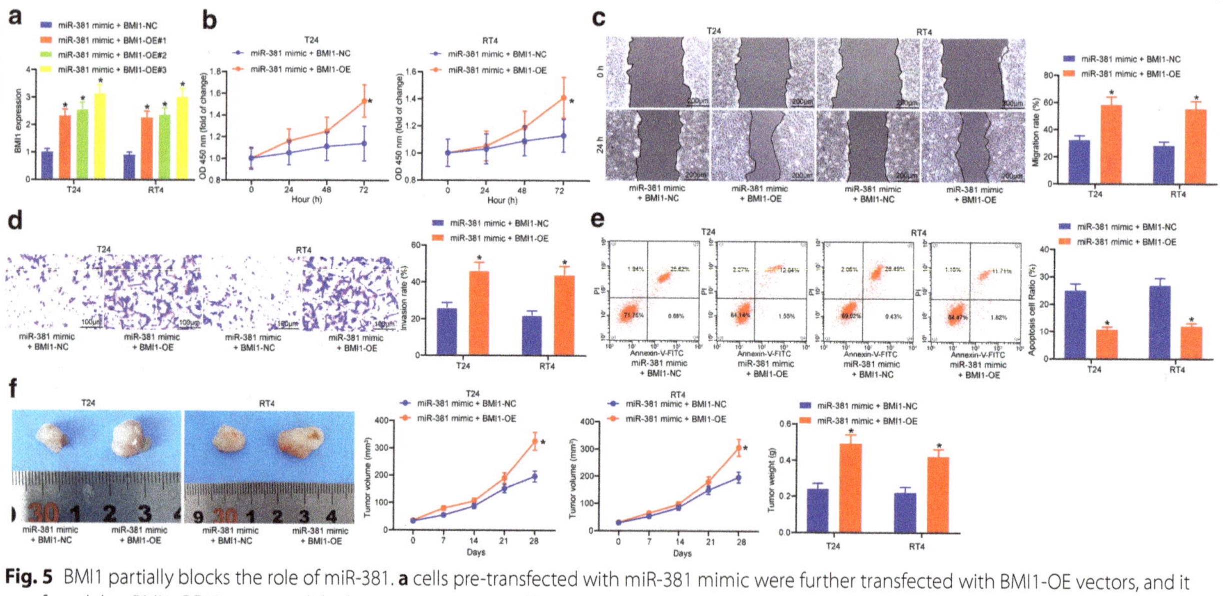

Fig. 5 BMI1 partially blocks the role of miR-381. **a** cells pre-transfected with miR-381 mimic were further transfected with BMI1-OE vectors, and it was found that BMI1-OE#3 presented the best overexpressing efficiency (*$p < 0.05$, two-way ANOVA); **b** optical density at 450 nm of each group of cells according the CCK-8 method (*$p < 0.05$, two-way ANOVA); **c** migration distance at the 24th hour measured by the scratch test (*$p < 0.05$, two-way ANOVA); **d** number of invaded cells at the 24th h determined by the transwell assay (*$p < 0.05$, two-way ANOVA); **e** number of PI-Annexin V-double positive cells detected by flow cytometry (*$p < 0.05$, two-way ANOVA); **f** tumor growth rate change and weight on the 28th day in nude mice (n = 8) (*$p < 0.05$, two-way ANOVA); Repetition = 3

findings suggested that BMI1 partially antagonized the effects of miR-381 mimic.

Inhibition of Rho/ROCK signaling blocks the functions of BMI1

To further validate the involvement of the Rho/ROCK signaling in the above events, we first determined the

Rho/ROCK2 activity in T24, RT4 and SV-HUC-1 cell lines. It was found that the phosphorylation of RhoA and protein level of ROCK2 was increased in BCa cell lines (Fig. 6a). Then, a Rho/ROCK-specific antagonist, Y-27632, was administrated into cells overexpressing BMI1, after which the phosphorylation of RhoA and protein level of ROCK2 was decreased (Fig. 6b). In addition, the CCK-8 and flow cytometry results showed that the increased cell growth and decreased cell apoptosis by BMI1 were blocked by Y-27632 (Fig. 6c, d), indicating this pathway is at least partially responsible for the BMI1-medeated cell growth.

Discussion

Treatment for BCa, especially for the invasive type MIBC remains great challenge owing to high recurrence following surgical resection and drug administration. Aside from the unfavorable prognosis, the huge economic cost in lifetime surveillance with periodic cystoscopy and evaluation of recurrence rate brings considerable burden to BCa patients [16–18]. It has been an emerging consensus that aberrant expression of some miRNAs, either extremely high or poor expression, is closely correlated with BCa pathogenesis [19]. Here, the current study evidenced that miR-381 could serve as a cancer suppressor in BCa with the involvement of BMI1 downregulation and the following Rho/ROCK inactivation.

The initial finding was that miR-381 was poorly expressed in the tumor tissues in BCa patients and was positively correlated with patient prognosis, preliminarily indicating a beneficiary role of miR-381 in BCa prognosis. miRNAs have been emerged as non-invasive biomarkers for BCa detection [20, 21] or even potential treating targets in clinical practice [22]. For instance, miR-3622a was noted to promote proliferation and invasion capacities of BCa through binding to LASS2 [12]. On the other hand, some miRNAs have been documented to exert suppressing functions in BCa. miR-502-5p, for example, has been recently found to suppress the malignant behaviors of BCa cells through the different miRNA targets including CCND1, NOP14 and DNMT3B [23]. Similar trends have also been seen in miR-124-3p [24] and miR-203a [25]. As for miR-381, it has been particularly suggested to play critical functions in overcoming cisplatin resistance in breast cancer treatment [26–28]. Likewise, its anti-tumor role has been increasingly revealed in other malignancies such as in cervical cancer [29] and in prostate cancer [30] through the different mRNA targets. Here our study found that miR-381 was poorly expressed in BCa cells. Overexpression of miR-381 inhibited the malignant behaviors of BCa T24 and RT4 cell lines, presenting as decreased cell viability, reduced cell migration and invasion, and increased cell apoptosis. In addition, similar results were found in animal experiments, where cells with stable miR-381 overexpression contributed to a significant inhibition in tumor growth in volume and weight regards.

Second, the findings above triggered us to further explore the downstream molecules of miR-381. A computer-based online prediction system suggested BMI1 as a target mRNA of miR-381, and this binding relationship was further validated by a luciferase assay. As a member of the polycomb group family, BMI1, owning stem cell characteristics, is prone to participate in the onset and development of tumors and is linked to tumor metastasis, recurrence and chemo-resistance as

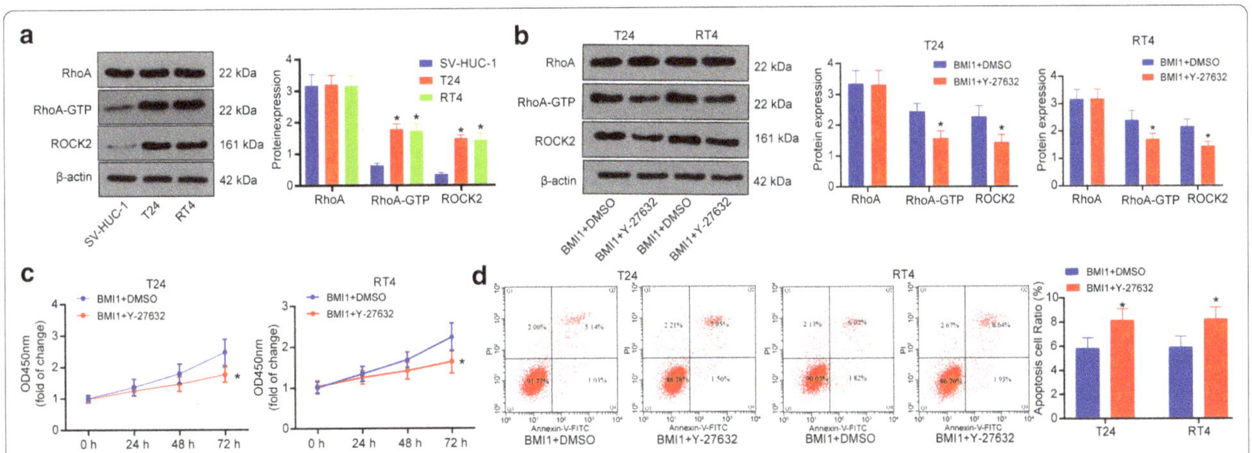

Fig. 6 Inhibition of Rho/ROCK signaling blocks the functions of BMI1. **a**, **b** Protein levels of ROCK2, RhoA and RhoA-GFP (phosphorylated RhoA) in each group of cells measured by western blot analysis (*$p < 0.05$, two-way ANOVA); **c** optical density at 450 nm of each group of cells according the CCK-8 method (*$p < 0.05$, two-way ANOVA); **d** number of PI-Annexin V-double positive cells detected by flow cytometry (*$p < 0.05$, two-way ANOVA). Repetition = 3

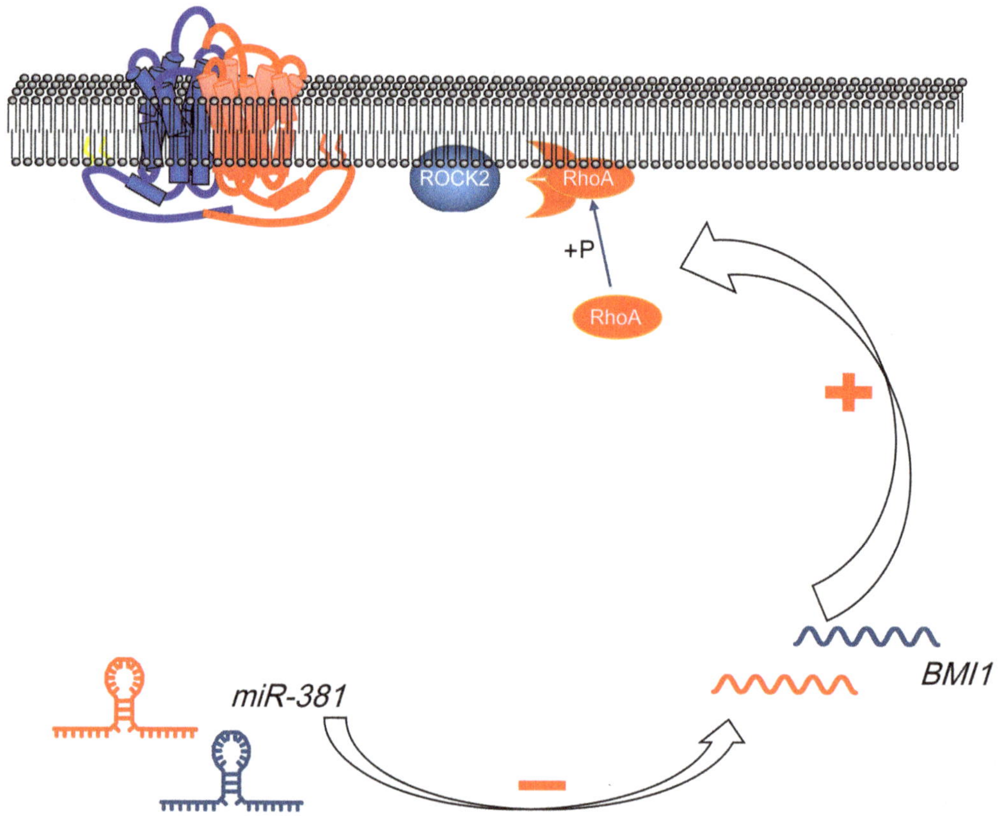

Fig. 7 A diagram for the molecular mechanism. In BCa cells, miRNA-381 directly binds to BMI1 expression to inhibit RhoA phosphorylation and ROCK2 expression, leading to suppressed malignant behaviors of bladder cells

well [31]. In addition, BMI1 is well-known to interact with another EMT and stemness promoter, TWIST1 [32, 33]. Not surprisingly, silencing of BMI1 has been suggested as a promising therapeutic target in many human cancer therapies [34, 35]. Here, our study found that artificial overexpression of BMI1 led to increased cell proliferation, migration, invasion and resistance to death in both T24 and RT4 cells. The involvement of BMI1 in BCa pathogenesis has been relatively largely studied. Its knockdown was noted to inhibit bladder cell growth, self-renewal and progression, and several upstream mediators of BMI1 such as miR-139-5p [36] and miR-200c [37] were identified. In the current paper, in order to further validate that BMI1 silencing holds accountable for the miR-381-mediated events, rescue experiments were performed where cells pre-transfected with miR-381 were further transfected with BMI1-OE. It was found that the malignant behaviors of cells inhibited by miR-381 mimic were partially recovered following BMI1 overexpression.

The Rho/ROCK signaling is well-known for its implication in cytoskeletal reorganization, which is elemental for cell migration and metastasis [38]. Specifically, this signaling was documented to be related to the invasion and metastasis and malignancy in BCa [15]. Here, our study identified that the phosphorylation of RhoA and ROCK2 expression was notably inhibited by miR-381, while overexpression of BMI1 led to reversed trends. A Rho-associated kinase inhibitor, Y-27632, has been suggested to inhibit the migration and metastasis of BCa [11]. Here, we further noticed that Y-27632 blocked the promoting roles of BMI1 in BCa cell growth. Therefore, it can be inferred that the Rho/ROCK pathway inactivation is possibly implicated in the miR-381/BMI1-mediated events.

Conclusion

To sum up, the present study evidenced that miR-381 could inhibit BCa progression through inhibiting BMI1, presenting as decreased cell proliferation, migration, invasion and resistance to death, as well as tumor growth in vivo. The Rho/ROCK pathway was found to be at least partially responsible for the above events (Fig. 7). However, this is a pre-clinical study with limited sample size, and the regulatory network by which BMI1 regulate the Rho/ROCK requires further investigation. Still, the findings of the present study need further validation. We hope these findings may offer novel insights into BCa treatment.

Abbreviations

ANOVA: Analysis of variance; BMI1: B-Cell-specific Moloney murine leukemia virus insertion region 1; CCK-8: Cell counting kit-8; EMT: Epithelial-mesenchymal transition; FBS: Fetal bovine serum; FITC: Fluorescein isothiocyanate; mean ± SD: Mean ± standard deviation; MIBD: Muscle invasive bladder cancer; miRNA: MicroRNA; NMIBD: Non-muscle invasive bladder cancer; PBS: Phosphate buffer saline; PI: Propidium iodide; RT-qPCR: Reverse transcription quantitative polymerase chain reaction; TNM: Tumor-Node-Metastasis; 3′UTR : 3′Untranslated region.

Acknowledgements

Not applicable.

Authors' contributions

DYC, LC proposed the protocol. DYC, LC, HFC, WSL were involved in data collection and management. HFC, WSL analyzed the data. DYC, LC contributed to manuscript writing and critically revised the manuscript. All authors read and approved the final manuscript.

References

1. Siegel RL, Miller KD, Jemal A. Cancer statistics, 2020. CA Cancer J Clin. 2020;70(1):7–30.
2. Fernandez MI, Brausi M, Clark PE, Cookson MS, Grossman HB, Khochikar M, et al. Epidemiology, prevention, screening, diagnosis, and evaluation: update of the ICUD-SIU joint consultation on bladder cancer. World J Urol. 2019;37(1):3–13.
3. Crabb SJ, Douglas J. The latest treatment options for bladder cancer. Br Med Bull. 2018;128(1):85–95.
4. Ringuette-Goulet C, Bolduc S, Pouliot F. Modeling human bladder cancer. World J Urol. 2018;36(11):1759–66.
5. Adams BD, Kasinski AL, Slack FJ. Aberrant regulation and function of microRNAs in cancer. Curr Biol. 2014;24(16):R762-776.
6. Iwakawa HO, Tomari Y. The functions of MicroRNAs: mRNA decay and translational repression. Trends Cell Biol. 2015;25(11):651–65.
7. Jin D, Guo J, Wu Y, Chen W, Du J, Yang L, et al. Metformin-repressed miR-381-YAP-snail axis activity disrupts NSCLC growth and metastasis. J Exp Clin Cancer Res. 2020;39(1):6.
8. Xie Y, Qi J, Zhu C, Zhao D, Liao G. MiR-381 functions as a tumor suppressor in gastric cancer by targeting ROCK2. Int J Clin Exp Pathol. 2019;12(1):164–72.
9. Li J, Ying Y, Xie H, Jin K, Yan H, Wang S, et al. Dual regulatory role of CCNA2 in modulating CDK6 and MET-mediated cell-cycle pathway and EMT progression is blocked by miR-381-3p in bladder cancer. FASEB J. 2019;33(1):1374–88.
10. M JR, S V. BMI1 and PTEN are key determinants of breast cancer therapy: A plausible therapeutic target in breast cancer. Gene 2018, 678:302–311.
11. Jiang L, Wen J, Luo W. Rhoassociated kinase inhibitor, Y27632, inhibits the invasion and proliferation of T24 and 5367 bladder cancer cells. Mol Med Rep. 2015;12(5):7526–30.
12. Fu S, Luan T, Jiang C, Huang Y, Li N, Wang H, et al. miR-3622a promotes proliferation and invasion of bladder cancer cells by downregulating LASS2. Gene. 2019;701:23–31.
13. Tang W, Zhou W, Xiang L, Wu X, Zhang P, Wang J, et al. The p300/YY1/miR-500a-5p/HDAC2 signalling axis regulates cell proliferation in human colorectal cancer. Nat Commun. 2019;10(1):663.
14. Jiang C, Zhu W, Xu J, Wang B, Hou W, Zhang R, et al. MicroRNA-26a negatively regulates toll-like receptor 3 expression of rat macrophages and ameliorates pristane induced arthritis in rats. Arthritis Res Ther. 2014;16(1):R9.
15. Kamai T, Tsujii T, Arai K, Takagi K, Asami H, Ito Y, et al. Significant association of Rho/ROCK pathway with invasion and metastasis of bladder cancer. Clin Cancer Res. 2003;9(7):2632–41.
16. Fankhauser CD, Mostafid H. Prevention of bladder cancer incidence and recurrence: nutrition and lifestyle. Curr Opin Urol. 2018;28(1):88–92.
17. Flannery K, Cao X, He J, Zhong Y, Shah AY, Kamat AM. Survival rates and health care costs for patients with advanced bladder cancer treated and untreated with chemotherapy. Clin Genitourin Cancer. 2018;16(4):e909–17.
18. Usuba W, Urabe F, Yamamoto Y, Matsuzaki J, Sasaki H, Ichikawa M, et al. Circulating miRNA panels for specific and early detection in bladder cancer. Cancer Sci. 2019;110(1):408–19.
19. Enokida H, Yoshino H, Matsushita R, Nakagawa M. The role of microRNAs in bladder cancer. Investig Clin Urol. 2016;57(Suppl 1):S60-76.
20. Tolle A, Jung M, Rabenhorst S, Kilic E, Jung K, Weikert S. Identification of microRNAs in blood and urine as tumour markers for the detection of urinary bladder cancer. Oncol Rep. 2013;30(4):1949–56.
21. Xiao S, Wang J, Xiao N. MicroRNAs as noninvasive biomarkers in bladder cancer detection: a diagnostic meta-analysis based on qRT-PCR data. Int J Biol Markers. 2016;31(3):e276-285.
22. Blanca A, Cheng L, Montironi R, Moch H, Massari F, Fiorentino M, et al. Mirna expression in bladder cancer and their potential role in clinical practice. Curr Drug Metab. 2017;18(8):712–22.
23. Ying Y, Li J, Xie H, Yan H, Jin K, He L, et al. CCND1, NOP14 and DNMT3B are involved in miR-502-5p-mediated inhibition of cell migration and proliferation in bladder cancer. Cell Prolif. 2020;53(2):e12751.
24. Wang JR, Liu B, Zhou L, Huang YX. MicroRNA-124-3p suppresses cell migration and invasion by targeting ITGA3 signaling in bladder cancer. Cancer Biomark. 2019;24(2):159–72.
25. Na XY, Shang XS, Zhao Y, Ren PP, Hu XQ. MiR-203a functions as a tumor suppressor in bladder cancer by targeting SIX4. Neoplasma. 2019;66(2):211–21.
26. Dou D, Ge X, Wang X, Xu X, Zhang Z, Seng J, et al. EZH2 contributes to cisplatin resistance in breast cancer by epigenetically suppressing miR-381 expression. Onco Targets Ther. 2019;12:9627–37.
27. Mi H, Wang X, Wang F, Li L, Zhu M, Wang N, et al. SNHG15 contributes to cisplatin resistance in breast cancer through sponging miR-381. Onco Targets Ther. 2020;13:657–66.
28. Yi D, Xu L, Wang R, Lu X, Sang J. miR-381 overcomes cisplatin resistance in breast cancer by targeting MDR1. Cell Biol Int. 2019;43(1):12–21.
29. Shang A, Zhou C, Bian G, Chen W, Lu W, Wang W, et al. miR-381-3p restrains cervical cancer progression by downregulating FGF7. J Cell Biochem. 2019;120(1):778–89.
30. Hu J, Wu X, Yang C, Rashid K, Ma C, Hu M, et al. Anticancer effect of icaritin on prostate cancer via regulating miR-381-3p and its target gene UBE2C. Cancer Med. 2019;8(18):7833–45.
31. Siddique HR, Saleem M. Role of BMI1, a stem cell factor, in cancer recurrence and chemoresistance: preclinical and clinical evidences. Stem Cells. 2012;30(3):372–8.
32. Ren H, Du P, Ge Z, Jin Y, Ding D, Liu X, et al. TWIST1 and BMI1 in cancer metastasis and chemoresistance. J Cancer. 2016;7(9):1074–80.
33. Wu KJ, Yang MH. Epithelial-mesenchymal transition and cancer stemness: the Twist1-Bmi1 connection. Biosci Rep. 2011;31(6):449–55.
34. Kim M, Lee S, Park WH, Suh DH, Kim K, Kim YB, et al. Silencing Bmi1 expression suppresses cancer stemness and enhances chemosensitivity in endometrial cancer cells. Biomed Pharmacother. 2018;108:584–9.
35. Li J, Vangundy Z, Poi M. PTC209, a specific inhibitor of BMI1, promotes cell cycle arrest and apoptosis in cervical cancer cell lines. Anticancer Res. 2020;40(1):133–41.
36. Luo H, Yang R, Li C, Tong Y, Fan L, Liu X, et al. MicroRNA-139-5p inhibits bladder cancer proliferation and self-renewal by targeting the Bmi1 oncogene. Tumour Biol. 2017;39(7):1010428317718414.
37. Liu L, Qiu M, Tan G, Liang Z, Qin Y, Chen L, et al. miR-200c inhibits invasion, migration and proliferation of bladder cancer cells through down-regulation of BMI-1 and E2F3. J Transl Med. 2014;12:305.
38. Tang Y, He Y, Zhang P, Wang J, Fan C, Yang L, et al. LncRNAs regulate the cytoskeleton and related Rho/ROCK signaling in cancer metastasis. Mol Cancer. 2018;17(1):77.

9

A prospective observational study of urinary cytokines and inflammatory response in patients with Overactive Bladder Syndrome

Kiren Gill[1*], Harry Horsley[2], Sheela Swamy[3], Rajvinder Khasriya[1] and James Malone-Lee[4]

Abstract

Background: Contemporary studies have discredited the methods used to exclude urinary tract infection (UTI) when treating overactive bladder (OAB). Thus we must revisit the OAB phenotype to check that UTI has not been overlooked.

Aims: To examine the differences in urinary cytokines IL6 and lactoferrin in OAB patients compared to controls, with references to microscopy of urine and enhanced quantitative urine culture.

Methods: A blinded, prospective cohort study with normal controls using six repeated measures, achieved two-monthly, over 12 months.

Results: The differences between patients and controls in urine IL6 ($F = 49.0$, $p < .001$) and lactoferrin ($F = 228.5$, $p < .001$) were significant and of a magnitude to have clinical implications. These differences were for lactoferrin correlated to symptoms (9.3, $p = .003$); for both to pyuria (IL6 $F = 66.2$, $p < .001$, Lactoferrin $F = 73.9$, $p < .001$); and for IL6 microbial abundance ($F = 5.1$, $p = .024$). The pathological markers had been missed by urinary dipsticks and routine MSU culture.

Conclusion: The OAB phenotype may encompass patients with UTI that is being overlooked because of the failure of standard screening methods.

Background

Overactive bladder syndrome (OAB) is characterized by urinary urgency, with or without urgency urinary incontinence, usually with increased daytime frequency and nocturia, if there is no proven infection or other obvious pathology [1]. The diagnosis is contingent on exclusion of urinary tract infection (UTI), usually achieved by bedside urinary dipstick testing and/or midstream culture analyses using Kass criterion for exclusion of infection [2]. Recently, dipstick and culture testing have been discredited due to poor sensitivity and ambiguous and misleading culture data [3, 4]. This raises the possibility that the OAB may need to be revaluated.

We have published data from fresh urine microscopy [5], routine culture and spun urinary sediment culture [3, 6]. We reported significant differences in the urinary white cell and urothelial cell counts and in the results of spun sediment culture between OAB patients and normal controls, over a period of 12-months. Like others [4, 7], we found that the dipsticks and routine culture failed to discriminate between the OAB patients and normal controls. However, other surrogate markers of infection and inflammation: Spun sediment cultures, microscopic pyuria (WBC), and urinary uroepithelial cell (EPC) counts, revealed significant between group differences [5]. These data suggest that standard screening for UTI in

*Correspondence: kiren.gill1@nhs.net
[1] Women's Health, Whittington Health NHS Trust, Magdala Avenue, London N19 5FN, UK
Full list of author information is available at the end of the article

the assessment of patients with OAB may be misleading when excluding infection.

Given the implications of these findings, we set out to validate our observations by comparing those three surrogate infection markers against the behaviour of two key urinary cytokines namely IL6 and Lactoferrin, in patients with OAB. We have already published on ATP in this context [8]. We chose IL-6 because it is a well-established inflammatory marker, and it has been reported to rise in association with increased bacterial loads in UTI. Lactoferrin acts to sequester iron and thereby deprive offending microbes of vital nutrition. Increases in urinary lactoferrin have been reported in association with UTI.

Aim

To explore the relationship between urinary cytokines and key urinary markers of bacterial cystitis; pyuria [9], and urinary spun sediment culture [10, 11] in women with OAB symptoms comparing them to normal controls, over a period of twelve months.

Methods

We conducted a prospective, blinded, observational cohort study of female outpatients with OAB symptoms, and asymptomatic control subjects. The study groups included patients who described OAB symptoms as defined by the ICS definition [12], including urinary urgency, increased day time frequency, nocturia with or without urge incontinence. Healthy female adults matched for age and menopausal status, with no urinary symptoms were recruited as controls. All participants provided written, informed consent. Women who were pregnant or planning a pregnancy were not eligible for inclusion. We did not include patients with structural disease of the urinary tract and other systemic diseases.

Study participants attended two monthly study visits over a one year. Patients and control subjects provided midstream urine (MSU) samples using the clean-catch method. All samples were subject to analysis by blinded researchers. We assessed the patient's symptoms, urinary cytology, microbiology and urinary immune response. Symptoms were assessed using standardised validated questionnaires including the ICIQ-FLUTS, a pain score and an urgency score [6]. Aliquots of spun urine were frozen at − 80 °C for cytokine analysis. Methods are discussed in detail below.

Symptom collection

Symptoms were collected using validated questionnaires which were self-administered [6, 13].

ICIQ Questionnaires

The International Consultation on Incontinence Questionnaires (ICIQ) was selected to evaluate symptoms [14].

Urgency Score

The symptoms of urinary urgency were measured using a validated ten-item scale, recording the characteristics and the degree of urinary urgency [15, 16].

Pain Score

The pain questionnaire, a validated, eight-item scale which recorded dysaesthesia/pain symptoms associated with the lower urinary tract [17].

Urine analyses

The methods of the assessment of pyuria and the microbiological assessment using the spun urinary sediment culture have been reported [3, 4, 7, 9, 10]. We used unspun fresh urine microscopy to obtain pyuria. Enhanced urinary sediment cultures were performed for quantitative and qualitative microbial analysis [3]. All specimens were subject to urinary dipsticks analysis and routine NHS culture with or without sensitivity where a positive culture was declared if $\geq 10^5$ cfu/ml. of a pure culture of a known urinary pathogen.

Urothelial cytokine response

Fresh urine samples were centrifuged and the supernatant was removed and aliquots frozen at -80 °C. For each cytokine analysis a separate aliquot was used and the urine samples only underwent one freeze / thaw cycle to ensure cytokine stability.

Quantification of Urinary IL-6

The Quantikine® High Sensitivity ELISA Human IL-6 Immunoassay was used to quantify urinary IL-6 (R&D Systems, Abingdon, UK), with a limit of detection of 0.09 pg ml^{-1} with an inter- and intra-assay coefficient of variation of less than 10%. Frozen urine samples underwent only one freeze thaw cycle ensuring stability of IL-6. The urine samples were thawed to room temperature and mixed thoroughly using a vortex mixer (Scientific Industries, New York, USA). Urinary IL-6 was determined using an Opsys MR fluorescence microplate reader (DYNEX Technologies, Worthing, UK). The minimum detectable dose (MDD) of the ELISA kit according to the manufacturers ranges from 0.016 to 0.110 pg ml^{-1}, with an average MDD of 0.039 pg ml^{-1}. All samples were analysed in triplicate to test the inter-assay precision and the mean value was taken. The intra-assay precision for urine assays suggested by the company was 5.5–9.8% and the inter-assay precision for this experiment was 5.5–11.2%.

Quantification of Urinary Lactoferrin

A separate aliquot of the frozen urine sample underwent one freeze thaw cycle to ensure stability of Lactoferrin. The Human Lactoferrin ELISA immunoassay was used to quantify urinary Lactoferrin (ICL, Portland, USA), with a range of detection of 3.125 ng ml^{-1} -100 ng ml^{-1}, with a sensitivity average of 0.725 ng ml^{-1}.

Lactoferrin concentration was determined using an Opsys MR fluorescence microplate reader (DYNEX Technologies, Worthing, UK). The reader produced standard curves, fit to a four-parameter logistics curve, which was used to calculate concentrates for each well. All samples were analyzed in triplicate to test the inter-assay precision and the mean value was taken.

Primary outcome measure

The primary outcome measure was urinary IL-6.

Secondary Outcome measures

The secondary outcome measures included the assessment of urothelial inflammation and immune activation, routine microbiological assessment and lower urinary tract symptoms. We studied the following measures:

1. Microscopic pyuria count
2. Urinary Lactoferrin
3. Qualitative and quantitative poly microbial growth using enhanced sediment cultures demonstrated on CPS3 agar
4. ICIQ-LUTS symptoms score
5. Whittington urgency score
6. Whittington pain score
7. Urine dipstick analysis
8. Routine NHS laboratory MSU culture

Statistical analysis

The primary statistical analysis was to determine the difference in urinary IL-6 in patients compared to controls. The secondary analyses similarly compared urinary lactoferrin and explored the relationship between these cytokines and pyuria, bacterial growth and lower urinary tract symptoms. The primary outcome data were assessed for normality using Q-Q plots, and parametric methods of analysis used as the data were normally distributed. Data from patients and controls were pooled to compare the performance of urine cytokines in relation to pyuria, bacterial growth by enhanced sediment culture and symptoms, in patients and controls. A linear mixed-effects models analysis (SPSS) was used to analyse the data to take into account the repeated measures. Urinary IL-6 and Lactoferrin were designated as the dependent variables, and other measures entered as independent covariates in the model. The categorical data were analysed by contingency tables and the $\chi 2$ test. The analysis was undertaken with the supervision of a statistician familiar with the analysis of multilevel models in SPSS.

Results

Between April 2011 and September 2013, 24 female patients with OAB (mean age = 63; $sd = 11$) and 22 asymptomatic control subjects (mean age 59; sd = 9) were recruited. The groups were matched for age, menopausal status and BMI. There was one drop-out from the patient group and one drop-out from the control group.

The results of the MSU cultures and dipsticks tests are reported in Tables 1 and 2. There were significant differences between the OAB patients and the normal controls in that the OAB patients were more likely to demonstrate a positive test.

The linear mixed-effects models procedure, used to analyse the longitudinal data, explored the relationship between urinary IL-6 / Lactoferrin and urgency score, pain score, LUTS score, pyuria and microbial growth on enhanced sediment culture. In the first model the independent covariate was the group (0 or 1 / control or patient), the dependant variable IL-6 / Lactoferrin and the repeated variables were indexed on visit number.

A second model examined the pooled data from 144 OAB patient visits and 132 control visits.

The dependant variable was log IL-6 / Lactoferrin and the independent covariates were the group number (0/1; controls/patients), urgency score, pain score, LUTS score, log pyuria and log total microbial growth.

There was a significant difference in urinary IL-6 between patients and controls (Table 3) and similar differences were found with Lactoferrin Table 4.

Table 5 shows the results of the mixed model repeated measures analysis applied to IL-6; it can be seen that pyuria count ($\log_{10}$ wbc μl^{-1}) and however total bacterial growth ($\log_{10}$ CFU ml^{-1}) proved a significant predictor of IL-6 however the symptoms scores did not.

Table 1 The results of the MSU cultures achieved over 6 two-monthly assessments

Group	Negative culture	Mixed growth	Positive culture
Normal controls	197 (89.5%)	22 (10.0%)	1 (0.5%)
OAB patients	231 (83.1%)	21 (7.6%)	26 (9.4%)

Chi. squared = 19.38, $df = 2$, $p < .001$

Table 2 The results of the dipsticks tests achieved over 6 two-monthly assessments

Group	Leucocyte negative	Leucocyte positive
Normal controls	206 (91.2%)	20 (8.8%)
OAB patients	172 (61.0%)	110 (39.0%)
Chi.squared = 58.35, *df* = 1, *p* < .001		
Group	**Nitrite negative**	**Nitrite positive**
Normal controls	226 (100.0%)	0 (0.0%)
OAB patients	275 (97.5%)	7 (2.5%)
Chi. squared = 4.008, *df* = 1, *p* = .05		

Table 3 Linear mixed models analysis with IL-6 as the dependant variable

Source	Numerator df	Denominator df	F	Significance
Group	1	247	49.0	$p < .001$

Dependent variable: LogIL6

Table 4 Linear mixed models analysis with Lactoferrin as the dependant variable

Source	Numerator *df*	Denominator *df*	F	Significance
Group	1	255	228.5	$p < .001$

Dependent variable: LogLactoferrin

Table 5 Mixed models analysis with IL-6 as the dependant variable

Dependent variable	Denominator df	F	Significance
LUTS score	205	0.w	$p = .658$
Urgency	233	1.0	$p = .317$
Pain	239	0	$p = .935$
Bacterial growth[§]	237	5.1	$p = .024$
Pyuria count[†]	258	66.2	$p = < .001$

*F is the test statistic: ratio of the variances and increase in magnitude of dependent variable demonstrated by patients compared with control subjects during the study; [§]Bacterial growth: log cfu ml^{-1}; [†]Pyuria count: wbc ul^{-1}

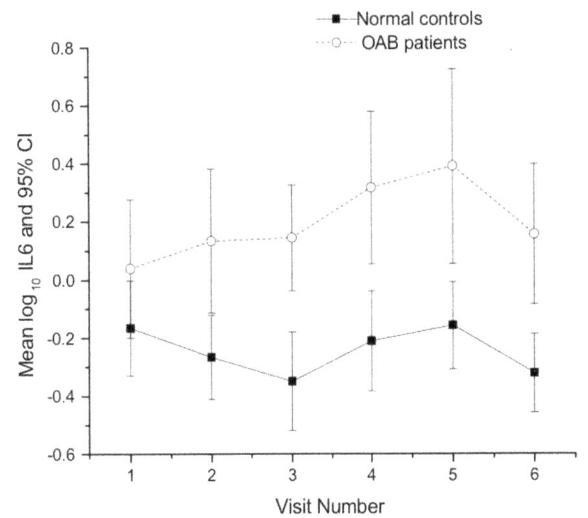

Fig. 1 Mean Log IL-6 in patients and controls at each visit

Mean urinary IL-6 was found to be significantly higher in patients when compared with controls across each visit (Fig. 1).

The linear mixed-effects models procedure was similarly used to explore the relationship between urinary Lactoferrin and urgency score, pain score, LUTS score, pyuria and microbial growth on enhanced sediment culture. In the first model the independent covariate was the group (0 or 1 / control or patient), the dependant variable Lactoferrin, and the repeated variables were indexed on visit number. There was a significant difference in urinary Lactoferrin between patients and controls (Table 4).

Table 6 Mixed models analysis with Lactoferrin as the dependant variable

Dependent variable	Denominator df	F	Significance
LUTS score	200	9.3	$p = .003$
Urgency	232	6.6	$p = .011$
Pain	208	0.2	$p = .622$
Bacterial growth[§]	231	0.1	$p = .793$
Pyuria count[†]	240	73.9	$p = < .001$

*F is the test statistic: ratio of the variances and increase in magnitude of dependent variable demonstrated by patients compared with control subjects during the study; [§]Bacterial growth: log cfu ml^{-1}; [†]Pyuria count: wbc ul^{-1}

A multiple mixed-effects model analysis was performed where the dependant variable was log Lactoferrin and the independent covariates were the group number (0/1), LUTS score, urgency score, pain score, log total microbial growth and log pyuria. Table 6 shows the results for each of these parameters. The predictors of Lactoferrin proved to be the LUTS symptoms, urgency and pyuria

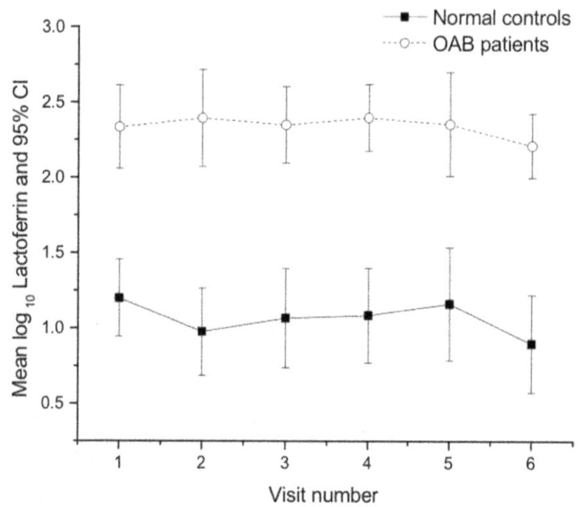

Fig. 2 Mean Log Lactoferrin in patients and controls at each visit

count ($\log_{10}$ wbc μl^{-1}) however total bacterial growth ($\log_{10}$ CFU ml^{-1}) did not.

Mean urinary Lactoferrin was found to be significantly higher in the patient group when compared with controls across each visit (Fig. 2).

Conclusion

This prospective, blinded comparative study addressed the role of inflammation in the urine of patients with overactive bladder symptoms, expressed as an increase in urinary cytokines. We also measured bacterial colonisation, and markers of infection, by pathogens in this group. The data demonstrate evidence of urinary tract inflammation and this was associated with increased evidence of microbial infection in women with OAB syndrome.

These data should be interpreted with caution due to the following limitations. We followed patients over a year whilst they were attending a centre for treatment. We made no attempt to measure the effect of treatment, whether by antimuscarinics or antibiotics; the study did not have that scope. Our purpose was to test for evidence of inflammation, ascertain whether there were any correlations with markers of infection and whether the findings were consistent and persisted over a twelve month period. Treatment effects in similar patients have been studied elsewhere [18, 19] but RCT data are still outstanding. In the context of this study; intervention studies that examine treatment effects on the variables we scrutinised are still necessary. Our measures are indirect markers of inflammation, we did not study the bladder histology or cystoscopic appearances. However, these patients had undergone normal cystoscopy and renal tract ultrasound prior to their diagnosis of OAB. The measures that we used to diagnose UTI -microscopy of fresh unspun urine and sediment culture are well validated. We emphasise that the gold standard criteria for the diagnosis or exclusion of UTI using MSU culture has been shown to be incompetent at this function. Enhanced culture studies and 16 s-rRNA genomics have shown that Kass' key assumption of a sterile normal bladder was incorrect and that his culture methods are overlooking a substantial number of infections [3, 10]. Determining causation is impossible given such a diverse microbiome with extensive overlap between patients and controls [3, 10, 20] thus we are limited to observations of association.

There is a growing body of evidence, from cross-sectional data, that bacterial infection may play a role in LUTS and OAB [6]. In this study, the patient group and controls were matched for age, BMI and menopause status and given the sample size, statistical power was maintained throughout. Inflammatory disease process in OAB patients compared to controls was clearly evident when we compared the microscopic pyuria, urinary IL-6 and Lactoferrin between the two groups. On the other hand urinary dipstick tests and MSU cultures, which are known to be insensitive [3], nevertheless differed between the two study groups. We noted a significant between groups difference in microbial abundance when we used a validated enhanced culture [10].

Urinary IL-6 association with pyuria and microbial growth did not come as a surprise; IL-6 acts as a pro-inflammatory agent attracting white cells into the tissues [21]. Increased urinary IL-6 secretion has been demonstrated in prospective studies of acute UTI [22]. Bacteria will trigger an innate immune response by parasitising uroepithelial cells. Like other mucosal surfaces, the lining of the urinary tract carries receptors capable of recognising invading microbes by binding to receptors to "Pathogen associated molecular patterns" (PAMPS). Of the various of these immune surveillance molecules the Toll-like receptor (TLR) family is the best characterised through studies of bacterial adherence and TLR4 signalling. In vivo studies, of a bacterial challenge to urothelial cells, have shown a rapid cytokine response with production of interleukin-1beta (IL-1beta), IL-6, and IL-8 (CXCL8). Type 1-fimbriated E. coli were found to activate IL-6 and IL-8 production more efficiently than the non-fimbriated[23]. IL-6 has been detected in the urine of a majority of patients with positive cultures, but it was only detected in the serum of symptomatic patients [24]. It has been argued that the cytokine response during UTI could have local and systemic components; epithelial cells are thought to be responsible for the local cytokine reaction [25]. Studies have shown that IL-6 production increases neutrophil migration and activation of IL8 [26, 27]. Uroepithelial cells also respond, not just to bacteria, but they can be stimulated by cytokines: IL-1alpha and TNFalpha induce secretion, by urothelial cells of IL-6 and IL-8 and the upregulation of mRNAs for IL-1alpha, IL-1beta, IL-6 and IL-8 [28]. There is a complex regulation of the production of IL-6 by membrane-bound and soluble receptors, which are modulated by numerous influences. Strains of *Escherichia coli* (*E.coli*) have developed strategies to evade immune response by suppressing cytokine reactions to infection [29].The studies discussed in this section have addressed acute UTI and its influence on urinary IL-6 secretion [22]; Our study takes a further step by implying a role for IL-6 in chronic disease.

Our data showed that urinary Lactoferrin was associated with pyuria and symptoms. Lactoferrin's primary role is to sequester free iron, so it inconveniences bacteria by removing a substrate essential for bacterial growth [30]. Lactoferrin has other antimicrobial properties, a key one is by binding to the lipopolysaccharide (LPS) of the bacterial wall and then generating peroxides; these oxidise membrane molecules causing bacterial lysis [30]. Lactoferrin will stimulate phagocytes. It has been reported to interfere with proton translocation through the cell membrane, disrupting microbial chemistry and neutralising cell attachment capacity [31, 32]. Specifically, Lactoferrin interacts with membrane-LPS *E. coli*, removing LPS from the membrane [33]. The susceptibility of the bacteria to Lactoferrin is thought to be dependent on their growth phase since bacteria are more open to killing by Lactoferrin when in early phase [32]. Lactoferrin has also been shown to modulate the activity of known antibacterial agents such as lysozymes and antibiotics [34]. It is thought that the dominant mechanism of action is via its iron binding properties and interaction with LPS on Gram-negative bacteria [35].

The data from this study were collected by application of a blinded, prospective, comparative protocol. The analysis of various measures that reflect different perspectives is called consilience and it strengthens the validity of the observations because of their coherence. This work has demonstrated strong evidence of inflammation of the urothelium associated with OAB and there is good evidence that infection is playing a significant part. For many years UTI has been excluded in OAB patients by deploying tests that are insensitive. Our data present a compelling case for us to re-evaluate our understanding of OAB, detrusor instability and detrusor hyperreflexia.

Acknowledgements

The authors would like to acknowledge and thank all the participates in the study.

Authors' contributions

KG and JML wrote the main manuscript. KG, HH, SS, RK and JML all contributed to data collection and processing, prepared figures and All authors read and approved the final manuscript.

Author details

[1] Women's Health, Whittington Health NHS Trust, Magdala Avenue, London N19 5FN, UK. [2] Bladder Infection and Immunity Group (BIIG), Department of Renal Medicine, Division of Medicine, University College London, Royal Free Hospital Campus, Rowland Hill Street, London NW3 2PF, UK. [3] Women's Health, St Thomas' Hospital, Westminster Bridge Road, London SE1 7EH, UK. [4] Bladder Infection and Immunity Group (BIIG), Department of Renal Medicine, Division of Medicine, University College London, 10 Harley Street, London W1G 9PF, UK.

References

1. Drake MJ. Do we need a new definition of the overactive bladder syndrome? ICI-RS 2013. Neurourol Urodyn. 2014;33(5):622–4.
2. Kass EH. Bacteriuria and the diagnosis of infection in the urinary tract. ArchInternMed. 1957;100:709–14.
3. Sathiananthamoorthy S, Malone-Lee J, Gill K, Tymon A, Nguyen TK, Gurung S, et al. Reassessment of routine midstream culture in diagnosis of urinary tract infection. J Clin Microbiol. 2019;57(3):e01452.
4. Kupelian AS, Horsley H, Khasriya R, Amussah RT, Badiani R, Courtney AM, et al. Discrediting microscopic pyuria and leucocyte esterase as diagnostic surrogates for infection in patients with lower urinary tract symptoms: results from a clinical and laboratory evaluation. Bju Int. 2013;112(2):231–8.
5. Gill K, Kang R, Sathiananthamoorthy S, Khasriya R, Malone-Lee J. A blinded observational cohort study of the microbiological ecology associated with pyuria and overactive bladder symptoms. Int Urogynecol J. 2018;29:1493.
6. Khasriya R, Barcella W, De Iorio M, Swamy S, Gill K, Kupelian A, et al. Lower urinary tract symptoms that predict microscopic pyuria. Int Urogynecol J. 2017;5:359.
7. Khasriya R, Khan S, Lunawat R, Bishara S, Bignal J, Malone-Lee M, et al. The inadequacy of urinary dipstick and microscopy as surrogate markers of urinary tract infection in urological outpatients with lower urinary tract symptoms without acute frequency and dysuria. JUrol. 2010;183(5):1843–7.
8. Gill K, Horsley H, Kupelian AS, Baio G, De Iorio M, Sathiananamoorthy S, et al. Urinary ATP as an indicator of infection and inflammation of the urinary tract in patients with lower urinary tract symptoms. BMC Urol. 2015;15:7.
9. Horsley H, Malone-Lee J, Holland D, Tuz M, Hibbert A, Kelsey M, et al. Enterococcus faecalis subverts and invades the host urothelium in patients with chronic urinary tract infection. PLoS ONE. 2013;8(12):e83637.
10. Khasriya R, Sathiananthamoorthy S, Ismail S, Kelsey M, Wilson M, Rohn JL, et al. Spectrum of bacterial colonization associated with urothelial cells from patients with chronic lower urinary tract symptoms. J Clin Microbiol. 2013;51(7):2054–62.
11. Sathiananthamoorthy S, Malone-Lee J, Gill K, Tymon A, Nguyen TK, Gurung S, et al. Reassessment of routine midstream culture in diagnosis of urinary tract infection. J Clin Microbiol. 2018;57:e01452.
12. Abrams P, Cardozo L, Fall M, Griffiths D, Rosier P, Ulmsten U, et al. The standardisation of terminology in lower urinary tract function: report from the standardisation sub-committee of the International Continence Society. Urology. 2003;61(1):37–49.
13. Abrams P, Avery K, Gardener N, Donovan J. The International Consultation on Incontinence Modular Questionnaire: www.iciq.net. J Urol. 2006;175(3 Pt 1):1063–6.
14. Abrams P, Andersson KE, Buccafusco JJ, Chapple C, de Groat WC, Fryer AD, et al. Muscarinic receptors: their distribution and function in body systems, and the implications for treating overactive bladder. BrJ Pharmacol. 2006;148(5):565–78.
15. Al-Buheissi SZ, Malone-Lee J. A simple well validated method for measuring urinary urgency. BJU Int. 2007;99:25.

16. Malone-Lee JG, Al-Buheissi S. Does urodynamic verification of overactive bladder determine treatment success? Results from a randomized placebo-controlled study. BJUInt. 2009;103(7):931–7.
17. Chaliha C A-BS, Khasriya R, Khan S, Lunawat R, Bishara S, Malone-Lee J. Characterising the phenotype of the painful bladder syndrome in patients presenting with lower urinary tract symptoms. International Urogynaecological Assocation Annual Meeting; Como Italy: Springer; 2009. p. 458.
18. Swamy S, Kupelian AS, Khasriya R, Dharmasena D, Toteva H, Dehpour T, et al. Cross-over data supporting long-term antibiotic treatment in patients with painful lower urinary tract symptoms, pyuria and negative urinalysis. Int Urogynecol J. 2018;30:409–14.
19. Swamy S, Barcella W, De Iorio M, Gill K, Khasriya R, Kupelian AS, et al. Recalcitrant chronic bladder pain and recurrent cystitis but negative urinalysis: What should we do? Int Urogynecol J. 2018;29:1035–44.
20. Wolfe AJ, Toh E, Shibata N, Rong R, Kenton K, Fitzgerald M, et al. Evidence of uncultivated bacteria in the adult female bladder. J Clin Microbiol. 2012;50(4):1376–83.
21. Wood MW, Breitschwerdt EB, Gookin JL. Autocrine effects of interleukin-6 mediate acute-phase proinflammatory and tissue-reparative transcriptional responses of canine bladder mucosa. Infect Immun. 2011;79(2):708–15.
22. Czaja CA, Stamm WE, Stapleton AE, Roberts PL, Hawn TR, Scholes D, et al. Prospective cohort study of microbial and inflammatory events immediately preceding Escherichia coli recurrent urinary tract infection in women. JInfectDis. 2009;200(4):528–36.
23. Samuelsson P, Hang L, Wullt B, Irjala H, Svanborg C. Toll-like receptor 4 expression and cytokine responses in the human urinary tract mucosa. InfectImmun. 2004;72(6):3179–86.
24. Hedges S, Anderson P, Lidin-Janson G, de Man P, Svanborg C. Interleukin-6 response to deliberate colonization of the human urinary tract with gram-negative bacteria. Infect Immun. 1991;59(1):421–7.
25. Agace W, Hedges S, Andersson U, Andersson J, Ceska M, Svanborg C. Selective cytokine production by epithelial cells following exposure to *Escherichia coli*. InfectImmun. 1993;61(2):602–9.
26. Sadik CD, Kim ND, Luster AD. Neutrophils cascading their way to inflammation. Trends Immunol. 2011;32(10):452–60.
27. Mihara M, Hashizume M, Yoshida H, Suzuki M, Shiina M. IL-6/IL-6 receptor system and its role in physiological and pathological conditions. Clin Sci (Lond). 2012;122(4):143–59.
28. Hedges S, Agace W, Svensson M, Sjogren AC, Ceska M, Svanborg C. Uroepithelial cells are part of a mucosal cytokine network. InfectImmun. 1994;62(6):2315–21.
29. Hunstad DA, Justice SS. Intracellular lifestyles and immune evasion strategies of uropathogenic Escherichia coli. AnnuRevMicrobiol. 2010;64:203–21.
30. Farnaud S, Evans RW. Lactoferrin–a multifunctional protein with antimicrobial properties. Mol Immunol. 2003;40(7):395–405.
31. Andrés MT, Fierro JF. Antimicrobial mechanism of action of transferrins: selective inhibition of H+-ATPase. Antimicrob Agents Chemother. 2010;54(10):4335–42.
32. Bortner CA, Arnold RR, Miller RD. Bactericidal effect of lactoferrin on Legionella pneumophila: effect of the physiological state of the organism. Can J Microbiol. 1989;35(11):1048–51.
33. Appelmelk BJ, An YQ, Geerts M, Thijs BG, de Boer HA, MacLaren DM, et al. Lactoferrin is a lipid A-binding protein. Infect Immun. 1994;62(6):2628–32.
34. Ellison RT 3rd, Giehl TJ. Killing of gram-negative bacteria by lactoferrin and lysozyme. J Clin Investig. 1991;88(4):1080–91.
35. Odell EW, Sarra R, Foxworthy M, Chapple DS, Evans RW. Antibacterial activity of peptides homologous to a loop region in human lactoferrin. FEBS Lett. 1996;382(1–2):175–8.

10

Clustering of patients with overactive bladder syndrome

James Gross[1], Joel M. Vetter[1] and H. Henry Lai[1,2*]

Abstract

Background: Overactive bladder is a heterogenous condition with poorly characterized clinical phenotypes. To discover potential patient subtypes in patients with overactive bladder (OAB), we used consensus clustering of their urinary symptoms and other non-urologic factors.

Methods: Clinical variables included in the k-means consensus clustering included OAB symptoms, urinary incontinence, anxiety, depression, psychological stress, somatic symptom burden, reported childhood traumatic exposure, and bladder pain.

Results: 48 OAB patients seeking care of their symptoms were included. k-means consensus clustering identified two clusters of OAB patients: a urinary cluster and a systemic cluster. The systemic cluster, which consisted of about half of the cohort (48%), was characterized by significantly higher psychosocial burden of anxiety (HADS-A, 9.5 vs. 3.7, $p<0.001$), depression (HADS-D, 6.9 vs. 3.6, $p<0.001$), psychological stress (PSS, 21.4 vs. 12.9, $p<0.001$), somatic symptom burden (PSPS-Q, 28.0 vs. 7.5, $p<0.001$), and reported exposure to traumatic stress as a child (CTES, 17.0 vs. 5.4, $p<0.001$), compared to the urinary cluster. The systemic cluster also reported more intense bladder pain (3.3 vs. 0.8, $p=0.002$), more widespread distribution of pain (34.8% vs. 4.0%, $p=0.009$). The systemic cluster had worse urinary incontinence (ICIQ-UI, 14.0 vs. 10.7, $p=0.028$) and quality of life (SF-36, 43.7 vs. 74.6, $p<0.001$). The two clusters were indistinguishable by their urgency symptoms (ICIQ-OAB, OAB-q, IUSS, 0–10 ratings). The two OAB clusters were different from patients with IC/BPS (worse urgency incontinence and less pain).

Conclusions: The OAB population is heterogeneous and symptom-based clustering has identified two clusters of OAB patients (a systemic cluster vs. a bladder cluster). Understanding the pathophysiology of OAB subtypes may facilitate treatments.

Keywords: Overactive bladder, Clustering, Phenotyping

Background

Overactive bladder (OAB) affects 1 in 6 adults in the United States and has an economic cost of $24.9 billion [1, 2]. Despite the enormous burden and negative impact on quality of life, our understanding of the underlying pathophysiology is poor. Treatment outcomes remain suboptimal overall. Most patients do not continue their medications one year after the prescription [3], and many patients are "refractory" to OAB treatments.

Recent research suggested that non-urologic factors such as anxiety, depression, psychological stress, somatic symptom burden, non-urologic pain, and increased hypersensitivity related to central sensitization might contribute to the symptomatology of OAB and other lower urinary tract symptoms (LUTS) [4–10]. This observation raises the possibility that the OAB population is heterogeneous and may be further sub-categorized based

*Correspondence: laih@wudosis.wustl.edu

[1] Division of Urologic Surgery, Department of Surgery, Washington University School of Medicine, 4960 Children's Place, Campus, Box 8242, St Louis, MO 63110, USA

Full list of author information is available at the end of the article

on their non-urologic factors in addition to their urinary symptoms.

Consensus clustering provides a means to discover patient subtypes in patient population with heterogeneous presentation. Unlike traditional comparative approach, clustering algorithms use empirical statistical methods to discover subtypes based on intrinsic patterns within the data without making any a priori assumption or preconceived notion on how the classification scheme should be constructed. This unbiased, data driven approach may provide novel insights and more precise classification of patient subtypes. To our knowledge, consensus clustering has not been reported for OAB patients. In this study, we incorporated patients' urinary symptoms and non-urologic factors into consensus clustering to identify potential patient subtypes within OAB.

Materials and methods

OAB participants

Male and female patients with OAB seen between October 2012 and July 2014 were approached to participate in this research study. The case definition of OAB was consistent with the 2002 International Continence Society terminology [11]. Specifically, OAB patients must have complaints of urinary urgency, with or without urgency urinary incontinence, usually with frequency and nocturia, in the absence of other causes. Exclusion criteria included: history of prostate surgery, incontinence surgery, urethral stricture, neurogenic bladder, urinary retention, pelvic radiation, cyclophosphamide cystitis, tuberculosis cystitis, urologic cancer, urinary stones, positive urine culture in the past 6 weeks, or residual volume $\geq$ 150 mL. The study was approved by Washington University Institutional Review Board. All participants signed an informed consent.

Assessment

Urinary symptoms, psychosocial symptoms, bladder pain, systemic pain, and quality of life were assessed using validated questionnaires.

OAB symptoms were assessed using the International Consultation on Incontinence—Overactive Bladder (ICIQ-OAB) [12] and OAB-q short form [13]. Urgency symptoms were assessed using the Indevus Urgency Severity Scale (IUSS) [14] and on a 0–10 numeric rating scale of urgency. Urinary incontinence symptoms were assessed using International Consultation on Incontinence—Urinary Incontinence short form (ICIQ-UI) [15] and Incontinence Impact Questionnaire Short Form (IIQ-7) [16].

The following psychosocial symptoms were assessed: (1) anxiety (Hospital Anxiety and Depression Scale, HADS) [17], (2) depression (HADS) [17], (3) psychological stress (Perceived Stress Scale, PSS) [18], (4) somatic symptom burden (Poly-Symptomatic, Poly-Syndromic Questionnaire, PSPS-Q) [19], and (5) reported exposure to various childhood trauma (Childhood Traumatic Events Scale, CTES) [20].

Intensity of bladder pain was assessed using a 0–10 numeric rating scale. Intensity of non-urologic pain was assessed using the Brief Pain Inventory (BPI) [21]. The distribution of pain was assessed using a whole body map as previously described [22]. Those reporting pain in 3 or more broader body regions outside the pelvis (left or right upper extremity, left or right lower extremity, head and neck, chest, lower back) were classified as having "widespread pain" [22].

Condition-specific quality of life was assessed using the OAB-q QOL subscale (OAB-q-HRQOL) [13]. Global quality of life was assessed using the SF-36.

Clustering analysis

Variables entering k-means consensus clustering included urinary incontinence (ICIQ-UI), OAB symptoms (ICIQ-OAB), anxiety (HADS), depression (HADS), psychological stress (PSS), somatic symptom burden (PSPS-Q), reported exposure to childhood trauma (CTES), and bladder pain (0–10). K-means uses Euclidean distance to group participants into clusters, while assigning observations to clusters in order to minimize the distance between observations and the mean or center of the cluster, or the total intra-cluster variation [23, 24]. The optimal number of clusters was estimated using the elbow method and compared to a number of different techniques for determining number of clusters using the *NbClust* package within the R statistical software to validate the choice [25]. We performed one-way ANOVA and chi-square tests for continuous and categorical variables respectively to test for differences between clusters. $p < 0.05$ was considered significant. All statistical analyses utilized the open source statistical package R v3.3.1.

Comparing the discovered oab clusters to interstitial cystitis/bladder pain syndrome

Since one of the identified OAB clusters had pain and psychosocial symptoms (see results below), in order to verify that our OAB population was distinct from interstitial cystitis/ bladder pain syndrome (IC/BPS), we compared the bladder pain and urinary incontinence scores of our two identified OAB clusters to an IC/BPS cohort that was previously described [26]. IC/BPS patients were required to have an unpleasant sensation (pain, pressure, discomfort) perceived to be related to the bladder, associated with lower urinary tract symptoms of more than 6 weeks duration, in the absence of infection or other identifiable causes, in accordance with the 2011 AUA Guideline [27]. The distinction between OAB and IC/BPS was based on the two published AUA Guidelines [27, 28], chief complaint, and overall clinical impression, taken into the account of their clinical evaluation and management (e.g., antimuscarinics for OAB, tricyclics for IC/BPS). Additionally, we assessed the likely diagnosis of the OAB patients by applying a previously described independent nomogram, which has a 94% accuracy for classifying or distinguishing patients as likely OAB versus likely IC/BPS based on GUPI, ICSI, and OAB-q [29]. Due to missing data, the Urge Incontinence Composite Index was based on only questions four and eight of the OAB-q.

Results

48 OAB patients (13 men, 35 women) had complete data for consensus clustering. Their characteristics are presented in Table 1. k-means clustering identified two OAB clusters: a urinary cluster and systemic cluster. The two clusters are illustrated in selected scatter plots in Fig. 1 (+ = systemic cluster, o = urinary) Comparisons between the two clusters are shown in Table 1.

There was a near equal percent split between the two clusters (52% urinary, 48% systemic). There were no age and sex differences between the two clusters.

The systemic cluster was characterized by significantly higher psychosocial burden of anxiety (HADS-A, 9.5 vs. 3.7, $p<0.001$), depression (HADS-D, 6.9 vs. 3.6, $p<0.001$), psychological stress (PSS, 21.4 vs. 12.9, $p<0.001$), somatic symptom burden (PSPS-Q, 28.0 vs. 7.5, $p<0.001$), and reported exposure to traumatic stress as a child (CTES, 17.0 vs. 5.4, $p<0.001$), compared to the urinary cluster. The systemic cluster also reported more intense bladder pain (3.3 vs. 0.8 on a 0–10 scale, $p=0.002$), more intense non-urologic pain (BPI, 3.1 vs. 1.7, $p=0.021$), and more widespread distribution of pain (34.8% vs. 4.0%, $p=0.009$). The systemic cluster had worse urinary incontinence (ICIQ-UI, 14.0 vs. 10.7, $p=0.028$), condition-specific quality of life (OAB-q-HRQOL, 56.0 vs. 40.3, $p=0.045$), and global quality of life (SF-36, 43.7 vs. 74.6, $p<0.001$). The two clusters were indistinguishable by their urgency symptoms (no differences in ICIQ-OAB, OAB-q, IUSS, and 0–10 urgency ratings, p all > 0.05).

Table 1 Comparisons between the two OAB clusters, mean ± SD

	Urinary cluster (n = 25, 52%)	Systemic cluster (n = 23, 48%)	p-value
Demographics			
Age (mean ± SD)	53.8 ± 13.9	54.2 ± 10.0	0.84
No. of females	16	19	0.20
Urinary symptoms: (mean ± SD)			
Urinary incontinence (ICIQ-UI, 0–21)^	10.7 ± 5.1	14.0 ± 4.1	0.028*
Incontinence impact (IIQ-7, 0–28)	6.5 ± 7.4	11.7 ± 8.6	0.027*
Overactive bladder (ICIQ-OAB, 0–16)^	8.8 ± 2.7	9.9 ± 2.6	0.20
Overactive bladder symptom severity (OAB-q SS, 6–36)	58.5 ± 20.0	69.3 ± 22.4	0.11
Psychosocial			
Anxiety (HADS-A, 0–21)^	5.5 ± 4.1	9.5 ± 3.7	< 0.001*
Depression (HADS-D, 0–21)^	3.7 ± 3.5	6.9 ± 3.6	< 0.001*
Psychological stress (PSS, 0–40)^	12.9 ± 6.4	21.4 ± 7.0	< 0.001*
Somatic symptom burden (PSPS-Q, 0–59)^	7.5 ± 6.6	28.0 ± 7.6	< 0.001*
Childhood traumatic exposure (CTES, 0–42)^	5.4 ± 6.0	17.0 ± 11.6	< 0.001*
Death in family	2.1 ± 2.8	3.7 ± 3.2	0.070
Parental upheaval	0.8 ± 1.8	2.7 ± 3.2	0.021*
Sexual trauma	0.6 ± 1.9	3.1 ± 3.2	0.004*
Victim of violence	0.6 ± 1.9	2.5 ± 3.2	0.017*
Major illness	0.2 ± 0.8	2.4 ± 2.9	0.001*
Other trauma	1.2 ± 2.4	2.6 ± 3.0	0.055
Quality of life			
Condition specific (OAB-q-HRQOL, 0–100, higher is worse)	40.3 ± 22.6	56.0 ± 26.9	0.045*
Global QOL (SF-36, 0–100, lower is worse)	74.6 ± 17.8	43.7 ± 18.4	< 0.001*

*$p<0.05$. ^ identifies variables that are used in the clustering algorithm

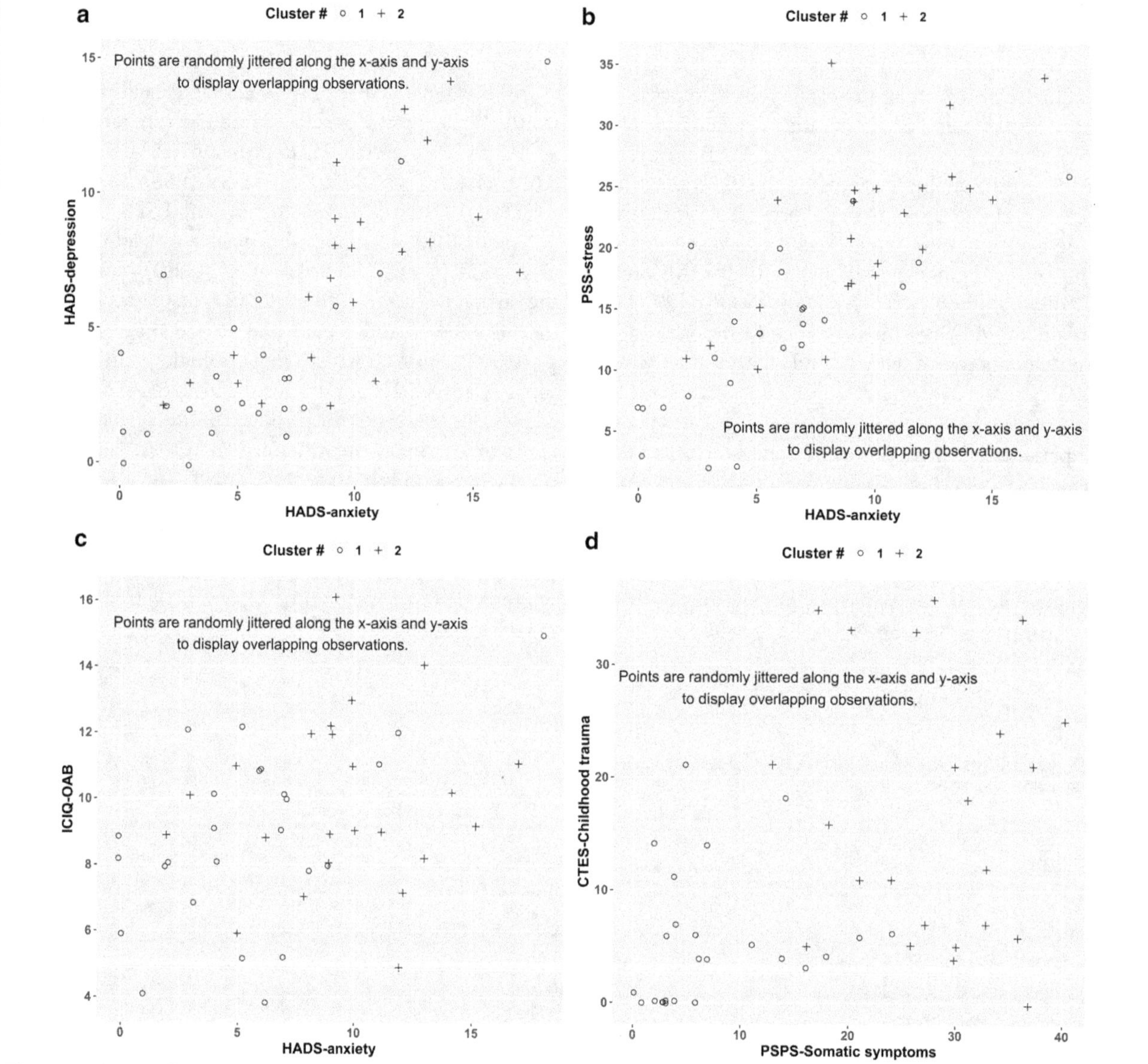

Fig. 1 Distribution of urinary and psychosocial measures. o = urinary cluster, + = systemic cluster

There were strong correlations between anxiety, depression, and stress across the two clusters (r = 0.78–0.62, see Table 2). This is illustrated in Fig. 1A, B. Correlations between psychosocial and urinary measures were weaker (r = 0.42 to 0.09, Fig. 1C). A combination of high somatic symptom burden and high childhood traumatic scores (blue dots in top right corner of Fig. 1D) appeared to separate the systemic cluster from the urinary cluster which has both low somatic symptom and low childhood traumatic scores (red dots in the bottom left corner).

We compared the bladder pain and urinary incontinence scores of our two identified OAB clusters to a known IC/BPS cohort to verify that our OAB population was not an IC/BPS population that was misclassified as patients with OAB. Results showed that the systemic cluster had significantly less bladder pain (3.3 vs. 6.6, $p < 0.001$) and more urinary incontinence (ICIQ-UI, 14.0 vs. 6.6, $p < 0.001$) compared to IC/BPS patients (Table 3). Additionally, we found that 46 of the 48 patients within our clinically diagnosed OAB cohort, which includes both the urinary and systemic cluster patients, were classified as likely OAB using the nomogram described by Ackerman et al. [29]. The additional 2 patients had insufficient data to use the nomogram.

Table 2 Correlation coefficients between urinary and psychosocial measures

	HADS-D (depression)	HADS-A	PSS	PSPS-Q	CTES	SHCU Q2	ICIQ-UI
ICIQ-OAB (overactive bladder)	0.30	0.37	0.24	0.17	0.11	− 0.09	0.43
ICIQ-UI (urinary incontinence)	0.39	0.42	0.40	0.40	0.09	0.16	
SHCU Q2 (bladder pain)	0.23	0.18	0.32	0.45	0.39		
CTES (childhood traumatic exposure scale)	0.07	0.16	0.20	0.44			
PSPS-Q (somatic symptom burden)	0.38	0.41	0.54				
PSS (stress)	0.62	0.78					
HADS-A (anxiety)	0.77						

Table 3 Comparisons of the two identified clusters to IC/BPS

	Urinary cluster (n = 25)	Systemic cluster (n = 23)	IC/BPS comparison group (n = 27)	p-value, urinary OAB versus IC/BPS	p-value, systemic OAB versus IC/BPS
Age (mean ± SD)	53.8 ± 13.9	54.2 ± 10.0	44.8 ± 16.6	0.036*	0.028*
No. of females	16	19	27	< 0.001*	0.038*
Bladder pain (0–10)	0.8 ± 1.7	3.3 ± 3.0	6.6 ± 2.1	< 0.001*	< 0.001*
Urinary incontinence (ICIQ-UI, 0–21)	10.7 ± 5.1	14.0 ± 4.1	6.6 ± 5.1	0.012*	< 0.001*

*p < 0.05

Discussion

We identified two subtypes of OAB patients using symptom-based consensus clustering: a urinary cluster and a systemic cluster. The systemic cluster, which consisted of about half of the cohort, was characterized by significantly higher psychosocial burden of anxiety, depression, psychological stress, somatic symptom burden, and reported exposure to traumatic stress as a child, compared to the urinary cluster. The systemic cluster also reported more intense bladder pain, more widespread distribution of pain, worse urinary incontinence, and poorer quality of life.

We believe that the systemic cluster was not simply an IC/BPS population mimicking OAB. Even though the systemic cluster had higher pain and psychosocial symptoms compared to the urinary cluster, the systemic cluster had significantly less bladder pain and more urinary incontinence compared to IC/BPS. Furthermore, the patients in both clusters were classified as OAB using a previously described independent nomogram, which had a diagnostic accuracy of 94% in their validation cohort [29]. These findings make it unlikely that patients in the systemic cluster had IC/BPS, which further supports this previously unrecognized cluster as a subtype of OAB.

Many of the differences between the two clusters were not only statistically different, but likely were clinically significant. The anxiety, stress, somatic symptom, and childhood trauma scores in the systemic cluster were 73%, 66%, 270% and 220% higher respectively than those in the urinary cluster. The systemic cluster had bladder pain in the mild pain category (mean 3.3 on a 0–10 scale) vs. minimal pain (mean 0.8) in urinary cluster. The systemic cluster was 7.7 times more likely to report widespread pain.

Even with different questionnaires (ICIQ-OAB, OAB-q, IUSS, and 0–10 urgency ratings), patients in our two identified clusters had indistinguishable urgency symptoms. This indicates that those patients belonging to the group with more systemic difficulties would be hard to distinguish from their counterparts in a setting where patients with OAB are only evaluated in regard to their syndrome defining urinary symptoms. Additional instruments (e.g., HADS and a body map) are needed to distinguish between these two groups in a clinical setting.

The identification of a systemic cluster in OAB is new. It appears that a subset of OAB patients (the systemic cluster) may not be "just" an OAB patient with "only" bladder symptoms. The finding of increased psychosocial burden and non-zero pain in OAB was relatively new in the literature. In a study comparing OAB and IC/BPS patients, 33% of OAB patients reported pain or discomfort associated with bladder filling [26]. A subset of OAB patients also reported urogenital pain and widespread pain [30]. The presence of pelvic pain was associated with worse psychosocial health [30]. High anxiety, depression, psychological stress, and somatic symptom burden were also associated with more severe urinary incontinence, and poorer quality of life [4–7, 10]. Our consensus clustering results have grouped these patients into a distinct systemic cluster. Notice that there were strong correlations among the various psychosocial measures, suggesting that individuals high in one psychosocial construct (e.g., anxiety) were more likely to have other psychosocial measures (e.g., depression, stress, see Fig. 1A, B).

Consideration of non-urologic factors such as psychological and pain profiles might be important in clinical phenotyping of OAB. Our results highlighted that the OAB population is heterogeneous and there may be different subtypes of OAB (a systemic cluster vs. urinary cluster). It is unclear whether the two identified clusters might have different underlying pathophysiology. Conceptually it is possible that the systemic cluster might have "top-down" or systemic mechanisms such as central sensitization, systemic inflammation, or psychosocial trauma. Central sensitization has recently been demonstrated in some OAB patients by Reynolds et al. [8, 9]. In future studies it is important to study the differences in pathophysiology among the OAB subtypes.

At this time, it is unclear what the therapeutic implications are in terms of treatments. We do not know whether there will be differential responses to OAB treatments between the two identified clusters. We hypothesize that the systemic cluster might be less responsive to traditional OAB treatments while those in the urinary cluster might respond more favorably. Theoretically one might consider the systemic cluster to be out of boundary of bladder-centric treatments and therefore might be less responsive or non-responsive to traditional treatments of OAB that focus on the bladder (e.g., oral antimuscarinics, beta-agonist, botox injection, pelvic floor therapy). This systemic cluster may explain why some OAB patients were "refractory" to traditional treatments of OAB. It may also explain why OAB as a whole can be difficult to treat effectively because it is a heterogeneous condition with many subtypes that are poorly understood.

Reynolds et al. have shown that patients requiring third line treatment for OAB ("refractory" patients) demonstrated higher rates of central sensitization when compared to patients who were first presenting for OAB treatment (treatment naïve) [9]. This observation lends credence to our hypothesis. It also supports the validity of this systemic cluster as a subgroup of patients within OAB that can be identified using clinical measures and potentially treated more effectively with different therapies than their counterparts in the urinary cluster. A larger cohort with longer term treatment data is necessary to investigate this hypothesis.

Further research is needed to validate the two identified OAB clusters, and to further assess whether or not the clusters identified here would respond differentially to OAB treatments. At this time we are not ready to advocate the use of additional questionnaires in clinical practice to assess non-urologic features in OAB patients. We need more research to assess the additional value of evaluating OAB patients with respect to their systemic profiles.

The limitations of this study are inherent to the use of clustering algorithms and the subjective nature of patient reported symptoms. The characteristics included in the model will impact how the patients can be grouped optimally. While these limitations exist, previous work supports the presence of an OAB subtype that fits the characteristics of our systemic cluster and suggests the potential for improvement in treatment algorithms if these subtypes could be identified in clinical practice. Another limitation is the small sample size. Future work should focus on establishing the reproducibility of these clusters in a larger data set, establishing the thresholds for membership between these clusters, assessing if there are treatment response differences between them, and examining their differences in pathophysiology. Moving clinical phenotyping research beyond symptom-based classification by incorporating other mechanistic data (e.g., biomarkers, functional MRI) in the future is also important.

Conclusions

The OAB population is heterogeneous and symptom-based clustering has identified two clusters of OAB patients (a systemic cluster vs. a urinary cluster). Understanding the pathophysiology of OAB subtypes may facilitate treatments.

Abbreviations

OAB: Overactive bladder; IC/BPS: Interstitial cystitis/bladder pain syndrome; ICIQ-UI: International consultation on incontinence—urinary Incontinence short form; IIQ-7: Incontinence impact questionnaire short form; ICIQ-OAB: International consultation on incontinence—overactive bladder; IUSS: Indevus urgency severity scale; HADS: Hospital anxiety and depression scale; PSS: Perceived stress scale; PSPS-Q: Poly-symptomatic, poly-syndromic questionnaire; CTES: Childhood traumatic events scale; BPI: Brief pain inventory; OAB-q-HRQOL: OAB-q QOL subscale.

Acknowledgements

We would like to thank all the subjects who participated in the study, Aleksandra Klim for recruiting the subjects, and Alethea Paradis for data management.

Authors' contributions

JG interpreted the analyzed data and drafted the main manuscript text. JV analyzed the patient data and prepared Fig. 1. HHL designed this study, acquired the patient data, interpreted the analyzed patient data, and drafted the main manuscript text. All authors read, provided revisions for, and approved the final manuscript.

Author details

[1] Division of Urologic Surgery, Department of Surgery, Washington University School of Medicine, 4960 Children's Place, Campus, Box 8242, St Louis, MO 63110, USA. [2] Department of Anesthesiology, Washington University School of Medicine, St Louis, MO, USA.

References

1. Onukwugha E, Zuckerman IH, McNally D, et al. The total economic burden of overactive bladder in the United States: a disease-specific approach. Am J Manag Care. 2009;15:S90–7.
2. Stewart WF, Van Rooyen JB, Cundiff GW, et al. Prevalence and burden of overactive bladder in the United States. World J Urol. 2003;20:327–36.
3. Chapple CR, Nazir J, Hakimi Z, et al. Persistence and adherence with mirabegron versus antimuscarinic agents in patients with overactive bladder: a retrospective observational study in UK clinical practice. Eur Urol. 2017;72:389–99.
4. Lai H, Gardner V, Vetter J, et al. Correlation between psychological stress levels and the severity of overactive bladder symptoms. BMC Urol. 2015;15:14.
5. Lai HH, Rawal A, Shen B, et al. The relationship between anxiety and overactive bladder or urinary incontinence symptoms in the clinical population. Urology. 2016;98:50–7.
6. Lai HH, Shen B, Rawal A, et al. The relationship between depression and overactive bladder/urinary incontinence symptoms in the clinical OAB population. BMC Urol. 2016;16:60.
7. Lai HH, Vetter J, Jain S, et al. Systemic nonurological symptoms in patients with overactive bladder. J Urol. 2016;196:467–72.
8. Reynolds WS, Brown ET, Danford J, et al. Temporal summation to thermal stimuli is elevated in women with overactive bladder syndrome. Neurourol Urodyn. 2017;36:1108–12.
9. Reynolds WS, Kowalik C, Cohn J, et al. Women undergoing third line overactive bladder treatment demonstrate elevated thermal temporal summation. J Urol. 2018;200:856–61.
10. Siddiqui NY, Wiseman JB, Cella D, et al. Mental health, sleep and physical function in treatment seeking women with urinary incontinence. J Urol. 2018;200:848–55.
11. Abrams P, Cardozo L, Fall M, et al. The standardisation of terminology of lower urinary tract function: report from the standardisation sub-committee of the international continence society. Neurourol Urodyn. 2002;21:167–78.
12. Jackson S, Donovan J, Brookes S, et al. The Bristol Female Lower Urinary Tract Symptoms questionnaire: development and psychometric testing. Br J Urol. 1996;77:805–12.
13. Coyne K, Revicki D, Hunt T, et al. Psychometric validation of an overactive bladder symptom and health-related quality of life questionnaire: the OAB-q. Qual Life Res. 2002;11:563–74.
14. Nixon A, Colman S, Sabounjian L, et al. A validated patient reported measure of urinary urgency severity in overactive bladder for use in clinical trials. J Urol. 2005;174:604–7.
15. Avery K, Donovan J, Peters TJ, et al. ICIQ: a brief and robust measure for evaluating the symptoms and impact of urinary incontinence. Neurourol Urodyn. 2004;23:322–30.
16. Uebersax JS, Wyman JF, Shumaker SA, et al. Short forms to assess life quality and symptom distress for urinary incontinence in women: the Incontinence Impact Questionnaire and the Urogenital Distress Inventory. Continence Program for Women Research Group. Neurourol Urodyn. 1995;14:131–9.
17. Zigmond AS, Snaith RP. The hospital anxiety and depression scale. Acta Psychiatr Scand. 1983;67:361–70.
18. Cohen S, Williamson G. Perceived stress in a probability sample of the United States. In: Spacapan S, Oskamp S, editors. The social psychology of health: Claremont symposium on applied social psychology. Newbury Parl: Sage; 1988. p. 31–67.
19. Lai HH, North CS, Andriole GL, et al. Polysymptomatic, polysyndromic presentation of patients with urological chronic pelvic pain syndrome. J Urol. 2012;187:2106–12.
20. Pennebaker JW, Susman JR. Disclosure of traumas and psychosomatic processes. Soc Sci Med. 1988;26:327–32.
21. Cleeland C. The brief pain inventory: user guide. Houston: MD Anderson Center; 2008.
22. Lai HH, Jemielita T, Sutcliffe S, et al. Characterization of whole body pain in urological chronic pelvic pain syndrome at baseline: a MAPP research network study. J Urol. 2017;198:622–31.
23. McLachlan G. Cluster analysis and related techniques in medical research. Stat Methods Med Res. 1992;1:27–48.
24. MacQueen J. Some methods for classification and analysis of multivariate observations. In: Proceedings of the 10th Berkeley symposium on mathematical statistics and probability. Berkeley: University of California Press; 1967, p. 281–297
25. Charrad M, Ghazzali N, Boiteau V, et al. NbClust: An R package for determining the relevant number of clusters in a data set. J Stat Softw. 2014;61:1–36.
26. Lai HH, Vetter J, Jain S, et al. The overlap and distinction of self-reported symptoms between interstitial cystitis/bladder pain syndrome and overactive bladder: a questionnaire based analysis. J Urol. 2014;192:1679–85.
27. Hanno PM, Burks DA, Clemens JQ, et al. AUA guideline for the diagnosis and treatment of interstitial cystitis/bladder pain syndrome. J Urol. 2011;185:2162–70.
28. Gormley EA, Lightner DJ, Burgio KL, et al. Diagnosis and treatment of overactive bladder (non-neurogenic) in adults: AUA/SUFU guideline. J Urol. 2012;188:2455–63.
29. Ackerman AL, Lai HH, Parameshwar PS, et al. Symptomatic overlap in overactive bladder and interstitial cystitis/bladder pain syndrome: development of a new algorithm. BJU Int. 2019;123:682–93.
30. Thu JHL, Vetter J, Lai HH. The severity and distribution of nonurologic pain and urogenital pain in overactive bladder are intermediate between interstitial cystitis and controls. Urology. 2019;130:59–64.

11

Unusual glomus tumor of the bladder: A rare case report and literature review

Li Chen[1], Bin Lai[2], Xiaoyan Su[3] and Jiwei Wang[1*]

Abstract

Background: Glomus tumor (GT), which are neoplasms of the glomus body, usually occur in the extremities, particularly under the nail bed. GT occurring in the bladder is very rare and has been reported as sporadic. In the present study, a rare case of bladder GT is reported and its clinical and histopathological characteristics are summarized by literature review.

Case presentation: A 57-year-old woman presented with intermittent gross hematuria for 2 years. Urinalysis displayed hematuria. The bladder ultrasound showed an avascular and homogeneous isoechoic polypoid mass with a maximum diameter of 6 mm at the right lateral wall of bladder. The bladder endoscopic examination showed a polypoid lesion, with a smooth surface, located in the right lateral wall. Then, a transurethral resection was performed, its histopathological features indicated a benign GT.

Conclusions: GT arising in the bladder is extremely rare, and only four cases have been identified in studies reported in English. It is difficult to diagnose bladder GTs according to their clinical features. The gold standard method used for their diagnosis is histopathology. However, it should also be considered in the differential diagnosis for bladder mass.

Keywords: Glomus tumor, Bladder, Urinary tract

Introduction

Glomus tumor (GT) is a mesenchymal neoplasm, composed of a mixture of glomus cells, blood vessels and smooth muscle cells arising from the glomus body. GT can occur in almost any part of the body, but it is most commonly seen in the extremities, particularly in the nail bed [1]. GT occurring in the bladder is very rare and has been reported sporadically. To the best of our knowledge, only 4 cases of bladder GT have been previously identified in studies reported in English [2–5]. The present study aimed to (1) present an extremely rare case of GT in the bladder and (2) summarize its clinical and histopathologic features by literature review.

*Correspondence: wangjiwei167@163.com
[1] Department of Ultrasound, The Second Affiliated Hospital of Nanchang University, Nanchang 330006, Jiangxi, China
Full list of author information is available at the end of the article

Case presentation

A 57-year-old woman presented with intermittent gross hematuria for 2 years. She did not report any other symptoms. Physical examination indicated no abnormal findings. Blood cell counts and biochemical tests were within the reference range. Urinalysis displayed hematuria. Therefore, it was suggested that she should undergo a urinary system ultrasound examination. The kidney and ureter ultrasounds indicated no abnormal findings, whereas the bladder ultrasound revealed an avascular and homogeneous isoechoic polypoid mass with a maximum diameter of 6 mm at the right lateral wall of the bladder (Fig. 1). She has no bladder tumors history or family history. So, the bladder of the patient was examined endoscopically and a polypoid lesion (6 mm in maximum diameter) was noted with a smooth surface, located in the right lateral wall (Fig. 2). Subsequently, a transurethral resection (TUR) was performed and the lesion was easily removed. Microscopic

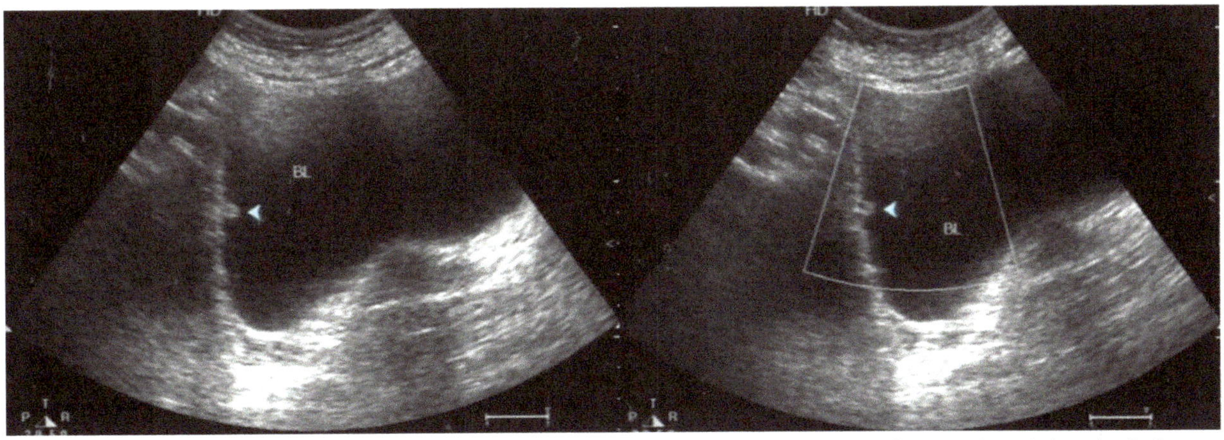

Fig. 1 Bladder ultrasound indicated a homogeneous isoechoic polypoid mass with a maximum diameter of 6 mm at the right lateral wall of bladder

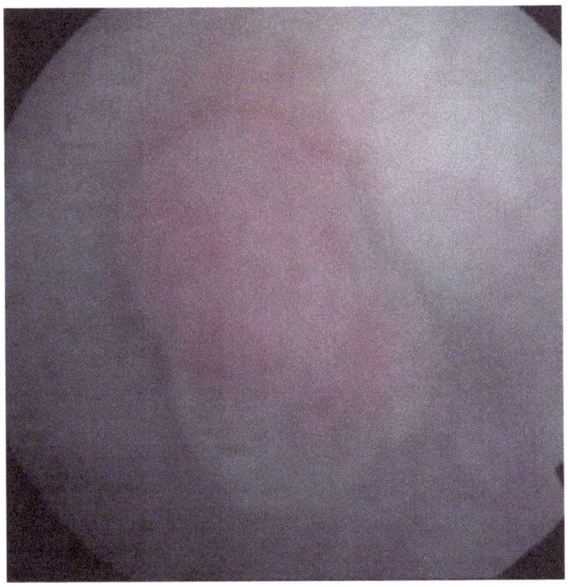

Fig. 2 Cystoscopy examination revealed a polypoid lesion with a smooth surface, located in the right lateral wall of bladder

examination indicated that the neoplasm was well circumscribed and composed of nests of monomorphic cells with bland nuclei and eosinophilic cytoplasm, clustered around dilated vessels. Atypia, mitoses, intravascular growth and necrosis were absent (Fig. 3). Immunohistochemical staining revealed that the neoplastic cells reacted positively to the smooth muscle actin (SMA) and vimentin, whereas they were negative to desmin (Fig. 4). A diagnosis of benign bladder GT was made. The patient remained asymptomatic and no recurrence was observed within a 2-year follow up.

Discussion and conclusions

GT, which are neoplasms of the glomus body, usually occur in the extremities, particularly under the nail bed. Localizations other than the extremities have been reported in various systems including the respiratory (e.g. nose, trachea, lung) [6–8] the digestive (e.g. larynx, esophagus, stomach, intestine, liver) [9–13], the reproductive (e.g. uterine cervix, ovary, testis) [14–16], the urinary (e.g. kidney, bladder, urethra) [2–5, 17, 18], the endocrine (e.g. thyroid, breast) [19, 20], the nervous (e.g.

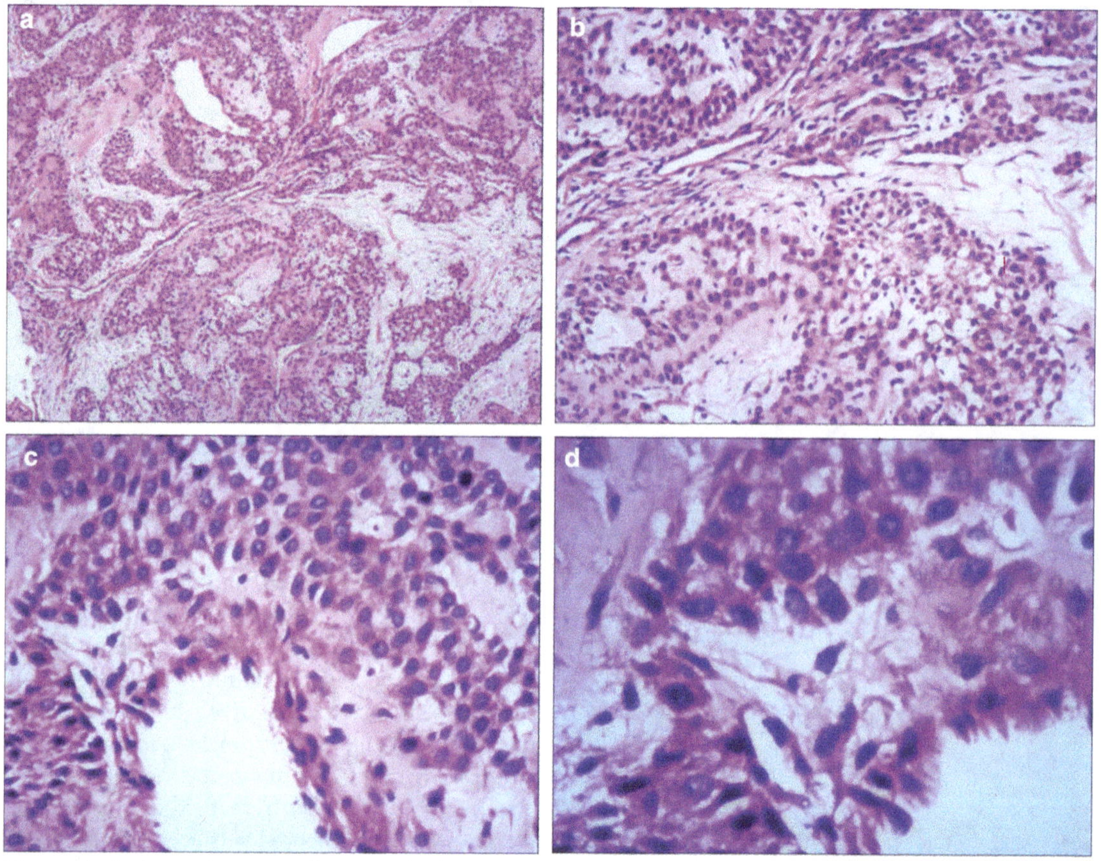

Fig. 3 Microscopically, the neoplasm was well circumscribed and composed of nests of monomorphic cells with bland nuclei and eosinophilic cytoplasm, clustered around dilated vessels (hematoxylin-eosin, original magnifications ×25 (**a**), ×100 (**b**), ×200 (**c**), and ×400 (**d**))

sciatic nerve) [21] and the cardiovascular (e.g. heart, carotid artery) [22, 23]. However, these are uncommon.

GT occurring in the bladder is very rare and has been reported as sporadic. To the best of our knowledge, only 4 cases of human bladder GT have been identified in the literature, indicating that the current case is the fifth. The clinical data of these five patients are presented in Table 1 and the histopathological data in Table 2. After reviewing of the clinical features of these patients, the following conclusions were made: (1) Bladder GT can occur in males (M) and females (F), no significant gender difference was evident; (2) Bladder GT mostly occurred in elderly subjects, with an age range from 56 to 84 years; (3) Bladder GT patients presented with hematuria or were asymptomatic; (4) Bladder GT patients usually exhibited no history of bladder tumor; (5) The size and location of bladder GT were flexible (the size ranged from 3 to 65 mm and the location could be anterior, lateral, or posterolateral wall); (6) Although the majority of GTs are benign, the bladder GTs were described in the present and previous studies were not always benign (2/5 cases were benign, 2/5 cases were atypical and 1/5 case

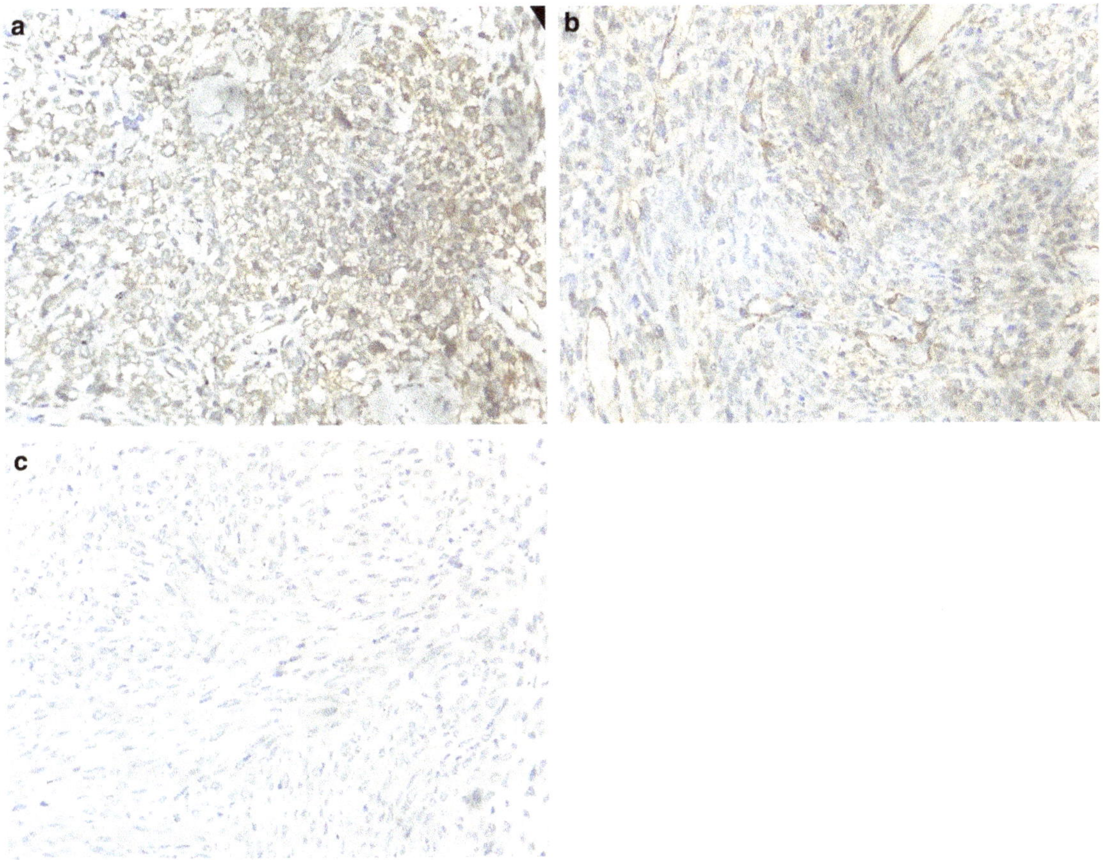

Fig. 4 Immunohistochemistry demonstrated that neoplastic cells exhibited positive reactivity to vimentin (**a**) and smooth muscle actin (**b**) and negative to desmin (**c**). (original magnifications ×200)

was malignant); (7) Transurethral resection is the most common treatment used for benign or atypical bladder GT, whereas for malignant bladder GT, comprehensive treatment could be performed according to patient condition. Although these findings are meaningful, no specific clinical feature was noted. The pathological and immunohistochemical examination are the standard methods used in the diagnosis of bladder GT.

GT is composed of a mixture of glomus cells, blood vessels and smooth muscle cells. GT is usually benign and rarely malignant or atypical. The criteria of malignancy GT are the following: (1) tumor with a deep location, (2) a size more than 2 cm, (3) atypical mitotic figures or apparent nuclear atypia, (4) 5 or more mitotic figures/50 high-power field [24]. The atypical GT was defined as a tumor with a high-grade nuclear pleomorphism in the absence of any other malignant features, such as large size, deep location, infiltrative growth, mitotic activity, or necrosis. The majority of the GTs are benign, whereas this not commonly noted for bladder GT. According to the present literature review, more than half of the patients with bladder GT were malignant or atypical cases.

In conclusion, GT arising in the bladder is extremely rare, and only four cases have been identified in studies reported in English. It is difficult to diagnose bladder GTs according to their clinical features. The gold standard method used for their diagnosis is histopathology. However, it should also be considered in the differential diagnosis for bladder mass.

Table 1 Clinical data from previous cases and the present case of glomus tumor in the bladder

Case no	Authors and reference	Age (yr.)	Sex	Cause of clinic visiting	Bladder tumor history	First-detected technique	Tumor size (mm)	Tumor location	Biochemistry and hematologic test	Diagnosis	Treatment	Follow-up/ clinical result
1	Shim HS, et al[4]	57	F	Gross hematuria	No	Magnetic resonance imaging	65	Left lateral wall	N/A	Malignant GT	TUR + chemotherapy	2 months/Died
2	Tripodi SA, et al[3]	63	M	Gross hematuria	No	Cystoscopy	12	Anterior wall	Within the reference range	Benign GT	TUR	1 year/Free
3	Lindsay LW, et al[5]	84	F	Incidental finding	low grade superficial urothelial carcinoma	Cystoscopy	3	Right posterolateral wall	N/A	Atypical GT	TUR	N/A
4	Palmisano F, et al[2]	58	M	Incidental finding	No	Computed tomography	25	Anterior wall	Within the reference range	Atypical GT	Robot- assisted Partial Cystectomy	7 months/Free
5	Jiwei W, et al. (present case)	56	F	Gross hematuria	No	Ultrasound	6	Right lateral wall	Within the reference range	Benign GT	TUR	1 year/Free

F, female; M, male; N/A, not mentioned in literature; GT, glomus tumor; TUR, transurethral resection

Table 2 Pathological data from previous cases and the present case of glomus tumor in the bladder

Case No	Authors and reference	Pathologic features	Immunohistochemically stains	
			Positive	**Negative**
1	Shim et al[4]	A large number of tumor cells had infiltrated into the subepithelial connective tissues and proper muscles, which were primarily perivascular in distribution. The cells showed diffuse cytologic atypia with spindle morphology and marked nuclear atypia with high mitotic activity (50/10HPF); Multifocal tumor necrosis and hemorrhage were also noted	SMA	Cytokeratins, Epithelial membrane antigen, S100 protein, Desmin, CD31, CD34
2	Tripodi et al[3]	The neoplasm was well circumscribed and composed of nests of monomorphic cells with bland nuclei and eosinophilic cytoplasm. Atypia, mitoses, intravascular growth, and necrosis were absent	SMA, CD34	p63, Cytokeratin AE1/AE3
3	Lindsay et al[5]	Abnormal proliferation of ovoid cells in the lamina propria, uniform ovoid nuclei with indistinct eosinophilic cytoplasm, sheet-like growth pattern with a prominent capillary network, mild nuclear atypia and mototic index accounted to 2 mitosis/HPF	SMA, Smooth muscle myosin	CD 34
4	Palmisano et al[2]	The neoplasm was composed of uniform small oval to spindle cells, without nuclear atypias, disposed in a vaguely storiform pattern, separated by a vascular stroma; numerous cells with bizarre nuclei were scattered throughout the lesion; mototic index accounted to 2 mitosis/50HPF	SMA, Vimentin, bcl-2	Citokeratins, p63, Desmin, Calponin, CD34, S100, HMB-45, CD68R, c-kit, DOG-1, ALK-1, Chromogranin, a-Inhibin
5	Jiwei et al. (present case)	The tumor cells were uniform small oval and clustered around dilated vessels. Atypia, mitoses, intravascular growth, and necrosis were absent	SMA, Vimentin	Desmin

HPF, high power fields; SMA, Smooth muscle actin

Abbreviations

GT: Glomus tumor; TUR: Transurethral resection; HPF: High power fields; SMA: Smooth muscle actin; F: Female; M: Male; N/A: Not mentioned or available.

Acknowledgements

Not applicable.

Authors' contributions

LC first discovered the bladder mass by ultrasound and wrote the manuscript. BL conceptualized the case report. XS diagnosed the case by histopathology. JW revised and edited the manuscript. All authors read and approved the final manuscript.

Author details

[1]Department of Ultrasound, The Second Affiliated Hospital of Nanchang University, Nanchang 330006, Jiangxi, China. [2]Department of Gastrointestinal Surgery, The Second Affiliated Hospital of Nanchang University, No1 Mingde Road, Nanchang 330006, Jiangxi, China. [3]Department of Pathology, The Second Affiliated Hospital of Nanchang University, Nanchang 330006, Jiangxi, China.

References

1. Vieira, F. G., Nakamura, R., Costa, F. M., Canella, C., & Marchiori, E. (2016). Subungual glomus tumor. J Clin Rheumatol 22(6), 331.
2. Palmisano F, Gadda F, Spinelli MG, et al. Symplastic glomus tumor of the urinary bladder treated by robot-assisted partial cystectomy: a case report and literature review. Urologia. 2018;85(3):130–2.
3. Tripodi SA, Rocca BJ, Mourmouras V, et al. Benign glomus tumor of the urinary bladder. Arch Pathol Lab Med. 2013;137(7):1005–8.
4. Shim HS, Choi YD, Cho NH. Malignant glomus tumor of the urinary bladder. Arch Pathol Lab Med. 2005;129(7):940–2.
5. Waters LL, Zhai QH, Buie JS, et al. Atypical glomus tumor of uncertain malignant potential in the urinary bladder. Pathol Lab Med Int. 2010;10(2):141–4.
6. Meguro S, Kusama Y, Matsushima S, et al. Nasal glomus tumor: A rare nasal tumor with diffuse and strongly positive synaptophysin expression. Pathol Int. 2019;69(11):672–4.
7. Wang C, Ma Y, Zhao X, et al. Glomus tumors of the trachea: 2 case reports and a review of the literature. J Thorac Dis. 2017;9(9):E815–26.
8. Wan PZ, Han Q, Wang EH, et al. Glomus tumor of uncertain malignant potential of the lung: a case report and review of literature. Int J Clin Exp Pathol. 2015;8(11):15402–6.
9. Aslam N, Qazi ZU, Ahmad AH, et al. Malignant glomus tumour of larynx: first case report and literature review. J Laryngol Otol. 2012;126(7):743–6.
10. Segura S, Mansoor S, Gorelick AB, et al. Glomus tumor of the esophagus: a case report and review of the literature. Conn Med. 2015;79(2):93–5.
11. Masouminia M, Ghani HA, Foote D, et al. Rare presentation of the glomus tumor in the stomach. Exp Mol Pathol. 2018;104(1):9–11.
12. Campana JP, Goransky J, Mullen EG, et al. Intestinal benign glomus tumor: description and review of the literature. Dig Dis Sci. 2014;59(10):2594–6.
13. Aversa JG, Monroe C, Levi A, et al. The first malignant primary hepatic glomus tumor: a case report. Int J Surg Case Rep. 2020;11(70):197–200.
14. Aynardi JT, Kim SH, Barroeta JE. Epithelioid glomus tumor of the uterine cervix: a case report and review. Int J Gynecol Pathol. 2016;35(3):275–8.
15. Maeda D, Takazawa Y, Oda K, et al. Glomus tumor of the ovary: a case report. Int J Surg Pathol. 2010;18(6):557–60.
16. Tullie STE, Quraishi MK, Karawita T, et al. Rare presentation of a testicular glomus tumour. BMJ Case Rep. 2019;12(11):e230935.
17. Chen YA, Li HN, Wang RC, et al. Malignant glomus tumor of the kidney: a case report and review of the literature. Clin Genitourin Cancer. 2017;15(1):e151–3.
18. Ramsay S, Chan G, Zimmerman WB, Chee J. Glomus tumour of the male urethra: an unusual diagnostic. BMJ. 2019;12(11):e232261.
19. Liu Y, Wu R, Yu T, et al. Malignant glomus tumor of the thyroid gland: a case report. J Int Med Res. 2019;47(6):2723–7.
20. Mizutani L, Tanaka Y, Kondo Y, et al. Glomus tumor of a female breast: a case report and review of the literature. J Med Ultrason. 2014;41(3):385–8.
21. Nwankwo BO, Henshaw RM, Kumar D. Glomus tumor of the sciatic nerve: an extraspinal cause of sciatica. Orthopedics. 2018;41(1):e151–3.
22. Elkrinawi R, Usta E, Baumbach H, et al. Late recurrence of a cardiac glomus tumor. Thorac Cardiovasc Surg. 2012;60(4):305–6.
23. Satis S, Tuna M, Alparslan N. Jarcho-Levin syndrome and concomitant carotid glomus tumor: first reported case. World Neurosurg. 2019;132:236–8.
24. Gill J, Van Vliet C. Infiltrating glomus tumor of uncertain malignant potential arising in the kidney. Hum Pathol. 2010;41(1):145–9.

12

Evaluation of hTERT, KRT7, and survivin in urine for noninvasive detection of bladder cancer using real-time PCR

Reza Yahyazadeh[1], Davood Bashash[2], Parisa Ghaffari[3], Saeid Kord[3], Ava Safaroghli-Azar[2] and Seyed H. Ghaffari[3*]

Abstract

Background: Transitional cell carcinoma (TCC) of the bladder is the second most common genitourinary malignancy. Because of the low sensitivity of urinary cytology and the invasiveness and expense of frequent cystoscopies for the detection of low-grade superficial lesions, we aim to establish a sensitive molecular approach to detect bladder cancer noninvasively.

Methods: Voided urine samples were collected from 80 patients with bladder cancer at the time of diagnosis, in addition to 30 patients with non-bladder cancer urological diseases and 20 healthy volunteers. The level of hTERT, KRT7, and survivin (SVV) mRNAs were analyzed using a qRT-PCR assay.

Results: The optimal threshold values for hTERT, KRT7, and SVV in urine were calculated by ROC curves analysis. The overall sensitivity was 81.3%, 91.3%, and 68.8% for hTERT, KRT7, and SVV, respectively, which were significantly higher than urine cytology (22.2%, $p < 0.001$). A higher positive ratio was obtained using multi-marker detection in comparison to single marker detection. The combined use of markers increased the sensitivity of cytology from 22.2 to 100%. In contrast with the urine cytology method, the sensitivity of these biomarkers was not correlated with the grades and stages of the bladder tumors.

Conclusions: Our data indicate that urinary hTERT, KRT7, and SVV have superior sensitivities over cytology. The combined use of these markers offers a powerful potential assay and promising tool for a sensitive, noninvasive, and highly specific diagnostic method and follow-up of low-grade TCC of the bladder.

Keywords: Bladder cancer, Transitional cell carcinoma, hTERT, KRT7, Survivin, Urine cytology, Real-time PCR

Background

Transitional cell carcinoma (TCC) of the bladder is the second most common malignancy of the genitourinary tract and the third most common cause of death among people with genitourinary tumors [1]. TCC responds well to local resection and subsequent adjuvant intravesical treatment [2]. Nevertheless, the recurrence rate of TCC is 50–70%. While 10% of pTa and 30% of pT1 tumors progress to muscle-invasive disease, a majority (80%) of the cases present with non-muscle-invasive papillary tumors (stages pTa or pT1), which have a much more satisfactory prognosis [3].

The heterogeneous characteristics, diverse genetic architecture coupled with different clinical manifestations put unresolvable obstacles in the way of successful diagnosis of bladder cancer [4]. From the first description of bladder cancer, the silent clinical manifestation of the disease, especially in low-grade stages, was one of the main challenges that physicians

*Correspondence: shghaffari200@yahoo.com; shghaffari@tums.ac.ir
[3] Hematology, Oncology and Stem Cell Transplantation Research Center, School of Medicine, Shariati Hospital, Tehran University of Medical Sciences, Tehran, Iran
Full list of author information is available at the end of the article

confronted [5]. Of note, the longer the diagnosis is delayed, the greater the risk of metastasis, which in turn would alter non-lethal cancer to a life-threatening malignancy [6, 7]. This unique feature highlights the importance of applying accurate as well as effective strategies to diagnose bladder cancer, not only rapidly but also with acceptable sensitivity. As the list of the proposed techniques for the detection of this malignancy is continually growing, interest in applying more accurate and affordable methods has increased overwhelmingly. Apart from cystoscopy and urine cytology, which are the gold standard techniques for the diagnosis of this cancer [8], recent molecular investigations have declared the rewarding impact of mRNA expression analysis not only in the detection but also in the follow-up of patients with bladder cancer [9–11]. Attention in recruiting this method has emerged from recent disclosures indicating the remarkable results in both its sensitivity and specificity, which matters especially in low-grade patients [12]. Besides its accuracy, an appealing advantage to this technique is the possibility of examination of the urine specimen, which categorizes it as a non-invasive approach [12]. By opening a valuable avenue for bladder cancer detection, identifying a group of genes that can be exploited for better diagnosis is still a debatable issue. Wide varieties of genes with different functions have been suggested to evaluate urine samples of bladder cancer patients [13–15]. However, some of these genes lost their importance in clinical investigations due to their lack of sensitivity or correlation with the stage of the disease.

There is a pressing need for a non-invasive method to diagnose carcinoma of the urinary bladder. Invasive cystoscopy examination remains the gold standard; nonetheless, it is required not only for the diagnosis but also for the repeated 3-month follow-up intervals. This is due to the fact that no currently available method is adequately sensitive and specific [16]. A method that could replace cystoscopies or at least reduce their number in given situations as well as adhering to greater accuracy than cytology would be highly commended by both patients and clinicians. Therefore, identification of urinary biomarkers for the detection of bladder cancer recurrence would be beneficial to minimize the frequency of cystoscopy.

In the present study, we aim to establish a noninvasive sensitive molecular approach for the detection of bladder cancer. We sought to evaluate the diagnostic potential of measuring three molecular markers (hTERT, SVV, and Keratin7 mRNAs) in the voided urine samples from patients with primary bladder carcinomas.

Methods

Patients and samples collection

Eighty patients diagnosed with bladder cancer, who were admitted to the Urology Department, of Shariati Hospital, were included in this study after giving informed consent. The diagnoses were made via cystoscopy and histopathology. The standard evaluations included urine analyses, blood chemistries, and radiological assessments. Any patients who had undergone any previous treatments were excluded from this study. A group of 30 patients suffering from hematuria due to non-neoplastic causes was used as a control (urinary tract infections, stones, benign prostate hyperplasia, and combined disorders). A group of 10 healthy volunteers was also included in this study. All subjects except 10 healthy volunteers, underwent cystoscopy as a reference standard for the detection of bladder cancer, and all tumors or suspicious lesions were resected for histopathological examination. The final diagnosis of bladder cancer was based on a histological examination. Tumor staging and grading were determined according to the TNM and World Health Organization classification [17]. Voided urine was obtained from the patients before they received any treatment and before they underwent surgery. Approximately 40 ml of morning voided urine samples were collected from the patients and the samples were tested for urine cytology in addition to the detection of mRNA for the biomarker genes via quantitative Real-time RT-PCR (qRT-PCR).

RNA isolation and cDNA synthesis

The urine samples were centrifuged and the pellet cells were washed twice with PBS. Next, RNA extraction was carried out using the FastPure RNA kit (Takara Bio, Inc., Otsu, Japan). About 1 μg of total RNA was subjected to reverse transcription using the PrimeScript RT reagent kit (Takara Bio) according to the manufacturer's instructions.

Quantitative real-time PCR

Quantitative real-time RT-PCR was performed on a light cycler instrument (Roche, Germany) using SYBR Premix Ex Taq technology (Takara Bio). PCR was conducted in a 20 μl reaction mixture including; 10 μl of SYBR Green master mix, 2 μl of cDNA samples, 0.5 μl of forward and reverse primers (10 pmol) in water plus 7 μl of nuclease-free water (Qiagen, Hilden, Germany). Thermal cycling conditions involved an initial activation step for the 30 s at 95 °C, followed by 45 cycles including a denaturation step for 5 s at 95 °C and a combined annealing/extension step for 20 s at 60 °C. Melting curve analysis was applied to validate whether all the primers yielded a single PCR product.

The target gene expression levels were normalized to the hypoxanthine phosphoribosyl transferase1 (HPRT1) levels in the same reaction. Relative expression levels of the target genes within a sample was calculated using the $2^{-\Delta\Delta Cq}$ formula, $\Delta\Delta C_q = (C_{q\ Target} - C_{q\ HPRT1})$ experimental sample $-$ $(C_{q\ Target} - C_{q\ HPRT1})$ control samples, where Cq is the quantification cycle. The fold expression relative to the average calibrator ΔC_q value (20 samples from healthy individuals and 20 samples from patients with urological disorders other than bladder cancer) was normalized to a reference gene (*HPRT1*). Samples were classified as positive for a particular gene if the $2^{-\Delta\Delta Cq}$ was above the cut-off point. The validity of qPCR products was confirmed by gel electrophoresis and sequencing of the representative qPCR reactions (data not shown). The sequences of the gene-specific primers are summarized in Table 1.

Statistical analysis

Nonparametric receiver operating characteristic analysis (ROC), an area under the curve (AUC), sensitivity, specificity, as well as likelihood ratios were calculated to determine the levels of hTERT, SVV, and KRT7 biomarkers that best differentiate the bladder cancer cases from the control subjects. The optimal cut-off values were calculated as the marker level that maximized the sensitivity and specificity. The likelihood ratio was calculated based on the following formula: LR+ = sensitivity/1 − specificity. To evaluate the performance of the biomarkers in the voided urine samples from bladder cancer patients, we computed the sensitivity, specificity, positive predictive value (PPV), negative predictive value (NPV), and the accuracy for cytology, hTERT, KRT7, and SVV when tested independently or in combinations in the urine samples. The comparison of the clinicopathological factors was analyzed using the Student's t test, chi-square tests, and ANOVA. All the performed statistical tests were two-sided and the *P*-values of < 0.05 were considered to be of statistical significance. The statistical analyses were performed using the Statistical Package for the Social Sciences (SPSS 21, Chicago, IL).

Table 1 Nucleotide sequences of primers used for real-time RT-PCR

Gene	Forward primer (5′–3′)	Reverse primer (5′–3′)
hTERT	TGACACCTCACCTCACCCAC	CACTGTCTTCCGCAAGTTCAC
SVV	CCAGATGACGACCCCATAGAG	TTGTTGGTTTCCTTTGCAATTTT
KRT7	TGTGGATGCTGCCTACATGAGC	CAATCTCCTGCTTGGTGTTGCG
HPRT1	TGGACAGGACTGAACGTCTTG	CCAGCAGGTCAGCAAAGAATTTA

Results

Patients

Of the 80 patients with bladder cancer enrolled in this study, there were 20 females and 60 males, with a median age of 63 years (age range 31–81 years). From 20 patients with urological disorders other than bladder cancer and 10 healthy volunteers, there were 10 females and 30 males with a median age of 58 years (range 28–70 years). According to the pathological report of surgical specimens, the tumor was low-grade in 60 (75%) and high-grade in 20 (25%) patients. The stage of cancer was Ta in 50 (62.5%), T1 in 17 (21.25%), T2 in 7 (8.75%), and T3 in 6 (7.5%). Voided urine cytology was positive in 25 (31.3%) and negative in 56 (70.0%) (Table 2).

Overall sensitivity, specificity, PPV, and NPV

The biomarkers gene expression levels in the urine samples were determined using a relative quantification method. To quantify the relative level of mRNA in urine samples, the C_q values of all samples were normalized to

Table 2 Clinicopathologic characteristics of bladder cancer (80 patients)

Characteristics	No. pts
Sex	
Male	60 (75%)
Female	20 (25%)
Age; median (range), years	63 (31–81)
Grade	
Low	60 (75%)
High	20 (25%)
Stage	
Ta	50 (62.5%)
T1	17 (21.25%)
T2	7 (8.75%)
T3	6 (7.5%)
Cytology	
Pos	25 (31.3%)
Neg	56 (70.0%)
hTERT	
Pos	65 (81.2%)
Neg	15 (18.8%)
KRT7	
Pos	73 (91.3%)
Neg	7 (8.8%)
SVV	
Pos	58 (72.5%)
Neg	22 (27.5%)

the Ct value of HPRT1 transcripts. Then, fold changes were calculated relative to the average Cq value from the control groups, including 30 urine samples from patients suffering from hematuria due to non-neoplastic causes and 10 urine samples from healthy individuals. As shown in Fig. 1, the median mRNA levels of hTERT, KRT7, SVV were significantly higher in the malignant group when compared with the normal control groups ($p < 0.001$). Hematuria did not affect the level of markers in patients with no bladder cancer.

In an attempt to evaluate the ability of molecular discrimination between positive and negative results, we

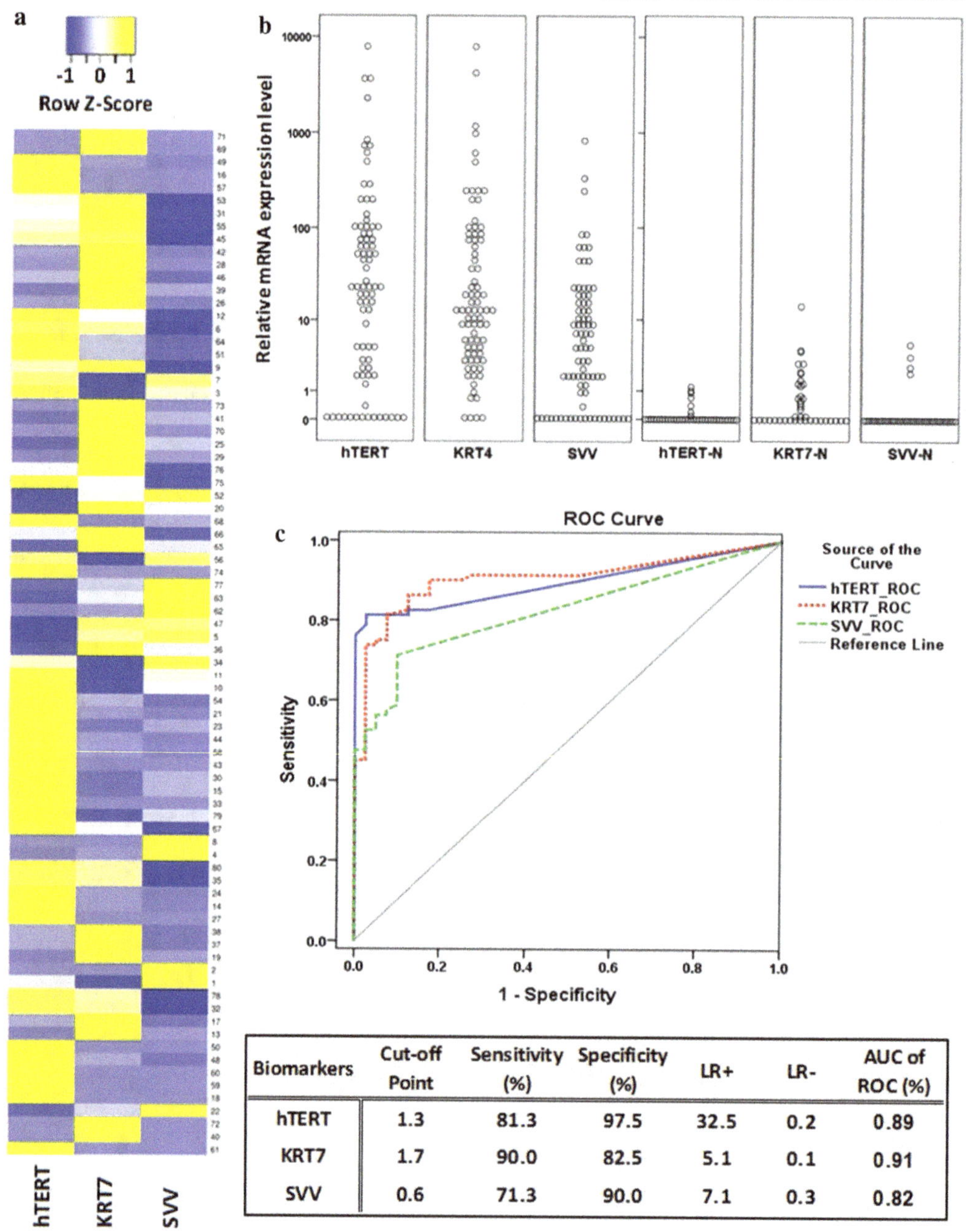

Biomarkers	Cut-off Point	Sensitivity (%)	Specificity (%)	LR+	LR-	AUC of ROC (%)
hTERT	1.3	81.3	97.5	32.5	0.2	0.89
KRT7	1.7	90.0	82.5	5.1	0.1	0.91
SVV	0.6	71.3	90.0	7.1	0.3	0.82

Fig. 1 Expression levels of hTERT, KRT7, and SVV mRNA in 80 bladder cancer patients. **a** Heat map representation of the three mRNA expression levels in the 80 bladder cancer urine samples. **b** Comparison of hTERT, KRT7, and SVV mRNA levels in the urine samples of bladder cancer and non-bladder cancer patients. **c** Receiver operating characteristic (ROC) curves were performed to determine the area under the ROC curve (AUC), sensitivity, specificity, as well as the likelihood ratios (LR^+ and LR^-) to determine the levels of the biomarkers that best differentiate the bladder cancer cases versus the control subjects. The optimal cut-off values were calculated as the marker level that maximizes the sensitivity and specificity

performed the Receiver Operating Characteristic (ROC) curves for each study variable. The area under curve (AUC) for hTERT (0.89), KRT7 (0.91) and SVV (0.82) was significantly larger than the reference line ($P<0.01$) (Fig. 1). The optimal cut-off values for the investigated biomarkers were determined based on the best balance of sensitivity and specificity along with larger increases in the likelihood ratios (LR+). The sensitivity, specificity, likelihood ratio, and AUC of ROC of all the three markers in the voided urine samples are shown in Fig. 1. The optimal cutoff values were 1.3, 1.7, and 0.6 for hTERT, KRT7, and SVV, respectively. Samples were classified as positive for a particular gene if the $2^{-\Delta\Delta Cq}$ was above the cut-off point.

We calculated overall sensitivity, specificity, PPV, NPV, and accuracy for cytology, hTERT, KRT7, and SVV when tested independently or in combinations in voided urine samples of bladder cancer patients. As shown in Table 3, the overall sensitivity and specificity were 81.3 and 97.5% for hTERT, 91.3 and 85% for KRT7, and 72.5 and 90% for SSV. The overall sensitivity for voided urine cytology was 31.3%; however, the voided urine cytology has a higher specificity than the other markers (100%). The PPV was 98.5, 92.4, 93.5, and 100% for hTERT, KRT7, SSV, and voided urine cytology, respectively. The NPV was 72.7, 82.9, 62.1, and 42.1% for hTERT, KRT7, SSV, and voided urine cytology, respectively. The overall accuracy was higher for KRT7 than hTERT, SSV, and voided urine cytology (89.2, 87.5, 78.3, and 54.2%).

The combination use of the markers was calculated (Table 3). The sensitivity of cytology was increased when it was combined with any other markers. The combination use of the two markers (hTERT and KRT7) gave the highest sensitivity and overall accuracy (100 and 95%), with a specificity of 85%. There was no significant difference in sensitivity of hTERT, KRT7, and SVV concerning sex, history of bladder cancer, tumor burden, and tumor stage.

Table 3 Overall sensitivity, specificity, positive predictive value (PPV), negative predictive value (NPV), and accuracy for cytology, hTERT, KRT7, and SVV when tested independently or in combinations in the voided urine samples of bladder cancer patients

	Sensitivity	Specificity	PPV	NPV	Accuracy
Cytology	31.3	100.0	100.0	42.1	54.2
hTERT	81.3	97.5	98.5	72.7	87.5
KRT7	91.3	85.0	92.4	82.9	89.2
SVV	72.5	90.0	93.5	62.1	78.3
Cyt + hTERT	85.0	100.0	100.0	74.1	88.3
Cyt + KRT7	95.0	85.0	92.7	89.5	91.7
Cyt + SVV	77.5	90.0	93.7	63.2	79.2
hTERT + KRT7	100.0	85.0	93.0	100.0	95.0
hTERT + SSV	95.0	90.0	94.9	87.8	92.5
KRT7 + SVV	93.8	75.0	88.2	85.7	87.5
Cyt + hTERT + KRT7	100.0	85.0	93.0	100.0	95.0
Cyt + hTERT + SSV	96.3	90.0	95.0	90.0	93.3
Cyt + KRT7 + SSV	96.3	75.0	88.5	90.9	89.2
hTERT + KRT7 + SVV	100.0	75.0	88.9	100.0	91.7
Cyt + hTERT + KRT7 + SVV	100.0	75.0	88.9	100.0	91.7

Comparison of hTERT, KRT7, and SVV detection in different grades of the tumor

The sensitivity of these tests was studied separately in high and low-grade bladder carcinomas (Table 4; Fig. 2). According to the results, in low-grade tumors, the cytology was positive in 9 out of 60 patients (15%) and negative

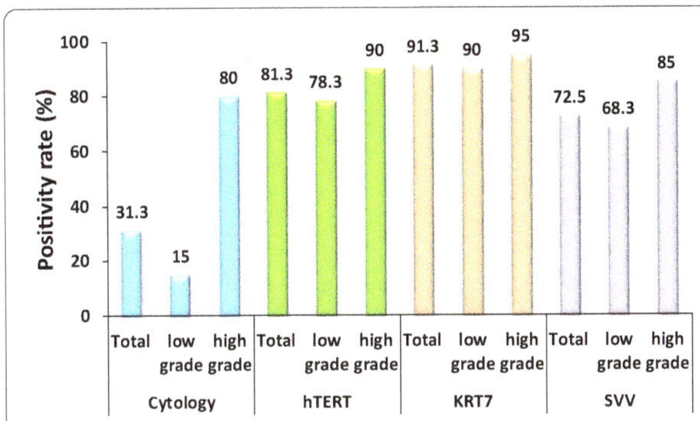

Fig. 2 The positivity rate of urine cytology, hTERT, KRT7, and SVV in the different grades of bladder cancer

Table 4 The positivity rate of urine cytology, hTERT, KRT7, and SVV in different grades of bladder tumors

Tumor stage	Cytology		hTERT		KRT7		SSV	
	Neg%	Pos%	Neg%	Pos%	Neg%	Pos%	Neg%	Pos%
Low (N: 60)	51 (85.0%)	9 (15.0%)	13 (21.7%)	47 (78.3%)	6 (10.0%)	54 (90.0%)	19 (31.7%)	41 (68.3%)
High (N: 20)	4 (20.0%)	16 (80.0%)	2 (10.0%)	18 (90.0%)	1 (5.0%)	19 (95.0%)	3 (15.0%)	17 (85.0%)
Total (N: 80)	55 (68.8%)	25 (31.3%)	15 (18.7%)	65 (81.3%)	7 (8.7%)	73 (91.3%)	22 (27.5%)	58 (72.5%)
	25/80 (31.3%)		65/80 (81.3%)		73/80 (91.3%)		58/80 (71.3%)	
p value	0.000		0.333		0.673		0.247	

in the rest of the 51 patients (85%). In high-grade tumors, cytology was positive in 16 out of 20 patients (80%) and negative in the rest of the 4 patients (20%). The sensitivity of urine cytology for the diagnosis of low-grade tumors was significantly lower than that of high-grade tumors ($p < 0.001$). As shown in Table 4, the result of the hTERT test was positive in 47 out of 60 patients suffering from low-grade tumors (78.3%) and negative in the rest of the 13 patients (21.7%). It was also positive in 18 out of 20 patients suffering from high-grade tumors (90%) and negative in the rest of the 2 patients (10%). Overall, there were not any statistically significant differences between the positive results of hTERT, KRT7, and SVV tests in high-grade and low-grade tumors ($p > 0.5$).

Comparison of hTERT, KRT7, and SVV detection in the different stages of tumors

As shown in Table 5; Fig. 3, when studying the different stages of the tumor, urine cytology was negative in 43 out of 50 patients suffering from stage Ta tumors (86.0%) and was just positive in 7 patients (14%). In 5 out of 17 patients suffering from stage T1, urine cytology was positive in 5 (29.4%), and it was negative in the rest of the 12 patients (70.6%). Urine cytology was positive for both T2 and T3 tumor stages in all 7 and 6 patients, respectively. These results show that with an increase in the stage of the tumor, we have a statistically significant increase in the sensitivity of urine cytology for the diagnosis of bladder carcinoma ($p < 0.001$). However, there was no statistically significant difference between the results of hTERT, KRT7, and SVV tests and the stages of the tumors ($p > 0.5$).

Discussion

For a long time, the combination of cystoscopy with urine cytology has constructed the gold standard method for the detection and surveillance of bladder cancer. However, the application of these methods in the clinical platform has been restricted due to some inextricable limitations [8]. Concerning cystoscopy, the invasiveness and cost of the whole process are prime reasons for the decline in its preference for diagnosis. [18]. On the other

Table 5 The positivity rate of urine cytology, hTERT, KRT7, and SVV in different stages of bladder tumor

Tumor stage	Cytology		hTERT		KRT7		SSV	
	Neg%	Pos%	Neg%	Pos%	Neg%	Pos%	Neg%	Pos%
Ta (N: 50)	43 (86.0%)	7 (14.0%)	12 (24.0%)	38 (76.0%)	5 (10.0%)	45 (90.0%)	15 (30.0%)	35 (70.0%)
T1 (N: 17)	12 (70.6%)	5 (29.4%)	1 (5.9%)	16 (94.1%)	1 (5.9%)	16 (94.1%)	4 (23.5%)	13 (76.5%)
T2 (N: 7)	0 (0%)	7 (100%)	1 (14.3%)	6 (85.7%)	0 (0%)	7 (100%)	2 (28.6%)	5 (71.4%)
T3 (N: 6)	0 (0%)	6 (100%)	1 (16.7.0%)	5 (83.3%)	1 (16.7%)	5 (83.3%)	1 (16.7%)	5 (83.3%)
Total (N: 80)	56 (70.0%)	25 (31.3%)	15 (18.8%)	65 (81.3%)	7 (8.8%)	73 (91.3%)	22 (27.5%)	58 (72.5%)
	25/80 (31.3%)		65/80 (81.3%)		73/80 (91.3%)		58/80 (72.5%)	
p value	0.000		0.329		0.903		0.507	

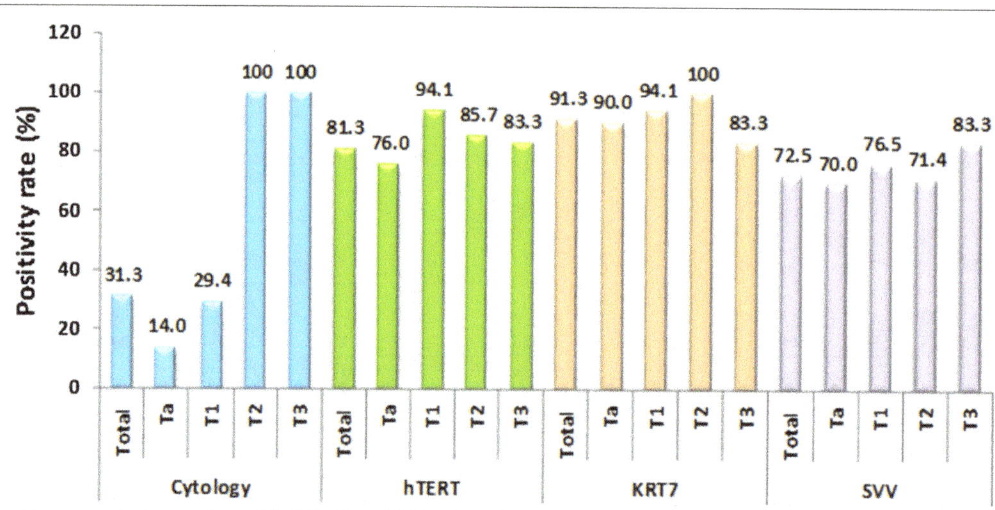

Fig. 3 The positivity rate of urine cytology, hTERT, KRT7, and SVV in the different stages of bladder cancer

hand, urine cytology, which is an important noninvasive technique with high specificity, has a restricted application due to its interpreter-dependent low sensitivity for low-grade tumors [19]. While this technique usually performs well with high-stage tumors (T2–T3), the sensitivity of urine cytology for the detection of early-stage tumors is relatively low with a range of 20–40%. This is probably because the Ta–T1 tumors shed fewer cancer cells into the urine [20, 21]. Hence, these challenges highlight the importance of the identification of new urine-based markers for the early as well as appropriate detection of bladder cancer, which is a well-known malignancy with a complicated molecular nature.

There are several FDA-approved immunochromatographic assays for bladder cancer detection. These tests include the measurement of soluble proteins such as bladder tumor-associated antigen (BTA), nuclear matrix protein 22 (NMP22), proteins detected on fixed urothelial cells (ImmunoCyt), and chromosomal aberrations detected by fluorescence in situ hybridization (UroVysion) [22]. Several molecular markers have been recently proposed to improve the diagnostic sensitivity of the urine. Among a wide variety of genes participating in the pathogenesis of human cancers, survivin (SVV) is one of the most studied ones due to its unique characteristics that not only plays a crucial role in the tumor progression but also are profoundly involved in the development of drug resistance. SVV is a member of the inhibitor of apoptosis proteins (IAPs) gene family. Its overexpression inhibits extrinsic and intrinsic pathways of apoptosis. Overexpression of SVV has been reported in almost all human malignancies, including, bladder cancer, lung cancer, breast cancer as well as stomach, esophagus, liver, ovarian and hematological cancers [23, 24]. Moreover, its use as a tumor biomarker has been well-established in some studies on different human cancers [25–27]. However, when it comes to bladder cancer, there are some concerns regarding its efficacy for early as well accurate detection of this type of cancer. The high expression of urinary SVV has been reported in bladder cancer [28]. Despite the positive correlation between the expression of SVV and the malignant degree of bladder cancer [29], conflicting results are reflecting the sensitivity of this gene for the detection of low-grade tumors. In this present study, by measuring the sensitivity and specificity of SVV in the urine specimens of bladder cancer patients using qRT-PCR analysis, we found a performance of 72.5% sensitivity, 90% specificity, and 78.3% accuracy. Notably, this technique was successful in the detection of low-grade bladder cancer patients with a sensitivity of 68.3%; suggesting that the measurement of SVV mRNA in urine may be useful for the detection of bladder cancer in both low- and high-grade cases.

There has been an increasing amount of attention focusing on the role of telomerase in the detection of bladder cancer [30]. Because of its expression in cancer and not in the normal tissues, urine telomerase is a suitable molecular marker for the detection of bladder cancer [31]. The catalytic subunit (hTERT) of telomerase is correlated with the telomerase activity [32]. In similarity with SVV, we found that hTERT, as a single biomarker, could provide an accuracy rate of 87.5% for the diagnosis of bladder cancer, thus, introducing this gene as another valuable prognostic biomarker for this malignancy. The well-established association between SVV and hTERT in the pathogenesis of a wide variety of human cancers proposes a possibility that the co-expression of these genes could serve as a novel biomarker for the early detection of this cancer. Notably, considering both the expression levels of SVV and hTERT in the patients resulted in an accuracy rate up to 92.5%. By combining these two biomarkers, suggests the successfulness of using these combinations in the diagnostics of bladder cancer.

KRT7, a member of the cytokeratin family, is highly expressed in a wide variety of human cancers such as ovarian cancer [33]and squamous cell carcinomas [34]. Recent studies using gene expression profiling of noninvasive primary urothelial tumors such as urothelial neoplasia (stage Ta) biopsies show that KRT7 is an early change in gene expression, which is found to be highly increased when compared to normal biopsies. Consequently, they suggested this expression could be detected in the urine sediments of bladder tumor patients [35]. In another study, the expression level of this gene in the circulating cells of patients undergoing radical cystectomy for urothelial cancer was linked to an increased risk of cancer recurrence and death [36]. Consistently, we found that the sensitivity of KRT7 detection for both low- and high-grade tumors was respectively 90 and 95%, as compared to the 15 and 80% obtained from cytology. Moreover, the sensitivity of KRT7 detection for the early stages of the tumor (Ta and T1) was as high as for the late-stage of tumors (T2 and T3). More interestingly, by combining the results of KRT7 expression and hTERT, a sensitivity of 100% was achieved for bladder cancer patients. Conclusively, our results also showed that combining the expression results of all three genes for bladder cancer patients, either alone or in combination with cytology, provided a sensitivity and NPV of 100%, which was not obtained from any other investigations. Given the significant role of SVV, hTERT, and KRT7 in bladder cancer detection, we suggest that the simultaneous expression analysis of the aforementioned genes could go hand in hand with cytology to provide a better outlook for both the early and accurate diagnosis of patients with bladder cancer in the clinical practice.

Conclusions

In the present study, we investigated the diagnostic potential of measuring the urinary levels of hTERT, SVV, and KRT7 mRNA for the detection of bladder cancer. The detection of these markers in voided urine samples demonstrates superior sensitivities over cytology. The combined use of these markers offers a powerful potential assay and promising tool for a sensitive, noninvasive, and highly specific method for diagnosis and follow-up of low-grade TCC of the bladder.

Acknowledgements

The authors would like to express their gratitude to the Hematology, Oncology and Stem Cell Transplantation Research Center and the Department of Urology, Shariati Hospital, Tehran University of Medical Sciences.

Authors' contributions

RY contributed to the study conception, study design, and patient data. SK performed the qPCR analyses. DB, PG, and ASA contributed to the writing and review of the manuscript. SHG was involved in the supervision, data interpretation, statistical analysis, and revising of the manuscript. All authors read and approved the final manuscript.

Author details

[1] Department of Urology, Shariati Hospital, Tehran University of Medical Sciences, Tehran, Iran. [2] Department of Hematology and Blood Banking, School of Allied Medical Sciences, Shahid Beheshti University of Medical Sciences, Tehran, Iran. [3] Hematology, Oncology and Stem Cell Transplantation Research Center, School of Medicine, Shariati Hospital, Tehran University of Medical Sciences, Tehran, Iran.

References

1. Jemal A, Siegel R, Ward E, Murray T, Xu J, Thun MJ. Cancer statistics, 2007. CA Cancer J Clin. 2007;57(1):43–66.
2. Konety BR, Getzenberg RH. Urine-based markers of urological malignancy. J Urol. 2001;165(2):600–11.
3. Fornari D, Steven K, Hansen AB, Vibits H, Jepsen JV, Poulsen AL, Schwartz M, Horn T. Microsatellite analysis of urine sediment versus urine cytology for diagnosing transitional cell tumors of the urinary bladder. APMIS. 2004;112(2):148–52.
4. Kaufman D. Challenges in the treatment of bladder cancer. Ann Oncol. 2006;17:v106–12.
5. Latini DM, Lerner SP, Wade SW, Lee DW, Quale DZ. Bladder cancer detection, treatment, and outcomes: opportunities and challenges. Urology. 2010;75(2):334–9.
6. Hollenbeck BK, Dunn RL, Ye Z, Hollingsworth JM, Skolarus TA, Kim SP, Montie JE, Lee CT, Wood DP Jr, Miller DC. Delays in diagnosis and bladder cancer mortality. Cancer. 2010;116(22):5235–42.
7. Gore JL, Lai J, Setodji CM, Litwin MS, Saigal CS. Mortality increases when radical cystectomy is delayed more than 12 weeks: results from a surveillance, epidemiology, and end results–medicare analysis. Cancer Interdiscip Int J Am Cancer Soc. 2009;115(5):988–96.
8. Cheung G, Sahai A, Billia M, Dasgupta P, Khan MS. Recent advances in the diagnosis and treatment of bladder cancer. BMC Med. 2013;11(1):13.
9. Weikert S, Christoph F, Schrader M, Krause H, Miller K, Müller M. Quantitative analysis of survivin mRNA expression in urine and tumor tissue of bladder cancer patients and its potential relevance for disease detection and prognosis. Int J Cancer. 2005;116(1):100–4.
10. Wang H, Xi X, Kong X, Huang G, Ge G. The expression and significance of survivin mRNA in urinary bladder carcinomas. J Cancer Res Clin Oncol. 2004;130(8):487–90.
11. Yahyazadeh SR, Mehraban D, Ghaffari SH, Moghadam K, Ghavamzadeh A, Naderi GH, Kazemeyni SM, Rasteh M. Detection of bladder transitional cell carcinoma: urinary hTERT assay versus urine cytology. Tehran Univ Med J. 2009;67(1):49–54.
12. Kumar P, Nandi S, Tan TZ, Ler SG, Chia KS, Lim W-Y, Bütow Z, Vordos D, De la Taille A, Al-Haddawi M. Highly sensitive and specific novel biomarkers for the diagnosis of transitional bladder carcinoma. Oncotarget. 2015;6(15):13539.
13. Osman I, Bajorin DF, Sun T-T, Zhong H, Douglas D, Scattergood J, Zheng R, Han M, Marshall KW, Liew C-C. Novel blood biomarkers of human urinary bladder cancer. Clin Cancer Res. 2006;12(11):3374–80.
14. van der Heijden AG, Mengual L, Lozano JJ, Ingelmo-Torres M, Ribal MJ, Fernández PL, Oosterwijk E, Schalken JA, Alcaraz A, Witjes JA. A five-gene expression signature to predict progression in T1G3 bladder cancer. Eur J Cancer. 2016;64:127–36.
15. Fröhlich C, Albrechtsen R, Dyrskjøt L, Rudkjær L, Ørntoft TF, Wewer UM. Molecular profiling of ADAM12 in human bladder cancer. Clin Cancer Res. 2006;12(24):7359–68.
16. Di Carlo A, Terracciano D, Mariano A, Macchia V. Urinary gelatinase activities (matrix metalloproteinases 2 and 9) in human bladder tumors. Oncol Rep. 2006;15(5):1321–6.
17. Sobin LH, Gospodarowicz MK, Wittekind C. International union against cancer: TNM classification of malignant tumors. 7th ed. Chichester: Wiley-Blackwell; 2010.
18. Zhu C-Z, Ting H-N, Ng K-H, Ong T-A. A review on the accuracy of bladder cancer detection methods. J Cancer. 2019;10(17):4038.
19. Brown FM. Urine cytology: is it still the gold standard for screening? Urol Clin N Am. 2000;27(1):25–37.
20. Nakamura K, Kasraeian A, Iczkowski KA, Chang M, Pendleton J, Anai S, Rosser CJ. Utility of serial urinary cytology in the initial evaluation of the patient with microscopic hematuria. BMC Urol. 2009;9:12.
21. Kumar A, Kumar R, Gupta NP. Comparison of NMP22 BladderChek test and urine cytology for the detection of recurrent bladder cancer. Jpn J Clin Oncol. 2006;36(3):172–5.
22. Goodison S, Rosser CJ, Urquidi V. Bladder cancer detection and monitoring: assessment of urine- and blood-based marker tests. Mol Diagn Ther. 2013;17(2):71–84.
23. Fukuda S, Pelus LM. Survivin, a cancer target with an emerging role in normal adult tissues. Mol Cancer Ther. 2006;5(5):1087–98.
24. Jaiswal PK, Goel A, Mittal RD. Survivin: a molecular biomarker in cancer. Indian J Med Res. 2015;141(4):389–97.
25. Lu B, Gonzalez A, Massion P, Shyr Y, Shaktour B, Carbone D, Hallahan D. Nuclear survivin as a biomarker for non-small-cell lung cancer. Br J Cancer. 2004;91(3):537–40.
26. Ikeguchi M, Kaibara N. Survivin messenger RNA expression is a good prognostic biomarker for oesophageal carcinoma. Br J Cancer. 2002;87(8):883–7.
27. Khan S, Jutzy JM, Valenzuela MMA, Turay D, Aspe JR, Ashok A, Mirshahidi S, Mercola D, Lilly MB, Wall NR. Plasma-derived exosomal survivin, a plausible biomarker for early detection of prostate cancer. PloS One. 2012;7(10):e46737.
28. Moussa O, Abol-Enein H, Bissada NK, Keane T, Ghoneim MA, Watson DK. Evaluation of survivin reverse transcriptase-polymerase chain reaction for noninvasive detection of bladder cancer. J Urol. 2006;175(6):2312–6.
29. Ku JH, Godoy G, Amiel GE, Lerner SP. Urine survivin as a diagnostic biomarker for bladder cancer: a systematic review. BJU Int. 2012;110(5):630–6.
30. Bravaccini S, Casadio V, Amadori D, Calistri D, Silvestrini R. The current role of telomerase in the diagnosis of bladder cancer. Indian J Urol. 2009;25(1):40–6.
31. Bravaccini S, Sanchini MA, Granato AM, Gunelli R, Nanni O, Amadori D, Calistri D, Silvestrini R. Urine telomerase activity for the detection of bladder cancer in females. J Urol. 2007;178(1):57–61.
32. Simon M, Park T-W, Leuenroth S, Hans VH, Löning T, Schramm J. Telomerase activity and expression of the telomerase catalytic subunit, hTERT, in meningioma progression. J Neurosurg. 2000;92(5):832–40.
33. Wang P, Magdolen V, Seidl C, Dorn J, Drecoll E, Kotzsch M, Yang F, Schmitt M, Schilling O, Rockstroh A. Kallikrein-related peptidases 4, 5, 6, and 7 regulate tumor-associated factors in serous ovarian cancer. Br J Cancer. 2018;119(7):1–9.
34. Zhao H, Dong Y, Quan J, Smith R, Lam A, Weinstein S, Clements J, Johnson NW, Gao J. Correlation of the expression of human kallikrein-related

peptidases 4 and 7 with the prognosis in oral squamous cell carcinoma. Head Neck. 2011;33(4):566–72.

35. Aaboe M, Marcussen N, Jensen KM, Thykjaer T, Dyrskjot L, Orntoft TF. Gene expression profiling of noninvasive primary urothelial tumors using microarrays. Br J Cancer. 2005;93(10):1182–90.

36. Pagliarulo V, Ancona P, Petitti T, Salerno A, Spadavecchia R, Di Stasi S, Cormio L, Maurizio B, Carrieri G, Ditonno P. Detection and clinical significance of circulating tumor cells in patients undergoing radical cystectomy for urothelial bladder cancer. Clin Genitourin Cancer. 2017;15(4):455–62.

13

Protocol for development and validation of a prediction model for 5-year risk of incident overactive bladder in the general population: The Nagahama study

Satoshi Funada[1,2*], Yan Luo[2], Takashi Yoshioka[3,4], Kazuya Setoh[5], Yasuharu Tabara[5], Hiromitsu Negoro[6], Shusuke Akamatsu[1], Koji Yoshimura[7], Fumihiko Matsuda[5], Toshi A. Furukawa[2], Orestis Efthimiou[8,9] and Osamu Ogawa[1]

Abstract

Background: An accurate prediction model could identify high-risk subjects of incident Overactive bladder (OAB) among the general population and enable early prevention which may save on the related medical costs. However, no efficient model has been developed for predicting incident OAB. In this study, we will develop a model for predicting the onset of OAB at 5-year in the general population setting.

Methods: Data will be obtained from the Nagahama Cohort Project, a longitudinal, general population cohort study. The baseline characteristics were measured between Nov 28, 2008 and Nov 28, 2010, and follow-up was performed every 5 years. From the total of 9,764 participants (male: 3,208, female: 6,556) at baseline, we will exclude participants who could not attend the follow-up assessment and those who were defined as having OAB at baseline. The outcome will be incident OAB defined using the Overactive Bladder Symptom Score (OABSS) at follow-up assessment. Baseline questionnaires (demographic, health behavior, comorbidities and OABSS) and blood test data will be included as predictors. We will develop a logistic regression model utilizing shrinkage methods (LASSO penalization method). Model performance will be evaluated by discrimination and calibration. Net benefit will be evaluated by decision curve analysis. We will perform an internal validation and a temporal validation of the model. We will develop a web-based application to visualize the prediction model and facilitate its use in clinical practice.

Discussion: This will be the first study to develop a model to predict the incidence of OAB.

Keywords: Urinary bladder, Longitudinal analysis, Cohort study, Risk calculator

Background

Overactive bladder (OAB) is defined as "a symptom characterized by urinary urgency, with or without urgency incontinence, usually with urinary frequency and nocturia in the absence of infection or other obvious pathology" [1]. The prevalence of OAB is estimated from 10 to 20% and increases with age [2–4]. OAB might significantly decrease the HRQOL in patients [5] and increase the expenditure of medical cost [6]. The prevalence of OAB is increasing in an aging society and the negative impacts on HRQOL and medical cost are becoming even more serious.

*Correspondence: sfunada@kuhp.kyoto-u.ac.jp
[1] Department of Urology, Faculty of Medicine, Kyoto University Graduate School of Medicine, 54 Shogoinkawahara-cho, Sakyo-ku, Kyoto 606-8507, Japan
Full list of author information is available at the end of the article

Population-based prediction models would be helpful for population health planning and policy decision-making [7]. The same is expected for OAB prediction model because some good behaviors, such as healthy eating habit, keeping healthy weight, quitting smoking and pelvic floor muscle exercise, are efficient for keeping the bladder as healthy as possible [8]. If an accurate prediction model can be developed, high-risk subjects could be identified and encouraged to such good habits at an early stage, which might prevent incident OAB and save on the medical cost related to pharmacotherapy. If such a model could be made freely available to the general public online and encourage good habits for a healthy bladder, it could change user's behavior to prevent incident OAB and impact on health care providers within clinical practice guidelines to inform decision making in the clinical setting. However, to our knowledge, no model has been developed to predict the new-onset of OAB in the literature. This could be due to lack of sufficient data to develop such a prediction model in terms of sample size, retrospective study design, and/or important predictors. We have recently reported longitudinal analyses of voiding dysfunction using a large prospective cohort data from the general population [9, 10]. These data can be used to develop an adequate model to predict new-onset OAB in the general population.

In this study, we will use a large prospective Japanese general population cohort to develop a model to predict the new-onset OAB at 5-year. We will develop a model consisting of only questionnaires and will compare the performance with another model including blood test. If the performance of the two models is deemed to be comparable, we will choose the model without blood testing, aiming to make the model more easily accessible, even by the general population. As the mechanism of incident OAB could be different between male and female due to factors such as the prostate gland, menopause and delivery, we will develop separate models for each sex. In addition, we will develop a web-based application to visualize the results interactively.

Methods/design

We will follow the Transparent Reporting of a Multivariable Prediction Model for Individual Prognosis or Diagnosis (TRIPOD) checklist for developing and validating our prediction model [7].

Study design and source of data

We will use the Nagahama cohort [4, 9, 10], a prospective population-based cohort study in the Nagahama city, a Japanese rural city of 125,000 inhabitants. Recruitment was performed between Nov 28, 2008 and Nov 28, 2010, and the baseline characteristics were measured. Follow-up was performed every 5 years after baseline assessment, and the follow-up assessment was performed between July 28, 2013 and Feb 10, 2016. The cohort study was approved by the ethics committee of Kyoto University Graduate School of Medicine (no. G278) and by the Nagahama Municipal Review Board. Written informed consent was obtained from all participants.

Study population

Participants were recruited from the general community residents of Nagahama city. Inclusion criteria were as follows: age 30–74 years; ability to independently participate in health examinations; no difficulties in communicating in Japanese; no serious diseases, symptoms, or other health issues; and voluntary participation. From the total 9764 participants (male: 3208, female: 6556) at baseline, we will exclude 1475 participants who did not attend the follow-up assessment because of death (n = 137), moving from Nagahama City (n = 279) or some other unknown reason (n = 1059). From the 8289 follow-up participant, we will exclude 912 OAB participant and 2 missing data of OAB at baseline, and 7375 participants (male: 2289, female: 5086) will be used in this analysis. The study flow chart is shown in Fig. 1.

Study outcome

The outcome will be new-onset OAB at 5-year follow-up assessment. We will use OABSS, a self-report measure assessing of urinary urgency validated by Homma et al. [11]. The questionnaire consists of the following items: (i) How many times do you typically urinate from waking in the morning until sleeping at night? (ii) How many times do you typically wake up to urinate from sleeping at night until waking in the morning? (iii) How often do you have a sudden desire to urinate, which is difficult to defer? (iv) How often do you leak urine because you cannot defer the sudden desire to urinate? OAB will be defined as a total OABSS score ≥ 3, with an urgency score (iii) ≥ 2 [11]. The number of new-onset OAB at follow-up assessment will be 224 for male and 290 for female.

Sample size calculation

We calculated the minimum sample size needed to build a prediction model using the criteria recommended by Riley et al. [12]. For these calculations it is required to provide an expected R^2 value. As there has been no prediction model of incident OAB previously, we have set $R^2 = 0.10$ as a conservative choice in this study. Based on the number of events in our dataset (224 male, 290 female) and the selected value for R^2, we calculated the upper limit of the number of predictors to be 27 for the model for males and 35 for females.

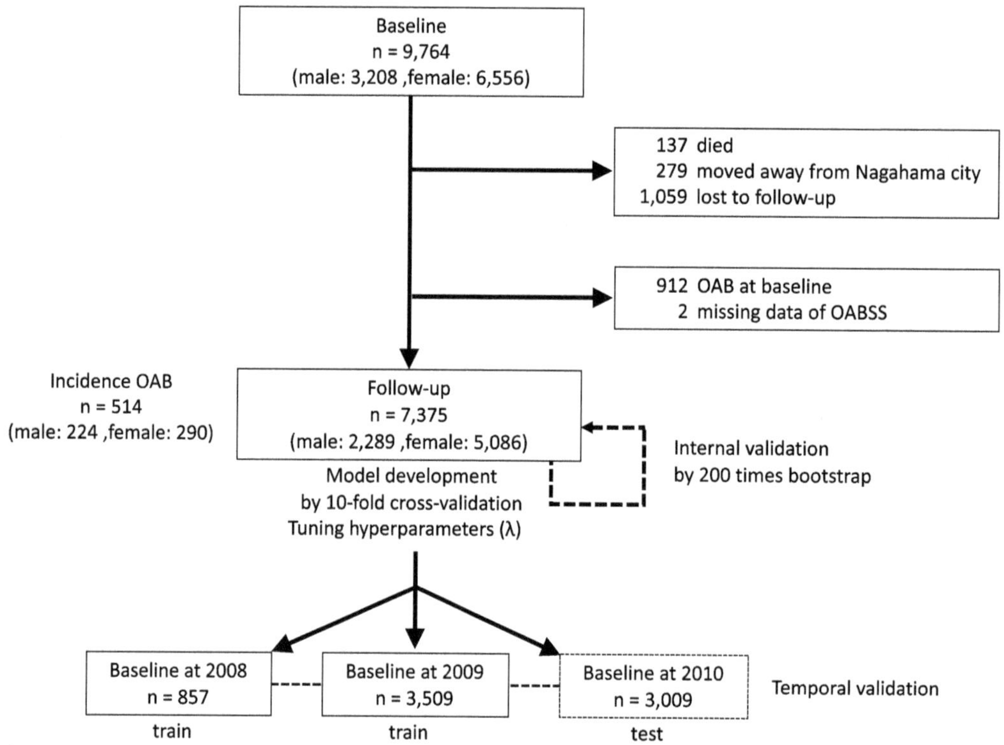

Fig. 1 Study flow chart

Candidate predictor variables

Based on previous reports [13–18] and expert opinion, we will initially include in the mode the following candidate predictors variables which were measured at baseline; demographic variables (age, body mass index [BMI], delivery, menopause, smoking status, alcohol habit, walking habit), history of comorbidities (hypertension, hyperlipidemia, diabetes, ischemic heart disease, stroke, kidney disease, cancer, depression, sleep disturbance, obstructive sleep apnea [OSA], benign prostate disease and prostate cancer [PCa]), questionnaires specific to OAB (OABSS question 1, question 2, question 3 and question 4) and blood test (HbA1c, B-type natriuretic peptide [BNP], the estimated glomerular filtration rate [eGFR]) and prostate specific antigen [PSA]). Trained physicians and research assistants administered the standardized questionnaire in which participants provided clinical background information, such as lifestyle and medical history. Anthropometric and physiological measurements were taken by trained nurses.

Age will be treated as continuous value. BMI will be calculated as continuous values using height and weight data. Smoking status will be categorized as a dichotomous variable either current or none smoker. Alcohol habit will be categorized as a dichotomous variable either current or none drinker. Walking habit will be categorized as a dichotomous variable by the questionnaire: walking for ≥ 1 h or < 1 h. Delivery will be categorized as a dichotomous variable either experienced or not. History and medical comorbidities (menopause, hypertension, hyperlipidemia, diabetes, ischemic heart disease, stroke, kidney disease, cancer, depression, sleep disturbance, OSA, benign prostate disease, prostate cancer) will be categorized as a dichotomous variable by the questionnaire: yes or no. OABSS question 1, question 2, question 3 and question 4 will be treated as continuous variables. Blood samples (HbA1c, BNP, creatine, PSA) will be used as continuous values. eGFR will be calculated from serum creatinine levels using the following formula: $194 \times \text{serum creatinine}^{-1.094} \times \text{age}^{-0.287}$ ($\times 0.739$ if female).

We will develop two models based on the sample size calculations as follows (Table 1a and b);

- Model 1 including demographic questionnaires (age, BMI, delivery and menopause), health behavior questionnaires (smoking status, alcohol habit and walking habit) and comorbidities questionnaires (hypertension, hyperlipidemia, diabetes, ischemic heart disease, stroke, kidney disease, cancer, depression, sleep disturbance, OSA, prostate disease and prostate cancer) and questionnaires

Table 1 Candidate predictor variables for new-onset OAB in (a) male, (b) female

Variable	Scale	Number of parameters	
		Model 1	Model 2
(a)			
Demographic			
Age	Continuous	1	1
BMI	Continuous	1	1
Health behavior			
Smoking status	Dichotomous	1	1
Alcohol habit	Dichotomous	1	1
Walking habit	Dichotomous	1	1
Comorbidity			
Hypertension	Dichotomous	1	1
Hyperlipidemia	Dichotomous	1	1
Diabetes	Dichotomous	1	1
Ischemic heart disease	Dichotomous	1	1
Stroke	Dichotomous	1	1
Kidney disease	Dichotomous	1	1
Cancer	Dichotomous	1	1
Depression	Dichotomous	1	1
Sleep disturbance	Dichotomous	1	1
Obstructive sleep apnea	Dichotomous	1	1
Prostate disease	Dichotomous	1	1
Prostate cancer	Dichotomous	1	1
OABSS			
Question 1	Continuous	1	1
Question 2	Continuous	1	1
Question 3	Continuous	1	1
Question 4	Continuous	1	1
Blood test			
HbA1c (%)	Continuous		1
BNP (pg/mL)	Continuous		1
eGFR (ml/min/1.73 m^2)	Continuous		1
PSA (ng/ml)	Continuous		1
Total		21	25
(b)			
Demographic			
Age	Continuous	1	1
BMI	Continuous	1	1
Delivery	Dichotomous	1	1
Menopause	Dichotomous	1	1
Health behavior			
Smoking status	Dichotomous	1	1
Alcohol habit	Dichotomous	1	1
Walking habit	Dichotomous	1	1
Comorbidity			
Hypertension	Dichotomous	1	1
Hyperlipidemia	Dichotomous	1	1
Diabetes	Dichotomous	1	1
Ischemic heart disease	Dichotomous	1	1
Stroke	Dichotomous	1	1
Kidney disease	Dichotomous	1	1
Cancer	Dichotomous	1	1
Depression	Dichotomous	1	1
Sleep disturbance	Dichotomous	1	1
Obstructive sleep apnea	Dichotomous	1	1
OABSS			
Question 1	Continuous	1	1
Question 2	Continuous	1	1
Question 3	Continuous	1	1
Question 4	Continuous	1	1
Blood test			
HbA1c (%)	Continuous		1
BNP (pg/mL)	Continuous		1
eGFR (ml/min/1.73 m^2)	Continuous		1
Total		21	24

specific OAB (OABSS question 1, question 2, question 3 and question 4)

- Model 2 consisting of Model 1 plus blood test (HbA1c, BNP, eGFR and PSA)

A total of 21 and 25 parameters of variables will be included in Model 1 and Model 2 for male, and 21 and 24 parameters will be included in Model 1 and Model 2 for female.

Data cleaning

We will create frequency tables for categorical variables and box plots for the continuous variables. We will identify values out of plausible range (i.e. values that are clearly erroneous), and we will classify them as missing data. We will exclude some categorical predictors with very small prevalence. Continuous variables will be standardized and categorical variables will be transformed into dummy variables.

Missing data

We will create 10 multiply imputed datasets using chained equations [19]. Each completed data set will be analyzed separately and the results will be combined by Rubin's rules to account for imputation uncertainty [20].

Model development

Logistic regression model will be used to develop Model 1 and Model 2 to predict a binary outcome, new-onset OAB. To avoid overfitting of data, we will employ a shrinkage method (LASSO) [21]. To find the optimal hyperparameter (λ) of penalization, a tenfold cross-validation will be performed.

Model performance

We will evaluate the predictive accuracy of each model by R^2 statistic. Model discrimination, i.e. the ability to classify the participants into high-risk or low-risk, will be evaluated using the C-statistic. Model calibration, agreement between observed outcomes and predictions, will be evaluated with calibration plots. To evaluate and compare the net benefit between models, decision curve analysis (DCA) will be performed [22].

Model validation

We will use internal validation and temporal validation to evaluate the model performance [23]. Internal validation will be performed via bootstrap procedure repeated 200 times to calculate optimism-corrected R^2, c-statistics and calibration slope. Temporal validity will be assessed by splitting the sample into 3 sets according to the year of baseline assessment (i.e. 2008, 2009 and 2010). We will use the first 2 sets (2008 and 2009) as the training set, and the 2010 set as the testing set, to evaluate discrimination and calibration.

Statistical software

We will use R version 4.0.2 for our analyses. We will program a Shiny application in R to present the prediction results interactively.

Discussion

We have described the protocol for developing a prediction model for OAB. To our knowledge, this is the first model to predict new-onset OAB based on a large-scale prospective cohort in the general population setting. Our prediction models have a large sample size and will incorporate various predictive variables based on previous studies and expert opinions. Moreover, we will develop a user-friendly web-based application to visualize the results of the prediction model. This may be very useful not only to healthcare providers but also to the general population, in interpreting and understanding the results. If we can develop an accurate prediction model for OAB and make it widely available through a web app, we will be able to detect high risk populations and thus intervene at an early stage, which may improve individual HRQOL and decrease the societal health care expenditure.

There are some limitations in this study. First, there may be a selection bias in the sample because the study participants were recruited not by random sampling but on a voluntary basis. However, compared with the previous study using randomly sampled Japanese population [24], Nagahama cohort showed similar prevalence of OAB [4], which may indicate absence of potential selection bias. Second, we will not be able to perform an external validation using an independent cohort, therefore we will not evaluate the general applicability of the models. Future studies will be necessary to demonstrate the external validity of the models with another cohort data.

As a future perspective, prediction models of incident OAB will need to be externally validated and there should be an investigation of their impact in clinical practice [25]. Our models will be developed by general population data and predictors of Model1 will include only self-reported questionnaires. This study aims to develop a model that is easy to use in the general population setting, and thus easy validate externally.

Abbreviations

BMI: Body mass index; BNP: B-type natriuretic peptide; DCA: Decision curve analysis; eGFR: The estimated glomerular filtration rate; HRQOL: Health-related quality of life; OAB: Overactive bladder; OABSS: OAB symptom score; OSA: Obstructive sleep apnea; PCa: Prostate cancer; PSA: Prostate specific antigen; TRIPOD: Transparent Reporting of a Multivariable Prediction Model for Individual Prognosis or Diagnosis.

Acknowledgements

We are extremely grateful to the Nagahama City Office and non-profit organization Zeroji Club for their help in performing the Nagahama Study. The Nagahama Study group executive committee is composed of the following individuals: Yasuharu Tabara, Takahisa Kawaguchi, Kazuya Setoh, Yoshimitsu Takahashi, Shinji Kosugi, Takeo Nakayama, and Fumihiko Matsuda from the Center for Genomic Medicine, Kyoto University Graduate School of Medicine (Ya.T, T.K., K.S., F.M.); and the Department of Health Informatics (Yo.T, T.N.) and, Department of Medical Ethics and Medical Genetics (S.K.), Kyoto University School of Public Health.

Authors' contributions

All authors contributed to the conception and conduct of this clinical trial. OO is the principal investigator of this study protocol. SF, YL, TY, SA, TAF, OE and OO designed the overall framework of the trial and KS, YT, HN, KY and FM helped with implementation. SF, YL, TAF and OE drafted the manuscript, and all co-authors read it and provided critical comments. All authors read and approved the final manuscript.

Author details

[1]Department of Urology, Faculty of Medicine, Kyoto University Graduate School of Medicine, 54 Shogoinkawahara-cho, Sakyo-ku, Kyoto 606-8507, Japan. [2]Department of Health Promotion and Human Behavior, Kyoto University School of Public Health, Kyoto, Japan. [3]Center for Innovative Research for Communities and Clinical Excellence (CiRC2LE), Fukushima Medical University, Fukushima City, Fukushima, Japan. [4]Department of Healthcare Epidemiology, Kyoto University Graduate School of Medicine and School of Public Health, Kyoto, Japan. [5]Center for Genomic Medicine, Faculty of Medicine, Kyoto University Graduate School of Medicine, Kyoto, Japan. [6]Department of Urology, University of Tsukuba, Ibaraki, Japan. [7]Department of Urology, Shizuoka General Hospital, Shizuoka, Japan. [8]Institute of Social and Preventive Medicine, University of Bern, Bern, Switzerland. [9]Department of Psychiatry, University of Oxford, Oxford, UK.

References

1. Abrams P, Cardozo L, Fall M, Griffiths D, Rosier P, Ulmsten U, et al. The standardisation of terminology of lower urinary tract function: report from the Standardisation Sub-committee of the International Continence Society. Neurourol Urodyn. 2002;21:167–78. https://doi.org/10.1016/S0090-4295(02)02243-4.
2. Irwin DE, Milsom I, Hunskaar S, Reilly K, Kopp Z, Herschorn S, et al. Population-based survey of urinary incontinence, overactive bladder, and other lower urinary tract symptoms in five countries: results of the EPIC Study. Eur Urol. 2006;50:1306–15.
3. Milsom I, Abrams P, Cardozo L, Roberts RG, Thüroff J, Wein AJ. How widespread are the symptoms of an overactive bladder and how are they managed? A population-based prevalence study. BJU Int. 2001;87:760–6. https://doi.org/10.1046/j.1464-410X.2001.02228.x.
4. Funada S, Kawaguchi T, Terada N, Negoro H, Tabara Y, Kosugi S, et al. Cross-sectional epidemiological analysis of the Nagahama study for correlates of overactive bladder: genetic and environmental considerations. J Urol. 2018;199:774–8. https://doi.org/10.1016/j.juro.2017.09.146.
5. Vaughan CP, Johnson TM, Ala-Lipasti MA, Cartwright R, Tammela TLJ, Taari K, et al. The prevalence of clinically meaningful overactive bladder: bother and quality of life results from the population-based FINNO study. Eur Urol. 2011;59:629–36. https://doi.org/10.1016/j.eururo.2011.01.031.
6. Irwin DE, Kopp ZS, Agatep B, Milsom I, Abrams P. Worldwide prevalence estimates of lower urinary tract symptoms, overactive bladder, urinary incontinence and bladder outlet obstruction. BJU Int. 2011;108:1132–8. https://doi.org/10.1111/j.1464-410X.2010.09993.x.
7. Moons KGM, Altman DG, Reitsma JB, Ioannidis JPA, Macaskill P, Steyerberg EW, et al. Transparent reporting of a multivariable prediction model for individual prognosis or diagnosis (TRIPOD): explanation and elaboration. Ann Intern Med. 2015;162:W1-73.
8. Prevention of Bladder Control Problems (Urinary Incontinence) & Bladder Health | NIDDK. https://www.niddk.nih.gov/health-information/urologic-diseases/bladder-control-problems/prevention. Accessed 12 Jan 2021.
9. Funada S, Tabara Y, Negoro H, Akamatsu S, Yoshino T, Yoshimura K, et al. Longitudinal analysis of bidirectional relationships between nocturia and depressive symptoms: the Nagahama Study. J Urol. 2020;203:984–90. https://doi.org/10.1097/JU.0000000000000683.
10. Funada S, Tabara Y, Setoh K, Negoro H, Akamatsu S, Yoshino T, et al. Impact of nocturia on mortality: the Nagahama Study. J Urol. 2020;204:996–1002. https://doi.org/10.1097/JU.0000000000001138.
11. Homma Y, Yoshida M, Seki N, Yokoyama O, Kakizaki H, Gotoh M, et al. Symptom assessment tool for overactive bladder syndrome-overactive bladder symptom score. Urology. 2006;68:318–23.
12. Riley RD, Snell KIE, Ensor J, Burke DL, Harrell FE, Moons KGM, et al. Minimum sample size for developing a multivariable prediction model: PART II—binary and time-to-event outcomes. Stat Med. 2019;38:1276–96.
13. Dallosso HM, McGrother CW, Matthews RJ, Donaldson MMK. The association of diet and other lifestyle factors with overactive bladder and stress incontinence: a longitudinal study in women. BJU Int. 2003;92:69–77.
14. Link CL, Steers WD, Kusek JW, McKinlay JB. The association of adiposity and overactive bladder appears to differ by gender: results from the Boston area community health survey. J Urol. 2011;185:955–63. https://doi.org/10.1016/j.juro.2010.10.048.
15. Ikeda Y, Nakagawa H, Ohmori-Matsuda K, Hozawa A, Masamune Y, Nishino Y, et al. Risk factors for overactive bladder in the elderly population: a community-based study with face-to-face interview. Int J Urol. 2011;18:212–8. https://doi.org/10.1111/j.1442-2042.2010.02696.x.
16. Ohgaki K, Horiuchi K, Kondo Y. Association between metabolic syndrome and male overactive bladder in a Japanese population based on three different sets of criteria for metabolic syndrome and the Overactive Bladder Symptom Score. Urology. 2012;79:1372–8. https://doi.org/10.1016/j.urology.2012.03.006.
17. Hirayama A, Torimoto K, Mastusita C, Okamoto N, Morikawa M, Tanaka N, et al. Risk factors for new-onset overactive bladder in older subjects: results of the Fujiwara-kyo study. Urology. 2012;80:71–6. https://doi.org/10.1016/j.urology.2012.04.019.
18. Kurita N, Yamazaki S, Fukumori N, Otoshi K, Otani K, Sekiguchi M, et al. Overactive bladder symptom severity is associated with falls in community-dwelling adults: LOHAS study. BMJ Open. 2013;3:e002413.
19. van Buuren S, Groothuis-Oudshoorn K. mice: multivariate imputation by chained equations in R. J Stat Softw. 2011;45:1–67.
20. Rubin DB, Schenker N. Multiple imputation in health-are databases: an overview and some applications. Stat Med. 1991;10:585–98. https://doi.org/10.1002/sim.4780100410.
21. Tibshirani R. Regression shrinkage and selection via the lasso. J R Stat Soc Ser B. 1996;58:267–88.
22. Vickers AJ, Elkin EB. Decision curve analysis: a novel method for evaluating prediction models. Med Decis Mak. 2006;26:565–74. https://doi.org/10.1177/0272989X06295361.
23. Steyerberg EW. Clinical prediction models. New York: Springer New York; 2009. https://doi.org/10.1007/978-0-387-77244-8.
24. Homma Y, Yamaguchi O, Hayashi K. An epidemiological survey of overactive bladder symptoms in Japan. BJU Int. 2005;96:1314–8. https://doi.org/10.1111/j.1464-410X.2005.05835.x.
25. Steyerberg EW, Moons KGM, van der Windt DA, Hayden JA, Perel P, Schroter S, et al. Prognosis Research Strategy (PROGRESS) 3: prognostic model research. PLoS Med. 2013;10:e1001381.

14

Down-regulation LncRNA-SNHG15 contributes to proliferation and invasion of bladder cancer cells

Aldhabi Mokhtar, Chuize Kong*, Zhe Zhang* and Yan Du

Abstract

Objectives: The aim of this study was to investigate the effect of lncRNA-SNHG15 in bladder carcinoma using cell lines experiments and the relationship between clinical characteristics and lncRNA-SNHG15 expression was analyzed.

Methods: Bladder cancer tissues and near-cancer tissues were collected. The real-time PCR (RT-PCR) was used to detect the expression of lncRNA-SNHG15 in tissues and cell lines. The expression of lncRNA-SNHG15 was downregulated by interference (siRNA), as detected by RT-PCR, that was used to determine the efficiency of the interference. CCK-8 and Transwell assays were used to evaluate the effect of lncRNA-SNHG15 on the proliferation and invasion capability of bladder cancer cells. The t-test was used for Statistical analyses, which were carried out using the Statistical Graph pad 8.0.1.224 software.

Result: The expression of lncRNA-SNHG15 was up regulated in 5637, UMUC3 and T24 cell lines compared with corresponding normal controls ($P < 0.05$). Up regulation was positively related to tumor stage ($P = 0.015$). And tumor size ($P = 0.0465$). The down-regulation of lncRNA-SNHG15 with siRNA significantly inhibited UMUC3 and T24 cell proliferation and invasion.

Conclusion: This study showed that lncRNA-SNHG15 is overexpressed in bladder cancer tissues and (5637, UMUC3 T24) cell lines. Up regulation was positively related to tumor stage ($P = 0.015$), and tumor size ($P = 0.0465$). Down-regulation of lncRNA-SNHG15 by siRNA significantly inhibited UMUC3 and T24 cell proliferation and invasion, indicating a potential molecular target for future tumor targeted therapy.

Keywords: Long noncoding RNA, SNHG15, Cell invasion, Cell proliferation, Bladder cancer

Background

Bladder cancer have a higher incidence in urinary malignancies. Because of its susceptibility to recurrence, progression, and metastasis, the current ideal treatment for bladder cancer is a comprehensive including surgery treatment, chemotherapy and Radiation therapy, but the overall effect is limited, and the invasion and metastasis are the main reasons of bladder cancer treatment failure [1]. Primary bladder tumors usually arise from the muscularis and mucosal epithelium, with the latter accounting for approximately 95% of cases, which about 90–95% are urothelial carcinoma. Bladder cancer has the characteristics of Polycentricity and recurrence over time, as well as the biological characteristics of local invasion and metastasis and a high postoperative recurrence rate. 70–80% of bladder cancer patients are initially diagnosed with noninvasive urinary epithelial papilloma. After active surgery and bladder perfusion treatment, 50% of patients are still diagnosed with non-invasive urinary papilloma.

*Correspondence: kongchuize_cmu@sina.cn; zhangzhe@cmu1h.com
Department of Urology, The First Hospital of China Medical University, 155 Nanjing North Street, Shenyang, Liaoning 110001, P.R. China

70% of the patients relapse within 5 years, and 10–30% of patients develop invasive urothelial cancer [2]. Following the sequencing of the human genome, it was found that the proportion of protein-coding genes in the entire human genome sequence was less than 3%, and that more than 80% of the sequences were frequently transcribed into RNA without protein-coding functions. Non-coding RNA is RNA that does not have protein-coding functions. Non-coding RNA is actually a complex network of gene expression regulation that plays a key role in regulating many important biological functions of cancer cells. It is classified into two types based on the length of the sequence: short non-coding RNA and long non-coding RNA. Long non-coding RNA (lncRNA) is a class of transcripts with more than 200 nucleotides, and those without protein-coding functions are mostly transcribed by polymerase II [3]. Although lncRNA cannot be translated into protein, it has effects on life activities such as gene transcription regulation, proteins post-translational modification, and epigenetic regulation of gene expression. It is closely related to pathophysiological changes, disease diagnosis and treatment [4]. LncRNA-SNHG15, an intergenic lncRNA found on chromosome 7p13, belongs to a non-coding class of RNAs that includes snoRNAs [5]. Increasingly, studies show that LncRNA-SNHG15 has abnormally expression in many types of tumors, such as renal cancer [6], lung cancer [7], colorectal carcinoma [8], prostate cancer [9]. Long non-coding RNASNHG 15 promotes cell proliferation in glioma microvascular endothelial cells [10], and also contributes to osteosarcoma cell proliferation, invasion and autophagy [11]. However, the expression and function of lncRNA-SNHG15 in bladder cancer is ambiguous. The aim of this study was to investigate the effect of lncRNA-SNHG15 in bladder carcinoma using cell lines experiments and the relationship between clinical characteristics and lncRNA-SNHG15 expression was analyzed. We investigated the role of lncRNA-SNHG15 in bladder carcinoma using data and cells line PCR, cck-8, and other experimental techniques to detect the expression of lncRNA-SNHG15 in bladder cancer tissues and cells line. The results showed that overexpression of lncRNA-SNHG15 was an associated molecular change in bladder carcinoma tissues, and cell lines (5637, UMUC3, T24). As a result, the effects of aberrant lncRNA-SNHG15 expression on the biological behavior of UMUC3 and T24 cell lines were also investigated. The results provided novel insights into the function and mechanisms of lncRNA-SNHG15 bladder carcinoma pathogenesis, and lncRNA-SNHG15 was identified as a potential therapeutic target for cancer intervention.

Methods

Cell lines

The human bladder cancer cell lines (5637, UMUC3, J82, T24) and the normal bladder epithelial SV-HUC-1 cell line (SV-HUC-1) were obtained from the Chinese Academy of Sciences, Type Culture Collection Cell Bank (Shanghai, China). The cells (SV-HUC-1) were cultured in Ham's F12 medium (Sigma, St. Louis, MO, USA). Fetal bovine serum (FBS),RNA extraction reagent Trizol and reverse transcription kit were purchased from japan (TaKaRa Co. Tokyo Japan), lncRNA-SNHG15interference RNA (siRNA lncRNA-SNHG15), and si-NC were obtained from Shanghai Jima Co(Shanghai, China), CCK-8 reagent were purchased from the Invitrogen Corporation (Carlsbad, CA, USA), Transwell chamber from the BD Biosciences (Franklin Lakes, NJ, USA).

Tissue samples

Between March and September 2018, 30 patients were diagnosed with bladder cancer and underwent surgical resection at the First Affiliated Hospital of China Medical University (Shenyang, China). Surgical bladder cancer tissues and matched near-cancer tissues were collected. The Ethics Committee on Human Research of China Medical University's First Affiliated Hospital approved the current study, and all patients provided written informed consent. Tissue samples were collected and stored at 80 °C before being used.

Real-time PCR

(1) Design the primer sequence as follows:

Reverse primer: ACCTGTACTCCGTACTCCGT.
Forward primer: GGCGGTGGATGACTAGACTG.

In addition, we use the Takara fluorescence quantitative PCR kit to set up 10 reaction systems using the TRIZOL method. Fill a 96-well plate with the above 10-L reaction system. Each sample had three auxiliary. When determining the expression level of LncRNA-snhg15, GAPDH was used as an inner. On a real-time quantitative PCR instrument, the green dye method was used to assess the expression of LncRNA-snhg15 in bladder cancer tissues and matched adjacent tissues, with GAPDH serving as an internal reference. Each sample was run at least three times, and the average CT value was calculated and analyzed.

Cell transfection assay

Cells were cultured in RPMI1640 medium containing, 10% FBS, placed in 5% CO2 incubator at 37 °C. When the cells were in the logarithmic growth phase, at a density of about 40% in 6-well plates. Each well received 5 μL Lipofectamine 2000 and 200 pmol siRNA lncRNA-SNHG15 mixture.

The siRNA sequence forLncRNA-SNHG15 was: GGA UUUAAAUAUGUGAAAA.

Cell proliferation by cck-8 assay

Cells were plant seeds in 96-well plates at a thickness 2×10^3 cells/well were transfected with SNHG15 NC siRNAs for 72 h in situ. Cell proliferation was evaluated using Cell Counting Kit-8 (CCK-8) assay (Dojindo Molecular Technologies, Inc., Shanghai, China) conforming to the manufacturer's protocol. The decadic was projected at 450 nm each 24 h utilizing a plate reader (Model 680; Bio-Rad Laboratories, Inc., Watford, UK).

Cell invasion with transwell assay

A Transwell chambers with a8-μm matrix gel coating hole is inserted into the 24 hole plate. Transwell kit without matrix gel was used for invasive test. After transfection of snhg15 and NC siRNAs for 72 h, the cells were trypsinized and suspended in RPMI-1640 containing 1% FBS. Subsequently, 0.2 ml of cell suspension (1 × 104/ml) was added to the upper cavity and 0.6 ml of RPMI-1640 containing FBS was added to the lower cavity. After incubation at 37 ℃ for 24 h, the remaining cells in the upper cavity were removed. The cells moving to the lower side were fixed with 4% paraformaldehyde for 10 min and stained with 1.0% crystal violet at room temperature for 10 min. The image was taken with EVOS™ XL core imaging system (Invitrogen; Thermo Fisher Scientific, Inc.).

Statistics

Statistical analyses were performed using the Statistical Graph pad 8.0.1.224 software, and the t-test was used.

Results

The expressions of lncRNA-SNHG15 in bladder cancer tissues and its relationship to clinical features

Interestingly, qRT-PCR results revealed that lncRNA-SNHG15 expression was higher in bladder cancer tissues than in adjacent tissues (*p* 0.05, Fig. 1a). The expression of lncRNA-SNHG15 is associated with clinical and pathological features. We investigated the relationship between increased lncRNA-SNHG15 expression levels and clinical characteristics in 30 bladder cancer cases to see if lncRNA-SNHG15 expression is related to clinical features. LncRNA-SNHG15 up-regulation was positively correlated with tumor stage ($P = 0.015$) and tumor size ($P = 0.0465$). However, lncRNA-SNHG15 expression levels were not related to other factors such as patient age, gender, tumor number, or nodal invasion. (See Table 1) This finding also suggested that lncRNA-SNHG15 was an important molecule in the development of bladder cancer.

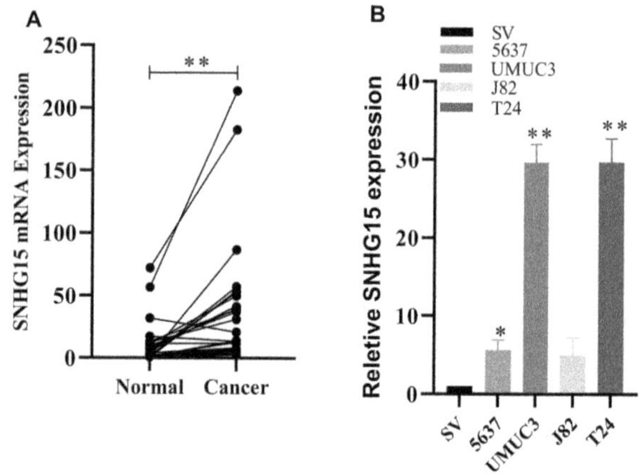

Fig. 1 Using the paired t test, $*P < 0.05$, LncRNA-SNHG15 Expression was found to be higher in bladder cancer tissues. LncRNA-SNHG15 Was up regulated in the bladder cancer cell lines. By RT-PCR, the relative Expression of LncRNA-SNHG15 was detected in tumor cells lines (5637, UMUC3, T24)and compared with the normal cell line (SV-HUC1) by RT-PCR $*P < (0.05)$

Table 1 The relationship between the expression of lncrna-snhg15 and clinical statistics

Factor	No	LncRNA-SNHG15		*p*
		High	low	
Total	30	19	11	
Gender				
Male	24	15	9	0.999
Female	6	4	2	
Age (year)				
≥ 50	25	17	8	0.3268
< 50	5	2	3	
Tumor size (cm)				
≥ 3	19	15	4	*0.0465
< 3	11	4	7	
Tumor stage				
Ta & T1	9	16	4	*0.015
≥ T2	21	3	7	

The expression level of LncRNA-SNHG15 was related to tumor size ($P = *0.0465$), degree of immersion ($P = *0.015$), metastases, but not related to gender and age

The effect of lncRNA-SNHG15 on bladder cancer cell proliferation, invasion and metastasis

The results of qRT-PCR showed that the expression of lncRNA-SNHG15 in bladder cancer (5637, UMUC3, T24) cell lines was higher than that in normal bladder epithelial (SV-HUC-1) cell line ($p<0.05$; Fig. 1b). To investigate the function of lncRNA-SNHG15, a siRNA targeting lncRNA-SNHG15 was transfected into UMUC3 and T24 cells. RT-qPCR revealed that lncRNA-SNHG15 was significantly downregulated 48 h after transfection of siRNA in the bladder cancer UMUC3 and T24 cell lines compared to the control group ($p<0.05$; Fig. 2). **CCK-8 assays** showed that siRNA lncRNA-SNHG15 could inhibit the proliferation of lncRNA-SNHG15 in bladder cancer bladder cancer UMUC3 and T24 cell lines ($p<0.05$; Fig. 3). In addition, a Transwell invasion assay was also used to examine the effect of lncRNA-SNHG15 on the migration capacity of UMUC3 and T24 cells. According to the Transwell invasion assay, down-regulation of lncRNA-SNHG15 expression significantly inhibits the invasion of bladder cancer (UMUC3 and T24) cell lines ($p<0.05$, Fig. 4).

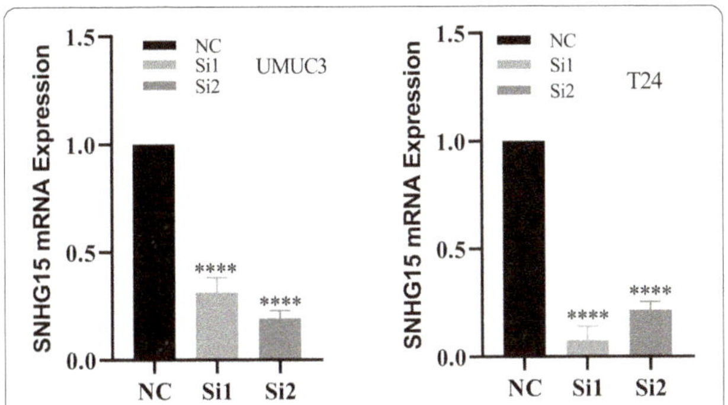

Fig. 2 (T24, UMUC3) Down regulation of LncRNA-SNHG15bysi RNA*$P<0.05$, compared to B with si-NC

Discussion

According to Antoni et al. reported that an estimated 430.000 new cases of bladder cancer were diagnosed in 2012, making bladder cancer the ninth most common cancer worldwide [12]. The 5-year recurrence-free survival rate for highly localized invasive bladder cancer after a radical cystectomy ranges between 62 and 89% [13]. Emerging evidence have suggests that lncRNAs act as oncogenic or suppressor genes in a variety of cancers, regulating transcription and post-transcription [14]. The underlying mechanism that regulates development of bladder cancer is largely unknown. The development of novel molecular biomarkers for the diagnosis and prognosis of bladder cancer is an urgent requirement. Long non-coding RNAs (long ncRNAs, lncRNA) are a type of RNA, defined as being transcripts with lengths exceeding 200 nucleotides that are not translated into protein. It is considered a byproduct of RNA transcription, and even "noise" in the transcription process of human genes, because it does not participate in protein coding and has no biological functions [15]. However, lately research found that LncRNA participates in the regulation of multiple signal pathways in cells through chromosome modification, transcription, and interference. Our team Du [6], has found that LncRNA-SNHG15 is highly expressed in renal cancer tissues, which is closely related to the proliferation, apoptosis, invasion and migration of renal cancer. The present study explored the expression of LncRNA-SNHG15 in bladder urothelial carcinoma using clinical characteristics in the 30 bladder cancer cases to determine whether and cell experiments. The results demonstrated that the expression was apparently localized in the adjacent tissues. The results show that the high expression of LncRNA-SNHG15, its effect the tumor malignant, more aggressive, strong invasion ability, and the possibility of recurrence after the surgery. In order to study the potential effect of LncRNA-SNHG15 on bladder cancer cell lines, In vitro cell experiments

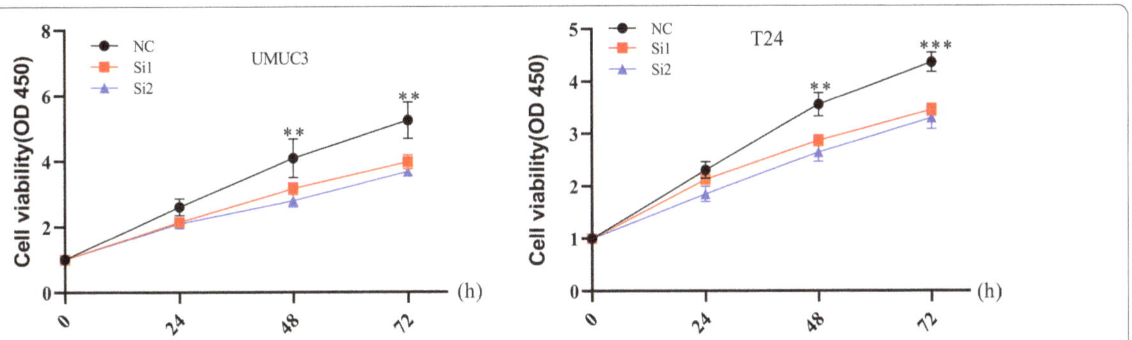

Fig. 3 TheCCK-8 assay was used performed to detect cell proliferation differences between si-NC and si-LncRNA-SNHG15*$P<0.05$, when compared with si-NC

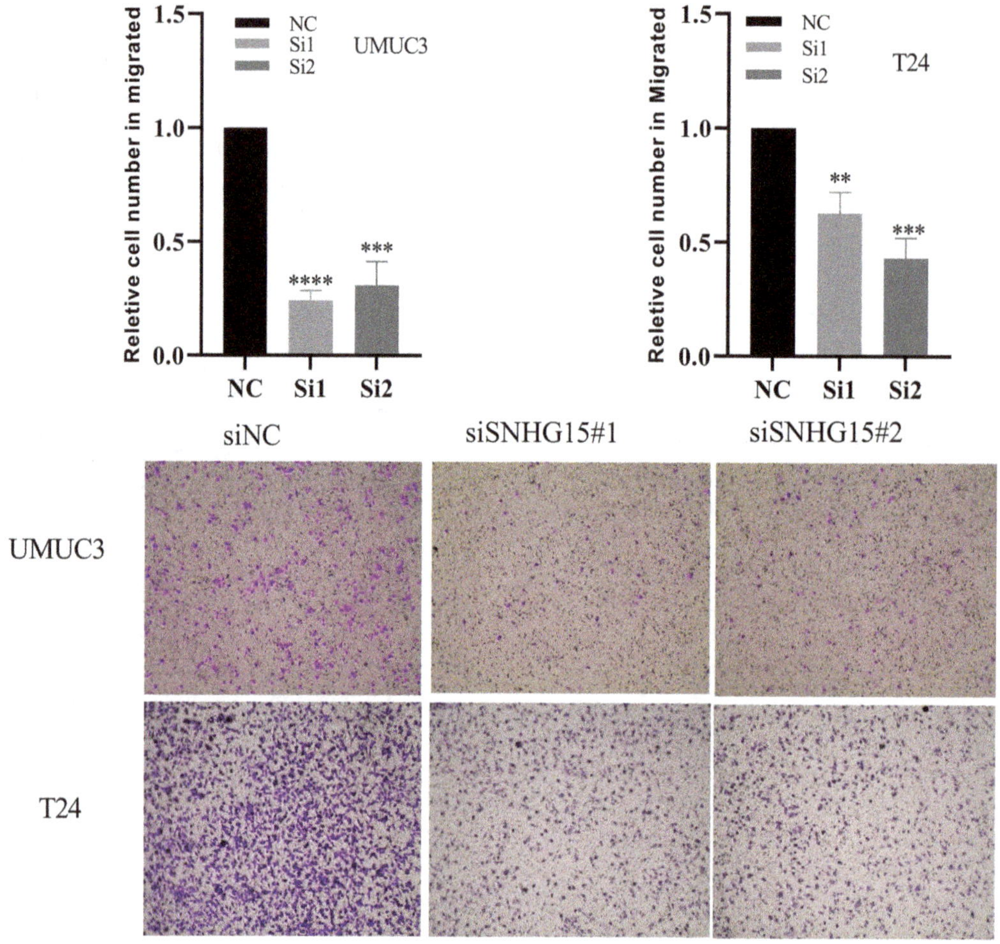

Fig. 4 Down-regulating the expression of LncRNA-SNHG15 can significantly inhibit the invasiveness of bladder cancer cells

in this study showed that the expression of LncRNA-SNHG15 in bladder cancer cells was significantly up-regulated in bladder cancer (5637, UMUC3,T24) cell lines. Transfection of specific si-RNA LncRNA-SNHG15 can inhibit the expression of LncRNA-SNHG15 in bladder cancer UMUC3, T24 cell lines. The data from the present study implied that LncRNA-SNHG15 distributed in the nucleus may serve its role by regulating the expression level of si-RNA. However, the underlying mechanisms require additional investigation. In summary, the present study demonstrated that LncRNA-SNHG15 has potential as a clinically promising biomarker for bladder urothelial carcinoma. LncRNA-SNHG15 regulated the proliferation and migration of 5637, UMUC3 and T24 cells, and these data may provide novel insights into molecular cancer therapy. We propose the following additional research on in vitro binding experiments: the p65 recombinant protein and snhg15 were co-incubated in vitro for an in vitro binding experiment to investigate the p65 functional region binding to snhg15.

Conclusion

In summary, this is the first study to investigate the lncRNA-SNHG15 in bladder carcinoma. This study discovered that lncRNASNHG15 is overexpressed in bladder cancer tissues and cells. Down regulation of lncRNA-SNHG15 can inhibit bladder cancer cell proliferation and invasion, making it a potential molecular target for future tumor targeted therapy. Certainly, additional potential functions and mechanisms must be investigated.

Abbreviations

FBS: fetal bovine serum; LncRNA: long non-coding RNA; miRNA: microRNA; PBS: phosphate-buffered saline; RT-PCR: real-time PCR; SNHG15: small nucleolar RNA host gene 15; Bcc: bladder cell; RPMI-1640: Roswell Park Memorial Institute; cck-8 assay: cell counting kit-8-cell proliferation and cytotoxicity assay; NC: normal cell.

Acknowledgements

Not applicable.

Authors' contributions

Z.Z. and C.K. conceived and supervised the study. A.M. and Y.D. performed the experiments, analyzed the experimental data. A.M. wrote the manuscript. "All authors made substantial contributions to conception and design, acquisition of data, or analysis and interpretation of data; took part in drafting the article or revising it critically for important intellectual content; agreed to submit to the current journal; gave final approval of the version to be published; and agree to be accountable for all aspects of the work". All authors read and approved the final manuscript.

References

1. Funt SA, Rosenberg JE. Systemic, perioperative management of muscle-invasive bladder cancer and future horizons. Nat Rev Clin Oncol. 2017;14(4):221–34.
2. Jacobs BL, Lee CT, Montie JE. Bladder cancer in 2010: how far have we come. CA Cancer J Clin. 2010;60(4):244–72.
3. Esteller M. Non-coding RNAs in human disease. Nat Rev Genet. 2011;12(12):861–74.
4. Orom UA, Derrien T, Beringer M, et al. Long noncoding RNAs with enhancer-like function in human cells. Cell. 2010;143(1):46–58.
5. Shen Y, Liu S, Fan J, et al. Nuclear retention of the lncRNA SNHG1 by doxorubicin attenuates hnRNPC-p53 protein interactions. EMBO Rep. 2017;18(4):536–48. https://doi.org/10.15252/embr.201643139.
6. Du Y, Kong C, et al. Knockdown of SNHG15 suppresses renal cell carcinoma proliferation and EMT by regulating the NF-κB signaling pathway. Int J Oncol. 2018;53:384–94.
7. Cui HX, Zhang MY, Liu K, et al. LncRNA SNHG15 promotes proliferation and migration of lung cancer via targeting microRNA-211-3p. Eur Rev Med Pharmacol Sci. 2018;22:6838–44.
8. Sun X, Bai Y, Yang C, et al. Long noncoding RNA SNHG15 enhances the development of colorectal carcinoma via functioning as a ceRNA through miR-141/SIRT1/Wnt/β-catenin. Artif Cells Nanomed Biotechnol. 2019;47(1):2536–44.
9. Zhang Y, Zhang D, et al. LncRNA SNHG15 acts as an oncogene in prostate cancer by regulating miR-338-3p/FKBP1A axis. Gene. 2019;705(15):44–50.
10. Ma Y, Xue Y, et al. SNHG15 affects the growth of glioma microvascular endothelial cells by negatively regulating miR-153. Oncol Rep. 2017;38:3265–77.
11. Liu K, Hou Y, et al. LncRNA SNHG15 contributes to proliferation, invasion and autophagy in osteosarcoma cells by sponging miR-141. J Biomed Sci. 2017;24:1–11.
12. Antoni S, Ferlay J, Soerjomataram I, Znaor A, Jemal A, Bray F. Bladder cancer incidence and mortality: a global overview and recent trends. Eur Urol. 2017;71:96–108.
13. Stein JP, Lieskovsky G, Cote R, Groshen S, Feng AC, Boyd S, Skinner E, Bochner B, Thangathurai D, Mikhail M, et al. Radical cystectomy in the treatment of invasive bladder cancer: long-term results in 1,054 patients. J Clin Oncol. 2001;19:666–75.
14. Guo W, et al. The coexpression of multi-immune inhibitory receptors on T lymphocytes in primary non-small-cell lung cancer. Drug Des Dev Ther. 2017;11:3367–76.
15. Li S, Yu Z, et al. The YAP1 oncogene contributes to bladder cancer cell proliferation and migration by regulating the H19 long noncoding RNA. Urol Oncol. 2015;33(10):427.e1-10.

15

Incidental diagnosis of nonfunctional bladder paraganglioma

Xi Tu[1†], Neng Zhang[1†], Xiyao Zhuang[2], Shulian Chen[1] and Xu Luo[1*]

Abstract

Background: Nonfunctional bladder paragangliomas is a rare urological disease. It may present clinical, radiology and pathological features similar to bladder cancer, Only scarce reports have been reported. Urologist must identify this generally benign neuroendocrine neoplasm to avoid misdiagnosis.

Case presentation: A 62-year-old female presented the outpatient department of our hospital with the symptoms of stomachache, frequent micturition, and urination pain for 20 days. Diagnosed with high blood pressure 1 year ago, administered Amlodipine besylate tablets 5 mg po qd occasionally, did not check blood pressure; denied any tumor observation in the family history. Color ultrasound of the urinary system showed a 38 mm × 34 mm hypoechoic mass on the right side of the bladder, CDFI: in the masses, blood supply was sufficient. Cystoscope showed bladder occupying lesion. Biopsy diagnosis: papillary polypoid cystitis was suspected as a malignant change (Fig. 3a). Then, the patient was admitted to our urological department. Further, computer tomography urography considered bladder cancer. Cystoscopy and biopsy failed to define the nature of the lesions in our outpatient department, which prompted a transurethral resection of the bladder tumor. histopathological and immunohistochemical results were diagnosed as bladder paragangliomas. For the reason, the tumor was removed by partial resection of the bladder. The postoperative recovery and follow-up were uneventful.

Conclusions: Nonfunctional bladder paragangliomas are occasionally found on imaging studies with the symptoms of urinary tract infection or/and intermittent painless hematuria. It may present clinical, radiology and pathological features similar to bladder cancer, so knowledge of this generally benign neuroendocrine neoplasm is of great importance to avoid misdiagnosis. It should be accompanied by the clinical and pathological characteristics of the patient and image changes. Partial resection of the bladder can effectively treat this disease.

Keywords: Paraganglioma, Bladder, Diagnosis, Treatment

Background

Paraganglioma of the urinary bladder (PUB) is a rare disease, accounting for 0.06% of all bladder tumors [1]. The PUB symptoms are correlated with over secretion of catecholamine or tumor impact. It is classified into functional and non-functional. Functional PUB usually exhibits symptoms such as headache, syncope, palpitation, and sweating. However, 10–15% of these tumors are nonfunctional and in 10%, hormone activity does not manifest clinically [2]. Non-functional PUB might have symptoms such as frequency and urgency of urination, intermittent painless whole course gross hematuria, and lumbar discomfort. In addition, histological characteristics such as the death of focal transparent cells and burnt

*Correspondence: 657167473@qq.com
†Xi Tu and Neng Zhang have contributed equally to this work
[1] Department of Urology, Affiliated Hospital of Zunyi Medical University, Zunyi 563000, Guizhou, China
Full list of author information is available at the end of the article

muscle infiltration might be easily diagnosed as bladder cancer [3]. The present study reported a case of a female patient who underwent bladder tumor resections two times due to the confusion of bladder cancer and whose histopathological and immunohistochemical results confirmed paraganglioma.

Case presentation

Chief complaints

A 62-year-old female presented the outpatient department of our hospital with the symptoms of stomachache, frequent micturition, and urination pain.

History of present illness

Patient's symptoms started 20 days ago, She had no symptoms such as lumbago, dizziness, headache, palpitation, chest tightness, nausea, vomiting, fever, chills, or other symptoms.

History of past illness

The patient was diagnosed with high blood pressure 1 year ago, administered Amlodipine besylate tablets 5 mg po qd occasionally, did not check blood pressure; terminal gross hematuria was observed once 4 months ago, the symptom disappeared, and no treatment was administered; denied any tumor observation in the family history.

Physical examination

After hospitalization, the patient's temperature was 36.5 ℃, 80 pulses/min, 20 breathing times/min, blood pressure was 159/108 mmHg and oxygen saturation in room air was 98%. no bulge, pressure pain or percussion pain in either of the kidney area; no pressure or percussion pain in both ways of the ureteral region; no bulge in the bladder area but light pressure-induced pain.

Supplementary examination

Fasting venous blood glucose was 8.34 mmol/L, and other indexes were normal. Chest X-ray showed mild interstitial changes in both lungs, ECG: 102 times/min. Color ultrasound of the urinary system showed a 38 mm × 34 mm hypoechoic mass on the right side of the bladder with an uneven surface and a large bottom; multiple strong echo masses were observed. CDFI: in the masses, blood supply was sufficient. Cystoscope showed bladder occupying lesion (Fig. 1). Biopsy diagnosis: papillary polypoid cystitis was suspected as a malignant change (Fig. 3a). Computer tomography urography(CTU) considered bladder cancer (Fig. 2).

Diagnosis and treatment process

Cystoscopy and biopsy failed to define the nature of the lesions. the urethral bladder tumor biopsy was performed. During the operation, the right bladder wall adjacent to the neck of the bladder showed vegetations with a size of about 4.5 cm × 4.5 cm, with a broad base, easy bleeding, and local surface tissue ulceration. The tumor was found to be hard and calcified during electrotomy. The histopathological studies revealed a large number of tumor cells proliferated with abundant cytoplasm, tumor cells were arranged in small nests or strips, and the blood sinusoids between tumor cells were abundant (Fig. 3b). The immunohistochemical study was positive for the expression for CD56, chromogranin A, neuron specific enolase and synaptophysin. Immunostaining for the polyclonal S-100 protein showed a sustentacular pattern, thereby confirming paraganglioma. Therefore, another operation was needed. The patient regularly administered phenoxybenzamine 10 mg po tid and metformin tablets 0.5 g po tid for 2 weeks. Before the operation, laboratory workup revealed elevated plasma renin activity to 8642.76 pg/mL, elevated angiotensin I to 16113.5 pg/mL, and an elevated angiotensin II level of 252.91 pg/mL. Partial resection of the bladder was conducted, and the focus was removed. After the operation, the patient stopped using phenoxybenzamine and continued with metformin tablets. Consecutively, blood pressure and blood sugar were monitored. the plasma renin activity, angiotensin I and angiotensin II were within normal range (56.83 pg/mL, 447.46 pg/mL, 79.04 pg/mL, respectively). When the

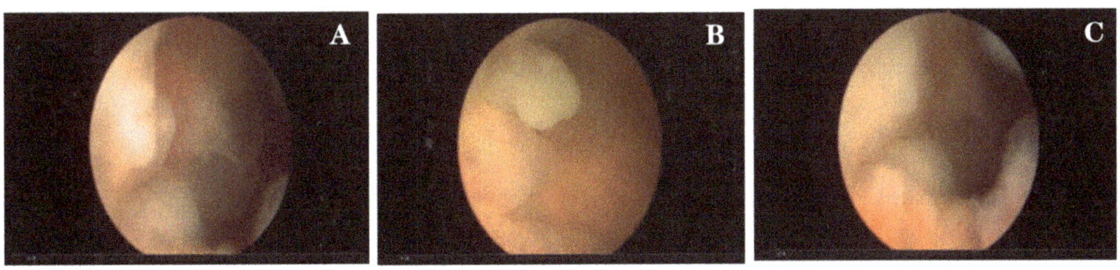

Fig. 1 Cystoscope. **a**, **b** Large tumor was observed in the right side of the bladder; a large number of growing follicles were observed; dead tissue and broad-based were seen; **c** the bottom of the tumor continued to the entrance of the right side

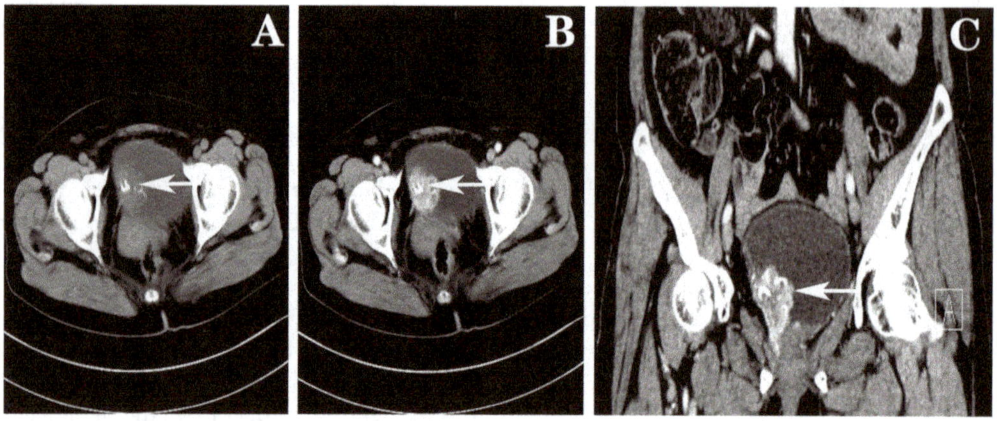

Fig. 2 CTU. **a** This images showed 34 mm × 37 mm low-density mass on the right side of the bladder with clear edges, and Calcium density shadow was seen inside; **b**, **c** the enhancement scanning was uneven

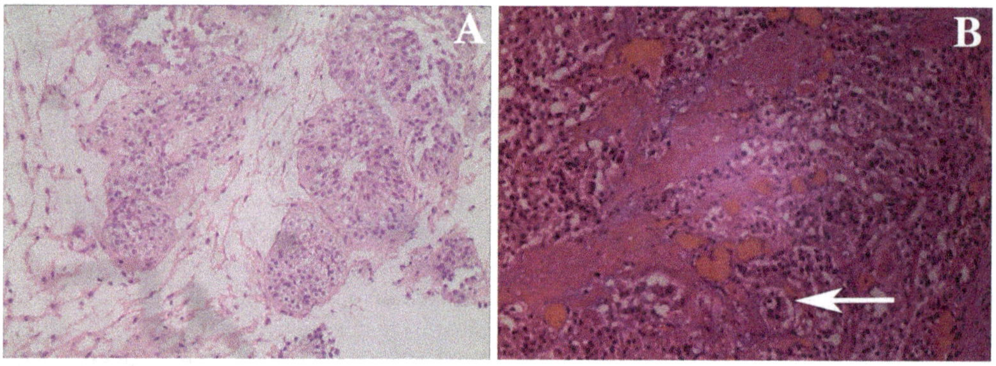

Fig. 3 Pathology. **a** This image showed papillary polypoid cystitis; **b** arrow showed tumor cells were arranged in small nests, the interstitial blood sinuses were also abundant

patient was ready to leave the hospital, her blood pressure was 128/86 mmHg, the blood sugar was 7.0–9.4 mmol/L, and the symptoms had improved.

Follow-up

Three and six months after the operation, no discomfort was reported. Blood sugar and blood pressure were at normal levels. No obvious abnormality was detected by cystoscopy. However, The patient was advised regular reexamination and lifelong follow-up, with respect to blood pressure, blood glucose, urinary catecholamine, ultrasound, CT, and cystoscopy.

Discussion and conclusion

PUB mainly occurs in young Caucasians, aged 20-40-years-old, with a male to female ratio of 1:3, mostly single, and common in the anterior wall, posterior wall, and top of the bladder. The triangle was rare [1, 4]. The cause of the disease was unknown. In the case of a familial paraganglioma, it may be related to the mutation in the succinate dehydrogenase coding gene [5]. Most of the PUB was located in the submucous or muscular layer of the bladder wall; about 37% could penetrate the whole bladder wall or the pelvic wall. In this case, the lesion is mainly located on the right lower wall of the bladder, and the tumor invades the lower part of the right ureter, causing the upper urinary tract to dilate and accumulate. The patient only showed symptoms of abdominal pain, frequent urination, and painful urination, and did not show symptoms of syncope, headache, palpitations, or sweating caused by increased catecholamine secretion. So it was considered non-functional bladder paraganglioma.

Color ultrasound of the urinary system is the first line of investigative modality to detect the silent as well as functioning ectopic lesions. Doppler demonstrates the vascular nature of these tumors, which was also observed in our case. the tumor showed a low-density shadow mass with clear edge, calcium density shadow and uneven enhancement on CT. On magnetic resonance imaging (MRI), these tumors are markedly hyperintense on T2-weighted (T2W) images. In addition to the monitoring of catecholamine or its metabolites, echocardiography, CT, magnetic resonance imaging (MRI), and radiotracer molecular imaging in the clinical suspicion of PUB is essential. The functional imaging technology of the tracer molecular may confirm that the tumor is paraganglioma (such as $^{123/131}$I-MIBG, ^{18} F-FDA, ^{18} F-FDG, ^{18} F-FDOPA, ^{11} C-ephedrine, ^{11} C-hydroxyethyl ephedra alkali.) [5]. The histological characteristics of paraganglioma are similar to those of bladder cancer. Paragangliomas commonly arise in the deep layers of the bladder wall, so when they develop they affect their own muscle layer, making it even more difficult to make the differential diagnosis with a tendency to diagnose urothelial carcinoma. Histologically, the paraganglioma is usually composed of cells with a "zellballen" pattern with abundant eosinophilic or amphophilic cytoplasm divided by delicate vascular stroma [3]. Biopsy of tumor tissue will confirm diagnosis with diffuse, strong positivity for neuron-specific enolase, synaptophysin, and/or chromogranin [6]. The case in this report was considered to be bladder cancer before the operation because the patient had no typical clinical symptoms related to hypersecretion of catecholamines. In addition, due to the lack of experience in diagnosis and treatment and the lack of in-depth combination with the patient's history of hypertension and high blood sugar after admission, the correct diagnosis was not made initially. In order to clarify the nature of the tumor, transurethral resection of the bladder tumor was carried out. histopathological and immunohistochemical results confirmed paraganglioma.

The PUB is not sensitive to radiotherapy and chemotherapy. The most common treatment is partial cystectomy. Other treatments include transurethral cystectomy and radical cystectomy. The symptoms can be controlled, and low incidence can be achieved by surgical resection. Adequate preoperative preparation can significantly reduce the risk of hypertension and the hazards of operation. In this case, the patient had been regularly taking phenoxybenzamine for 2 weeks. Her blood pressure was stable before, during, and after the operation. The surgical treatment of metastatic pheochromocytoma is rarely effective. Radical bladder surgery, bilateral pelvic lymphadenectomy, radiotherapy, and chemotherapy are feasible for the cases with wide pathological range, impossible bladder preservation, and lymph node metastasis. Reportedly, 76% of the patients with paraganglioma received > 40 Gy of external irradiation, and their clinical symptoms were significantly relieved for at least 1 year or until death [7]. Patients who did not benefit from the operation or local radiotherapy could choose ^{131}I-MIBG and cytotoxic chemotherapy. The study found that MIBG treatment was beneficial to 67% of the patients' biochemical reactions, and 89% of the patients' symptoms were improved [8]. However, the combination of external irradiation and ^{131}I-MIBG has a good effect on the local control and treatment of malignant paraganglioma [7]. Cytotoxic chemotherapy is feasible for patients with paragangliomas that cannot be resected as they progress rapidly or exhibit marked bone metastasis. The most widely used chemotherapy regimens include CVD (cyclophosphamide, vincristine, and dacarbazine). The survival rate of patients with malignant paragangliomas is variable. According to the study population, the overall 5-year survival rate is 35–60% [6].

Nonfunctional bladder paragangliomas are occasionally found on imaging studies with the symptoms of urinary tract infection or/and intermittent painless hematuria. It may present clinical, radiology and pathological features similar to bladder cancer, so knowledge of this generally benign neuroendocrine neoplasm is of great importance to avoid misdiagnosis. In our study, the patient underwent open surgery to remove the tumor completely. The prognosis was good.

Abbreviations

CT: Computed tomography; CDFI: Color doplor flow image; ECG: Electrocardiograph; PUB: Paraganglioma of the urinary bladder; CTU: Computer tomography urography; MIBG: Metaiodobenzylguanidine; MRI: Magnetic resonance imaging; 18F-FDA: 18 F-fluorodopamine; 18F-FDG: 18 F-fluoro-2-deoxy-D-glucose; 18F-FDOPA: 18 F-fluoro-dihydroxyphenylalanine; I-MIBG: Iodine-labeled meta-iodobenzylguanidine; CVD: Cyclophosphamide, vincristine, and dacarbazine.

Acknowledgements

There is no acknowledgment.

Authors' contributions

XT and NZ were the patient's Urologists, reviewed the literature and contributed to manuscript drafting; XYZ reviewed the literature and contributed to manuscript drafting; SLC and XL were responsible for the revision of the manuscript for important intellectual content; All authors read and approved the final manuscript.

Author details

[1]Department of Urology, Affiliated Hospital of Zunyi Medical University, Zunyi 563000, Guizhou, China. [2]Department of Internal Medicine, Chengdu Shuangliu Hospital of Traditional Chinese Medicine, Chengdu, Sichuan, China.

References

1. Kappers MH, van den Meiracker AH, Alwani RA, Kats E, Baggen MG. Paraganglioma of the urinary bladder. Neth J Med. 2008;66:163–5.
2. Sherwani P, Anand R, Narula MK, Siddiqui AA, Aggarwal S. Concurrent nonfunctional paraganglioma of the retroperitoneum and urinary bladder: a case report with literature review. Indian J Radiol Imaging. 2015;25(2):198–201.

3. Spessoto LC, Vasilceac FA, Padilha TL, Gatti M, De Arruda JGF, Pessutti D, et al. Incidental diagnosis of nonfunctional bladder paraganglioma. Urol Case Rep. 2016;4:53–4.
4. Beilan JA, Lawton A, Hajdenberg J, Rosser CJ. Pheochromocytoma of the urinary bladder: a systematic review of the contemporary literature. BMC Urol. 2013;13:22.
5. Malhotra AK, Yan R, Tabeshi R, Nadel H, Tran H, Masterson J. Case—Bladder paraganglioma in a pediatric patient. Can Urol Assoc J. 2018;12(5):108–16.
6. Chaaya G, Morales J, Castiglioni A, Subhani N, Asmar A. Paraganglioma of the urinary bladder: a rare cause of hypertension and urinary tract infections. Am J Med Sci. 2018;355(2):191–4.
7. Fishbein L, Bonner L, Torigian DA, Nathanson KL, Cohen DL, Pryma D, et al. External beam radiation therapy (EBRT) for patients with malignant pheochromocytoma and non-head and -neck paraganglioma: combination with 131I-MIBG. Horm Metab Res. 2012;44(5):405–10.
8. Gedik GK, Hoefnagel CA, Bais E, Olmos RA. 131I-MIBG therapy in metastatic phaeochromocytoma and paraganglioma. Eur J Nucl Med Mol Imaging. 2008;35(4):725–33.

16

Cross-talk and clinical value of m[superscript 6] A regulatory gene in bladder cancer

Ben-zheng Zhou[1], Qin Luo[2] and Ye Zhang[1*]

Abstract

Background: RNA modification is a regulation at the post-transcriptional level. RNA methylation modification accounts for more than 60% of all RNA modifications, and m[superscript 6]A(6-methyladenine) is the most common type of RNA methylation modification on mRNA of higher organisms. The modification level of transcription m[superscript 6]A is dynamically regulated by methyltransferase (reader), binding protein (writer) and demethylase (eraser). Furthermore, m[superscript 6]A methylation has been found to have an impact on tumor initiation and progression through various mechanisms.

Methods: 13 genes related m[superscript 6]A from all the gene expressions in The Cancer Genome Atlas (TCGA) were screened. Gene Ontology (GO) and KEGG analysis were applied to explore the functions of genes identified in study. We clustered the related regulators of m[superscript 6]A into three subgroups with "ConsensusClusterPlus". 13 genes were used for univariate Cox analysis to find genes associated with prognosis, and the risk model was constructed based on lasso regression. According to the median risk score of each patient, the patients were divided into high and low risk groups for survival analysis. The ROC curve evaluates the model. Then the risk group and clinical characteristics were analyzed.

Results: The three subgroups had different clinical characteristics. Our tumor clusters were related to grade, survival status. Moreover, we observed a significantly longer overall survival (OS) in the cluster 1 than the cluster 2 and cluster 3. Three m[superscript 6]A-related genes related to prognosis were used to construct a prognostic risk model. We found age are independent prognostic marker. What's more, risk score can also be an independent prognostic factor.

Conclusion: Revealing the regulation and functional mechanism of cross-talk among m[superscript 6]A writers, erasers, and readers, and determine its role in bladder cancer may help in developing novel and efficient strategies for the diagnosis, prognosis and treatment of bladder cancer.

Keywords: N6-methyladenosine (m[superscript 6]A), RNA modification, Bladder cancer, Prognostic, Clinical feature

Background

RNA methylation has been found in various RNAs including messenger RNA (mRNA) [1, 2], microRNA (miRNA) precursor [3, 4] and long non-coding RNA (lncRNA) [5] transfer RNA [6], ribosomal RNA [7], small nuclear RNA [8].

m[superscript 6]A(6-methyladenine) is the most common type of RNA methylation modification on mRNA of higher organism RNA. M[SUPERSCRIPT 6]A patterns are involved in various aspects of mRNA metabolism including mRNA export, translation, decay and perform an significant function in post-transcriptional regulation of gene expression and protein translation [9].

The m[superscript 6]A patterns involve a series of proteins identified as methyl-transferase (m[superscript 6] A writer), binding proteins (m[superscript 6]A readers) and demethylase (m[superscript 6]A eraser) enzymes of

*Correspondence: 460972083@qq.com
[1] Department of Urology, Xiangyang No.1 People's Hospital, Hubei University of Medicine, Xiangyang, Hubei, People's Republic of China
Full list of author information is available at the end of the article

m[superscript 6]A [10]. Readers such as YTH domain-containing 1 (YTHDC1), YTH domain-containing 1 (YTHDC2), YTH N6-methyl-adenosine RNA binding protein 1 (YTHDF1), YTH N6-methyladenosine RNA binding protein 2 (YTHDF2) and heterogeneous nuclear ribonucleoprotein C (HNRNPC). Writers, composed of methyltransferase-like 3 (METTL3), methyl transferase-like 14 (METTL14), Wilms-tumor associated protein (WTAP), KIAA1429, RNA binding motif protein 15 (RBM15) and zinc finger CCCH domain-containing protein 13 (ZC3H13). Erasers such as fat mass- and obesity-associated protein (FTO) and α-ketoglutarate-dependent dioxygenase alkB homolog 5 (ALKBH5) [11–15].

N6-methyladenosine (m[superscript 6]A) which is dynamic and reversible plays significant roles in tumor initiation and progression. Moreover, accumulating evidence supports the fact that the aberrant level of m[superscript 6]A is strongly associated with a variety of cancers, such as cervical cancer, renal cell carcinoma, Gastric Cancer, acute myeloid leukemia [11, 16–18].

A study demonstrated that METTL3 plays an oncogenic role in growth and invasion of bladder cancer cell via AFF4/NF-κB/MYC signaling pathway [19]. METTL3 promote tumor proliferation of bladder cancer by accelerating pri-miR221/222 maturation in m[superscript 6]A-dependent manner [20]. They found METTL3 affected the tumor formation by the regulation the m[superscript 6]A modification in non-coding RNAs.

Although m[superscript 6]A has been found to play a role in the initiation and development of various cancers mechanisms. Given the dual role and specific regulatory of m[superscript 6]A in cancer, many specific regulatory mechanisms and their correlation to clinical characteristics are unclear. In our study, we analyzed clinical data and microarray data of bladder cancer from TCGA database, evaluated 13 genes related to m[superscript 6]A regulation in bladder cancer, and analyzed the correlation between genes and clinicopathological characteristics. To explore new independent prognostic indicators.

Results

Differential expression of m[superscript 6]A related genes

433 transcription flies, of which 19 files were normal tissues and 414 files were cancer tissues and 412 patient clinical information were obtained from the TCGA database. The expression level of 13 genes related to m[superscript 6]A (Table 1)are presented as heatmaps (Fig. 1A). We found from the heat map that there were statistically significant differences between the six genes in bladder cancer and normal tissues. METTL3, TYTHDF1, YTHFDF2 and HNRNPC were highly expressed in cancer tissues and low in normal control tissues. Whereas, ZC3H13 and FTO were highly expressed in normal tissues and low expressed in cancer tissues. The violin plot more intuitively shows the expression levels of these 6 different genes (Fig. 1B). To better understand the interactions among the thirteen m[superscript 6]A RNA methylation regulators, the Correlation heat map was constructed (Fig. 1C). We found that YTHDC1 and METTL14 have positive correlation. Similarity, YTHDC1 and YTHDF2 have positive correlation. WTAP was significantly correlated with RBM15, METTL14 and HNRNPC.

Table 1 Differential expression of 13 genes in bladder

Gene	conMean	treatMean	logFC	*p* value
ZC3H13	8.166508	5.894558918	−0.470335451	0.00179274
YTHDC1	12.39476384	11.54114272	−0.102944707	0.13340077
HNRNPC	45.19322095	54.80889763	0.278303736	0.006283505
YTHDF1	16.04730916	24.2889248	0.597967224	1.67E−06
METTL3	4.331225737	6.980737576	0.688604112	1.27E−05
RBM15	2.489039	2.996865201	0.267865357	0.190334729
ALKBH5	30.26376411	28.81526188	−0.070758305	0.22049202
FTO	3.711241526	2.915021917	−0.348395164	0.004210122
YTHDC2	2.862321684	3.010217152	0.072681745	0.709773978
WTAP	15.78561205	14.06913859	−0.1660762	0.139320296
YTHDF2	17.15391163	22.08248668	0.364365048	0.002676947
METTL14	3.163150579	2.908623639	−0.121025605	0.070851609
KIAA142	5.036854421	6.082507481	0.272143156	0.129563833

WTAP is a key gene from the PPI network of key regulatory factors of m[superscript 6]A, which is closely related to METLL3, KIAA149, ZC3H13, RBM15, METTL14, ALKBH5 and YTHDC1 (Fig. 1D). That means the cross-talk among m[superscript 6]A writers, erasers, and readers and determine its role in bladder cancer. There are several separate genes in reader, suggesting that different readers may have different functions.

Functional characteristics of the identified m[superscript 6]A regulators and regulators correlation mRNAs

To better predict the functions of 13 m[superscript 6]A regulator genes identified in our study. We matched each m[superscript 6]A regulator to the top 20 related mRNAs as key genes for functional analysis. In total, 260 genes were obtained. We performed GO enrichment and KEGG pathway analysis. Top 10 dysregulated GO processes for each subgroup (biological process, cellular component and molecular function) were analyzed. Genes associated with biological processes were RNA splicing, RNA transport. Nuclear speck, chromosomal region, spliceosomal complex were related to the cellular component. Helicase activity, single-stranded DNA binding were related to molecular mechanism (Fig. 2). These genes were enriched in RNA transport, mRNA

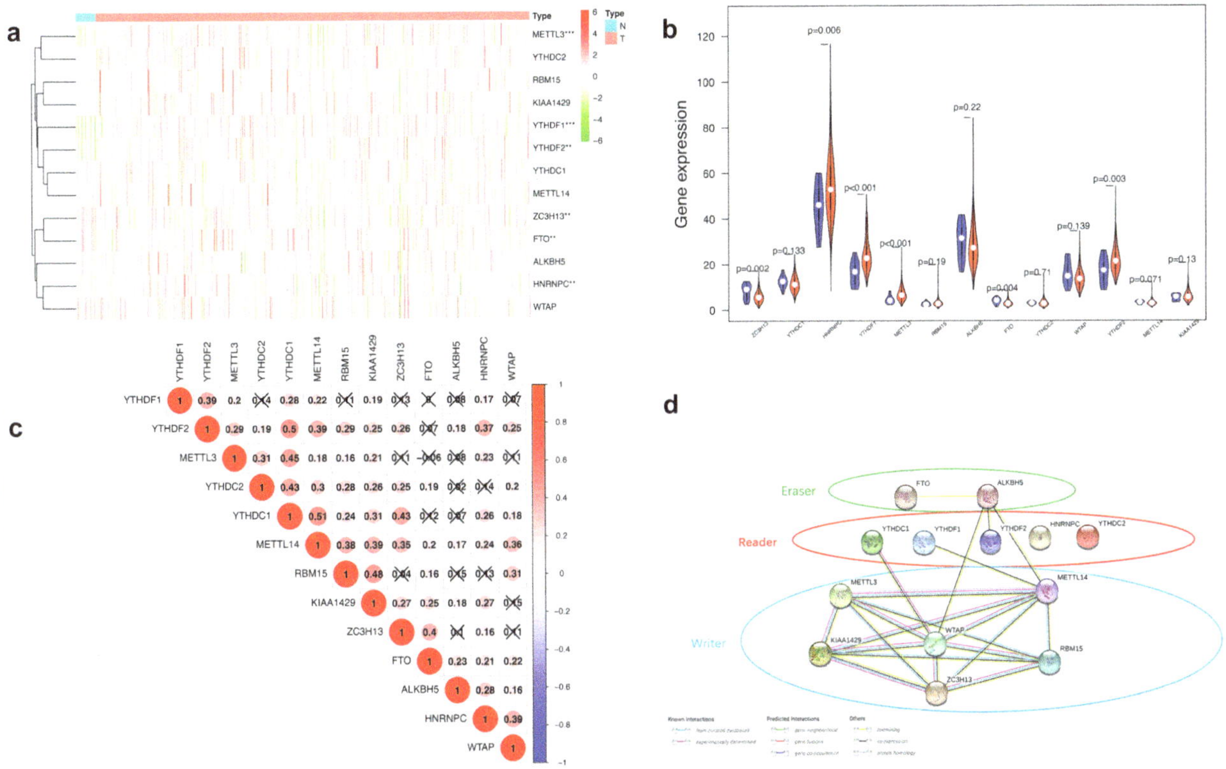

Fig. 1 Interaction of m[superscript 6]A regulators in bladder cancer. **A** A heat map of the proportion of 13 related m[superscript 6]A regulator genes. X-axis display sample name and sample classification, Y axis showing sample clustering information and 13 genes. ***$p<0.001$, **$p<0.05$. **B** The violin map of 13 m[superscript 6]A regulator genes. The X-axis represents 13 m[superscript 6]A regulator genes, and the Y-axis indicates the fraktion of genes. Blue represent normal tissue, and red represent cancer tissue. **C** Correlation matrix of 13 regulator genes. Variables have been ordered by average linkage clustering. Red colour means positive correlation, blue colour means negative correlation. The cross means no correlation. The darker the color, the higher the correlation. **D** PPI network for m[superscript 6]A regulator genes

surveillance pathway, signaling pathways regulating pluripotency of stem cells, cell cycle, basal transcription factors (Fig. 3).

m[superscript 6]A RNA methylation related genes identified three clusters of BC with distinct clinical features

According to the regulatory gene of m[superscript 6]A, tumor types were classified. We found from the figure that when the tumor was divided into 3 types, the growth rate of CDF slowed down significantly (Fig. 4A, B). Although, when the tumor was classified as 3 type, the correlation between groups was higher than that of type 2. Therefore, we compared the clinical characteristics of the datasets divided into three groups, namely cluster 1, cluster 2 and cluster 3 (Fig. 4C). There was a significant correlation between our tumor type and bladder cancer grade (Fig. 5A). What's more, there was also a significant correlation between our tumor typing and survival status. We observed a significantly longer overall survival (OS) in the cluster 1 than the cluster 2 and cluster 3 (Fig. 5B). Principal component analysis (PCA) was further used to compare the transcriptional profile between cluster 1, cluster 2 and cluster 3. The results showed a clear distinction between cluster 2 and cluster 3.

Three m[superscript 6]A-related genes related to prognosis were used to construct a prognostic risk model

To investigate the prognostic value of m[superscript 6]A RNA methylation regulatory gene in bladder cancer. Univariate Cox regression analysis was constructed with the TCGA data set (Fig. 6A). $P<0.1$ as the reference standard, we found that three genes were correlated with the prognosis of bladder cancer, namely YTHDC1, FTO, WTAP.

In order to further predict clinical outcomes of m[superscript 6]A RNA methylation regulatory factors in bladder cancer, lasso regression algorithm was used to calculate 3 prognostic genes in the TCGA data set. Three genes to construct the risk signature based on the minimum criteria, and get the coefficients from the LASSO algorithm (Fig. 6B). ROC curves showed the predictive efficiency of the risk signature (Fig. 7).

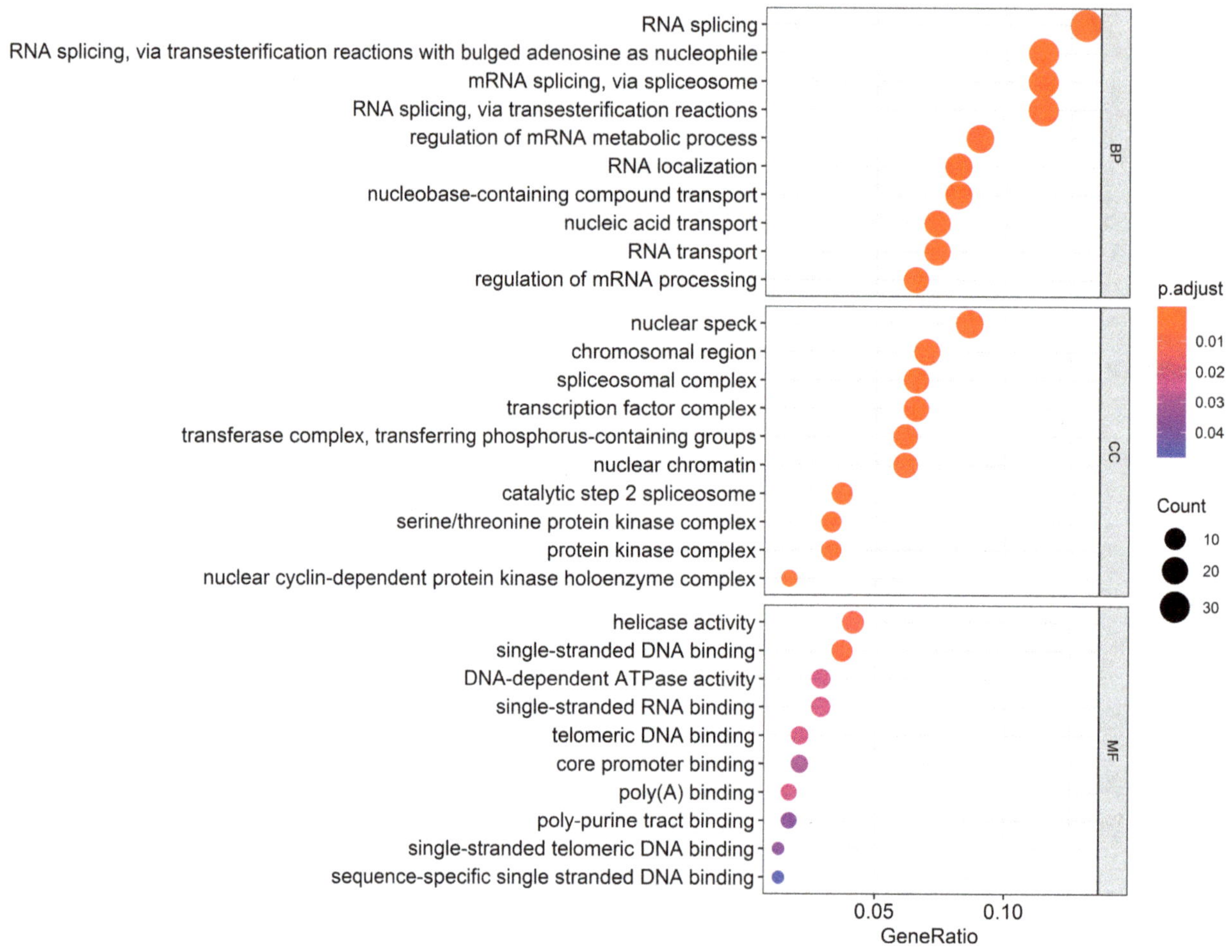

Fig. 2 Top 10 GO terms of each subgroup (biological process, cellular component and molecular function) (260 related m[superscript 6]A regulator genes) in bladder cancer. The size of the spot indicated the gene_numbers enriched in the GO, and the color of the spot indicated the significance level of the enriched GO

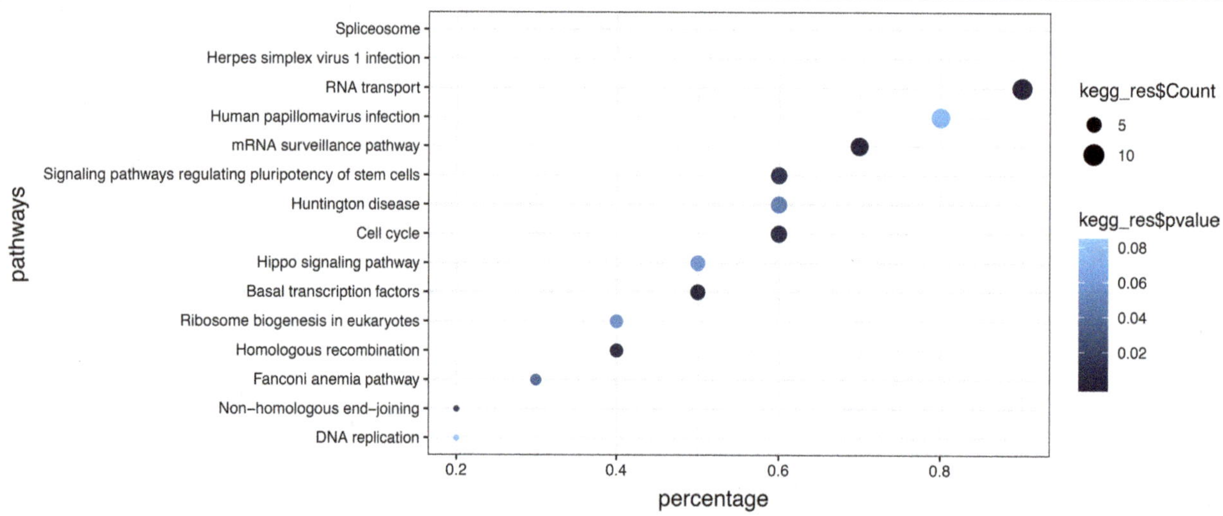

Fig. 3 Top 15 KEGG terms of DEGs (260 related m[superscript 6]A regulator genes) in bladder cancer. The size of the spot indicated the gene_numbers enriched in the pathway, and the color of the spot indicated the significance level of the enriched pathway

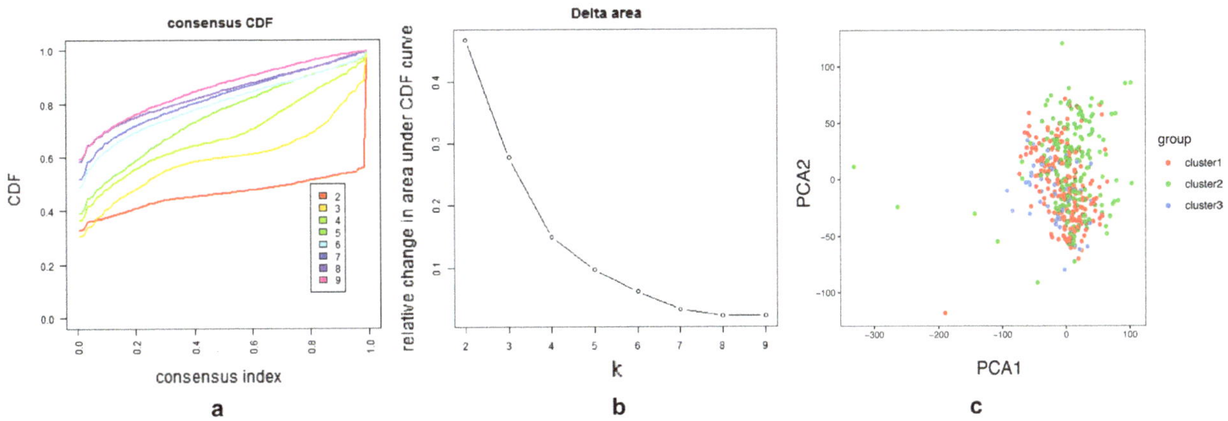

Fig. 4 Clustering the related regulators of m[superscript 6]A into three subgroups with "ConsensusClusterPlus". **A** Consensus clustering cumulative distribution function (CDF) for k = 2 to 9. **B** Relative change in area under CDF curve for k = 2 to 9. **C** Principal Component Analysis of all RNA expression of bladder cancer

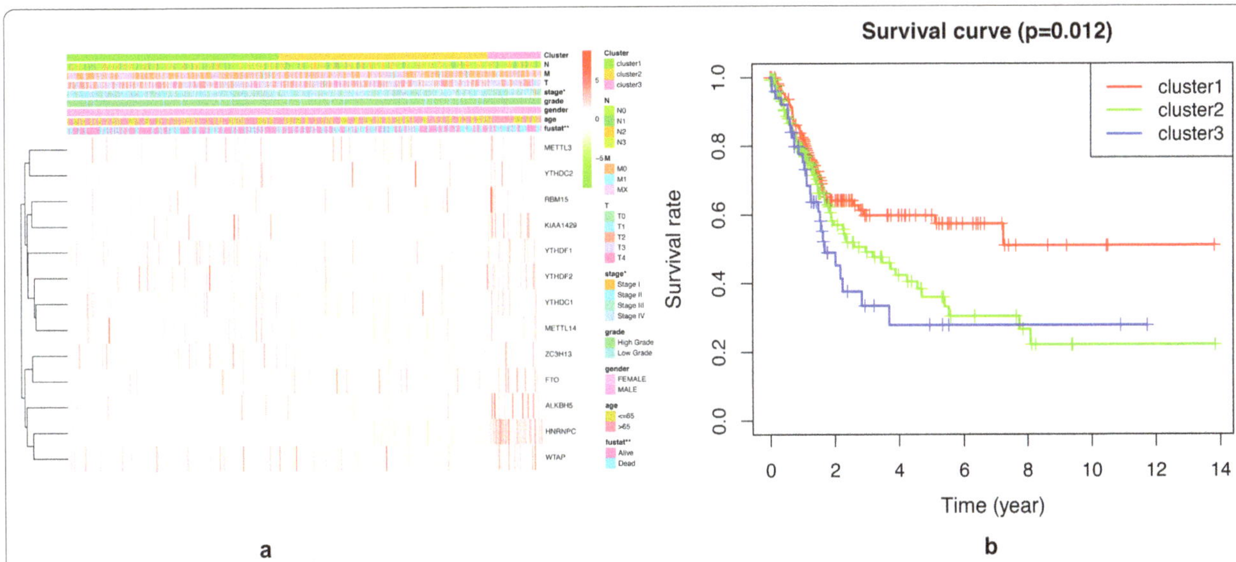

Fig. 5 **A** The heatmap shows the expression levels of the thirteen m[superscript 6]A RNA methylation regulators in cluster1, cluster2 and cluster 3 in bladder cancer with clinical charateristics. **B** Kaplan–Meier survival curves were generated from the comparison of cluster 1, cluster 2 and cluster 3 using the level of the bladder cancer

Cross-validation suggested that there was no correlation between the three selected genes. We used the expression levels and clinical characteristics of the three genes to calculate the risk signature for each patient.

To investigate the prognostic role of the three-gene risk signature, we separated the bladder cancer patients in the TCGA datasets into low and high-risk groups based on the median risk score and observed significant differences in overall survival (OS) (Fig. 8). We also used the immunohistochemical results of Human Protein Atlas database to explore the expression of independent prognostic factor in bladder cancer and found that YTHDC1 and FTO levels in normal bladder tissues were significantly higher than in bladder cancer tissues. However, the antibody staining levels of WTAP in bladder cancer tissues were relatively increased (Fig. 9).

YTHDC1, FTO and WTAP mRNA expression in different stages (TNM) of bladder cancer samples

We analyzed the RNA-Seq data for YTHDC1, FTO and WTAP in different stages (TNM) of bladder cancer samples from TCGA (412 bladder cancer and 19 normal

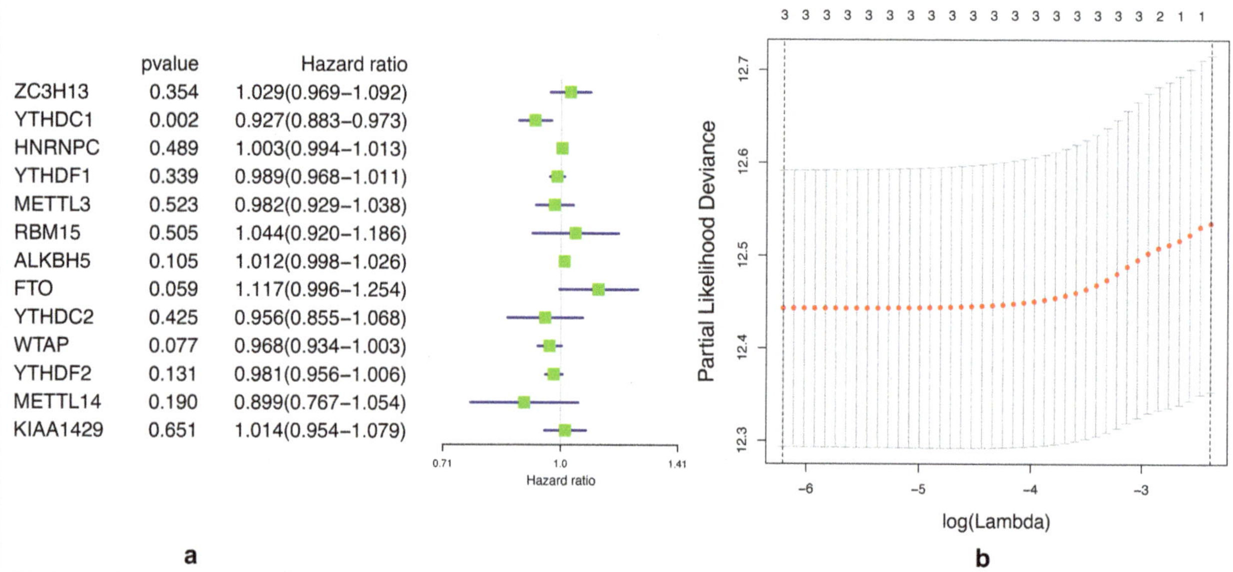

Fig. 6 13 related m[superscript 6]A regulator genes calculated by univariate Cox regression (**A**) and the coefficients calculated by multivariate Cox regression with LASSO (**B**)

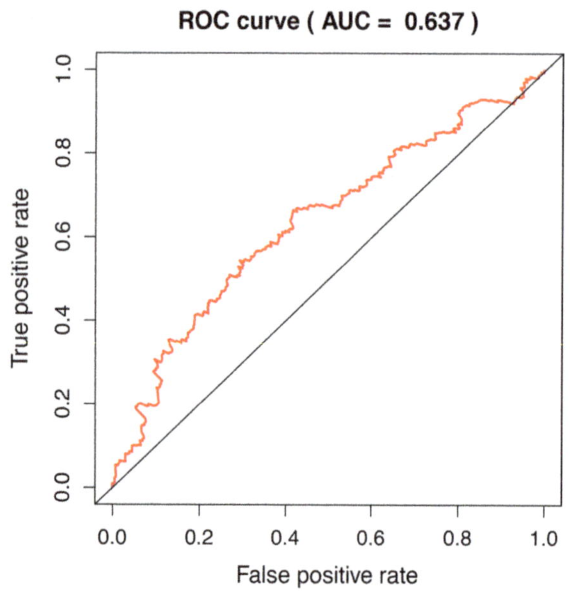

Fig. 7 ROC curves showed the predictive efficiency of the risk signature

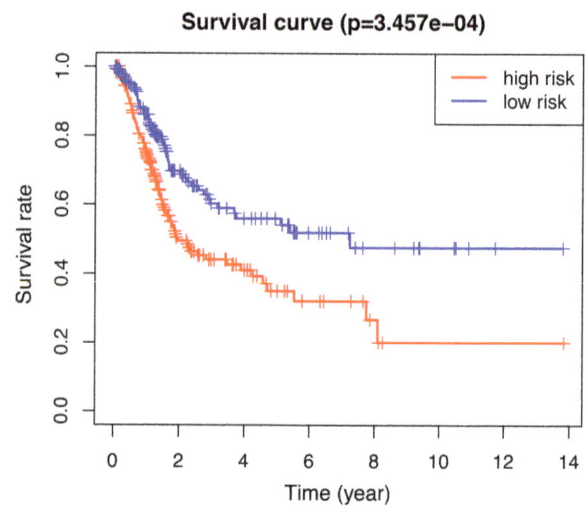

Fig. 8 Kaplan–Meier survival curves were generated from the comparison of high risk and low risk expression group for bladder cancer using the risk scores

samples). Among the 412 cancer samples, there were 2 without stage described, 2 of stageI, 131of stageII, 141 of stageIII and 136 of stageIV. For the limitation of sample size, stageI was excluded for analysis of YTHDC1, FTO and WTAP mRNA expression between bladder cancer and the normal controls. The expression level of YTHDC1and WTAP mRNA was significantly down-regulated in stageIV of bladder cancer tissues compared with the normal controls respectively ($p=0.043$ and $p=0.012$ for stageIV). The expression level of FTO mRNA was significantly down-regulated in stageII–IV of bladder cancer tissues compared with the normal controls ($p=0.00025$ for stageII, $p=0.047$ for stageIII and $p=0.0055$ for stageIV, Fig. 10).

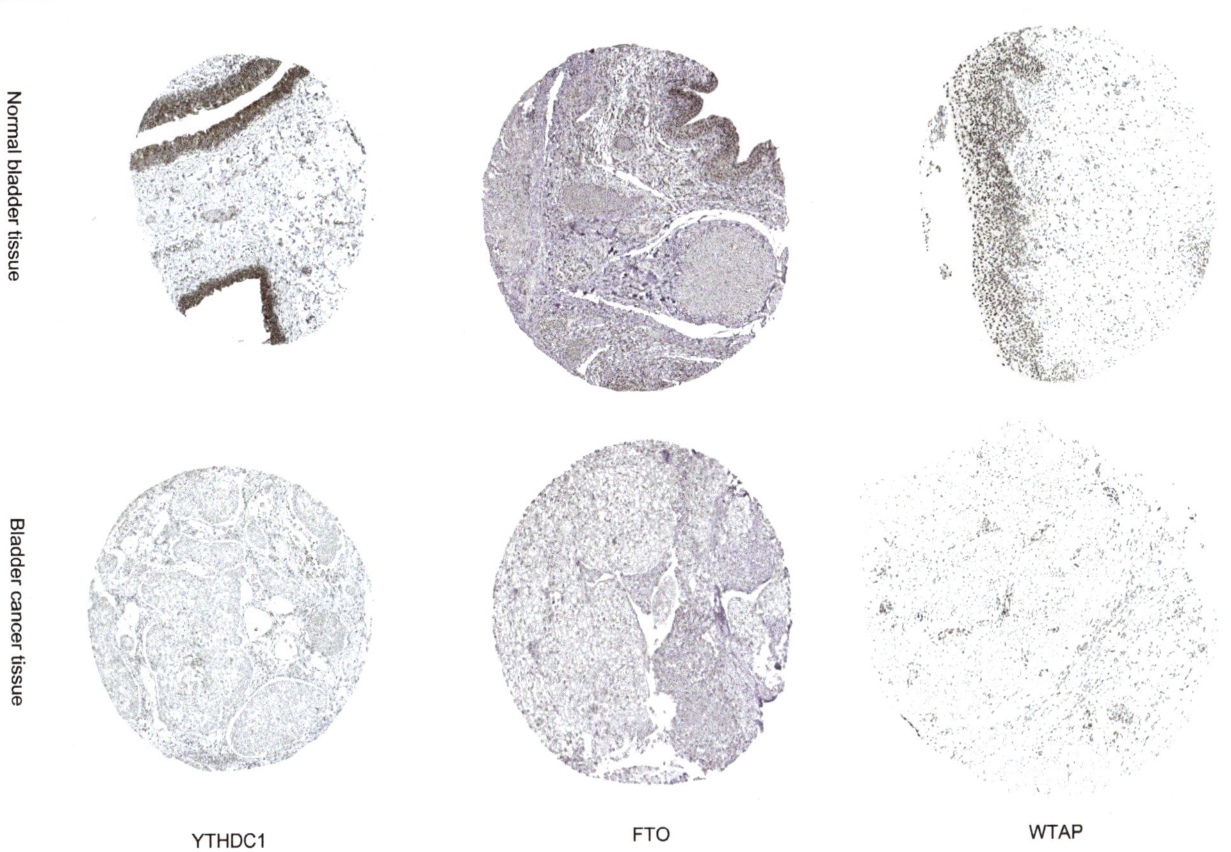

Fig. 9 Validation of independent prognostic factor expression in bladder cancer and normal bladder tissue

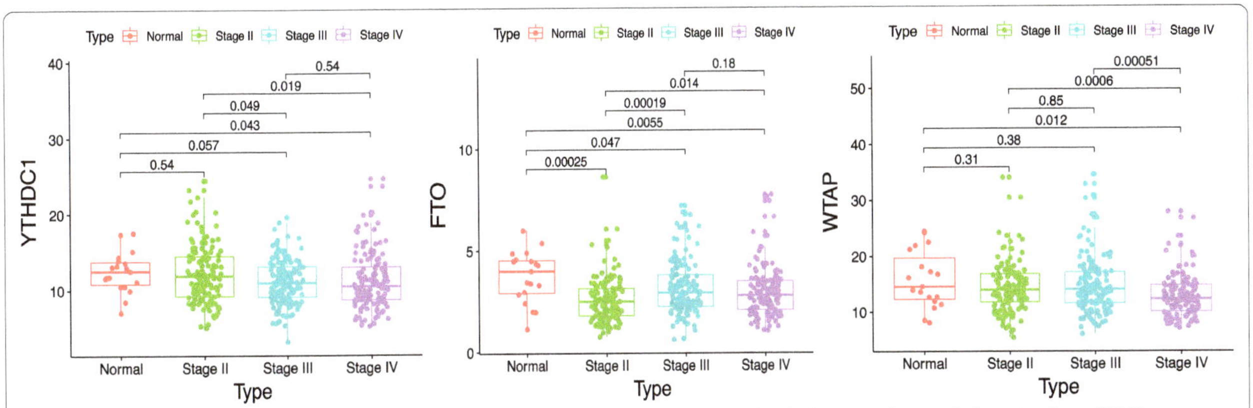

Fig. 10 Expression of YTHDC1, FTO and WTAP mRNA in bladder cancer tissues compared with the normal controls from the data of TCGA

Risk scores by median identified low group and high group with clinical features

The heat map reveals the expression of three selected m[superscript 6]A RNA methylation regulators and clinical traits in high-risk and low-risk patients in the TCGA data set. We found that as the expression level of FTO gene increased, the risk value of patients also increased. Whereas, WTAP and YTHDC1 are low-risk genes. As gene expression increased, patients' risk values decreased.

We also examined the association between the risk scores and each clinicopathological feature (Fig. 11). The relationship between patient risk values and clinical traits was not significant from our results, but patient

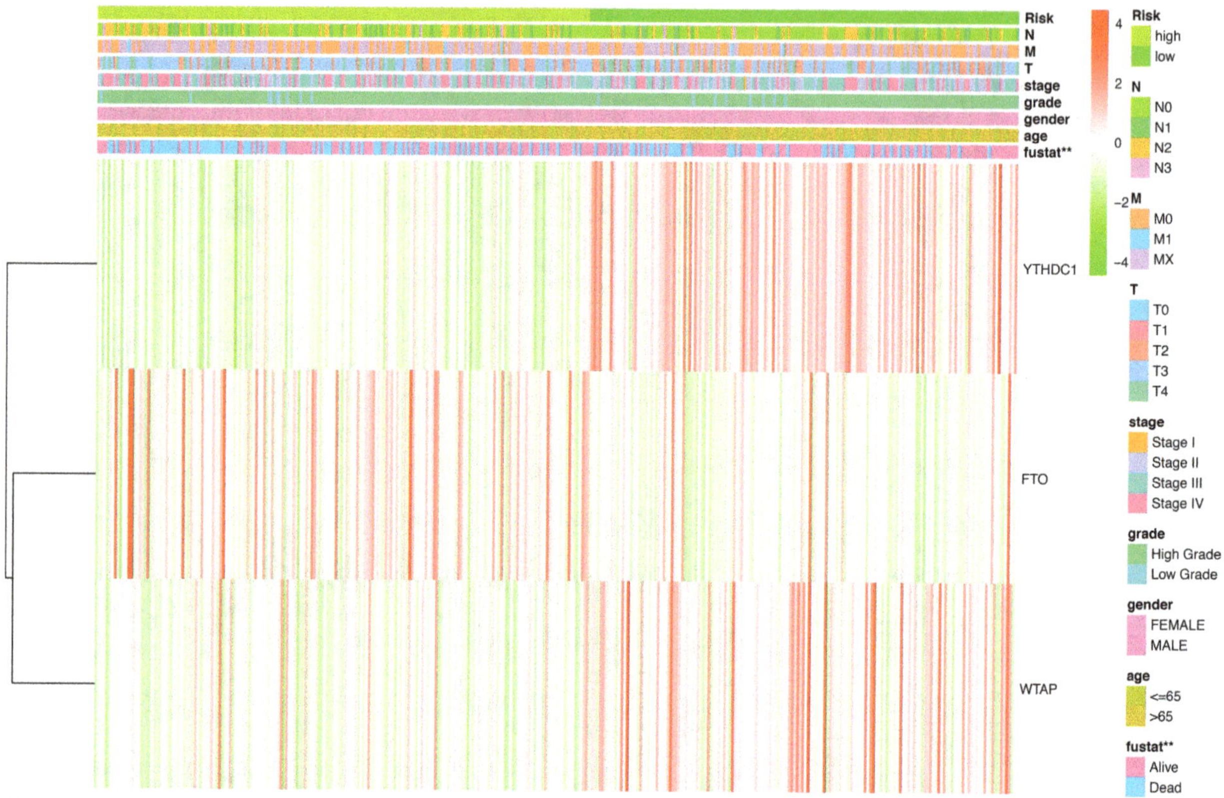

Fig. 11 The heatmap shows the expression levels of the three m[superscript 6]A RNA methylation regulators in low- and high-risk bladder cancer with clinical charateristics

risk values and patient survival status were statistically significant.

Then, univariate and multivariate Cox regression analysis was performed on the TCGA data set to determine independent prognostic indicators. Through univariate analysis, age, stage, T level and risk score were all correlated with OS (Fig. 12). With these factors were included into multivariate Cox regression, risk score and age were still significantly correlated with OS ($p < 0.001$) (Fig. 13).

We confirmed that age, stage, T, N and risk scores were associated with patient survival in univariate Cox regression. However, among multivariate Cox regression, only age and risk scores were statistically significant. We believe that in addition to age as an independent prognostic factor. More importantly, we revealed risk score can also be an independent prognostic factor.

Methods

Screening datasets with 13 related regulators of m[superscript 6]A

Data from The Cancer Genome Atlas (TCGA) were obtained in May 2019. A total of 433 transcription files were included, of which 19 cases were normal tissues and 414 cases of bladder cancer. At the same time, the clinical data of 412 patients with bladder cancer was obtained from TCGA. We first performed a gene expression matrix on 433 transcripts from the TCGA database. Thirteen genes related to m[superscript 6]A methylation were screened out for subsequent analysis.

Analysis of 13 genes related to m[superscript 6]A methylation

In order to investigate the expression matrices of 13 genes, we showed the expression, correlation and difference of m[superscript 6]A regulators through heat map, correlationmap and violin map. Data analysis was performed using package pheatmap, corrplot, vioplot.

Protein–Protein interaction (PPI) was conducted with string database (https://string-db.org/).

GO and KEGG enrichment analysis

Gene Ontology (GO) analysis was applied to explore the functions of genes identified in study. GO analysis organizes genes into hierarchical categories and can uncover gene regulatory networks on the basis of biological process, molecular functions and Cellular Component.

KEGG pathway analysis was performed to reveal the function and interactions among genes. The

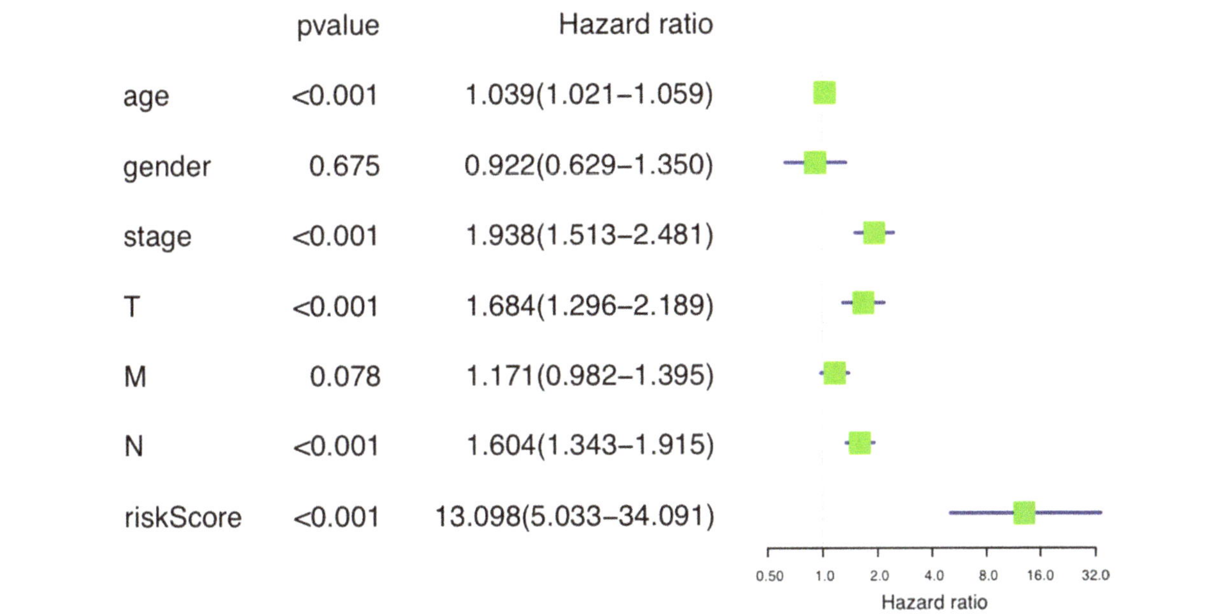

Fig. 12 Univariate Cox regression analyses of the association between clinicopathological factors (including the risk score) and overall survival of patients

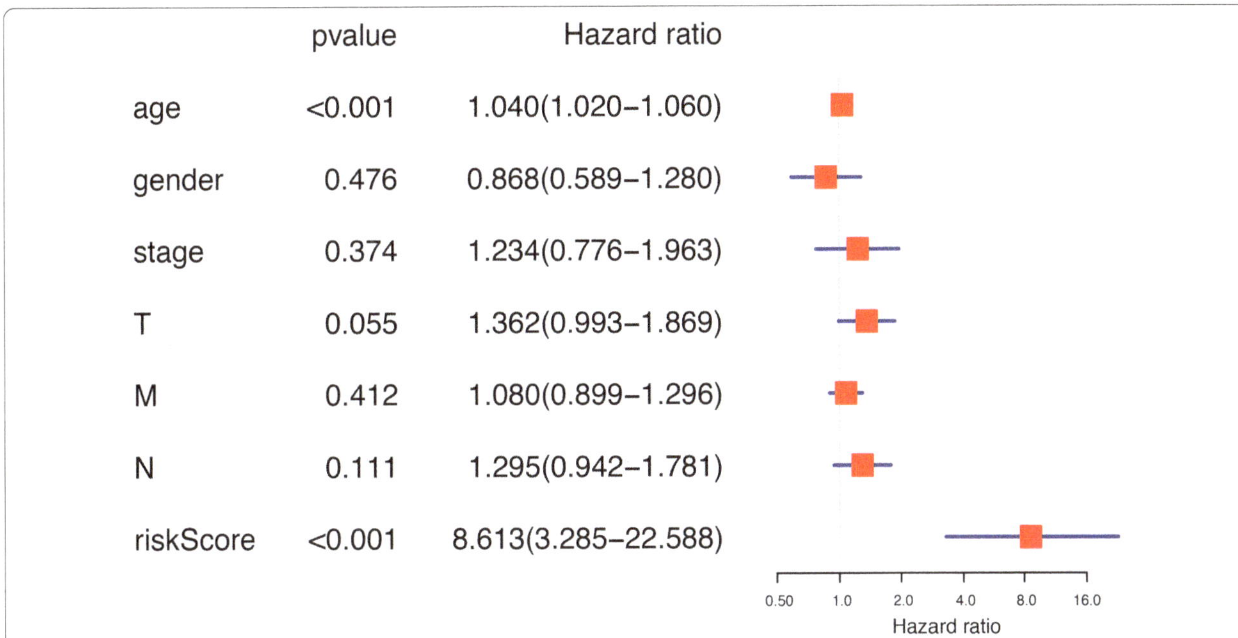

Fig. 13 Multivariate Cox regression analyses of the association between clinicopathological factors (including the risk score) and overall survival of patients

enrichment Gene Ratio was the value ratio between the sequenced gene and all annotated genes enriched in the pathway.

Data analysis was performed using package stringi and ggplot2. The enrichment significance $p < 0.05$ was set as the cut-off for significantly enriched functional GO terms and KEGG pathways.

Analysis the relationship between m[superscript 6]A regulators with clinical characteristic, survival

To investigate the function of m[superscript 6]A RNA methylation regulators in bladder cancer survival and clinical characteristics, we clustered the bladder cancer into different subgroups with "ConsensusClusterPlus". PCA graph was used to verify the accuracy of cluster of 13 genes related to m[superscript 6]A with the package limma, ggplot2.

To reveal the prognostic value of m[superscript 6] A RNA methylation regulators, univariate Cox regression analyses of their expression in the TCGA was constructed. Therefore, we identified three genes ($p < 0.1$) that were significantly related to survival. We selected these three genes for functional analysis and established a potential risk model by using LASSO Cox regression algorithm. Finally, three genes and their coefficients were determined by the minimum criteria. The online database Human Protein Atlas (http://www.proteinatlas.org/) was utilized to explore the expression of independent prognostic factor at a translational level.

We downloaded gene expression data by RNA-seq and the corresponding clinical data for a total of 412 bladder cancer and 19 normal samples from TCGA. All RNA expression levels of the samples were normalized. The significance of differences of YTHDC1, FTO and WTAP mRNA expression between different stages of bladder cancer and the normal controls was assessed using a one-way ANOVA with Tukey's tests. The differential expression levels of FTO mRNA between the bladder cancer and adjacent tissues were analyzed with t-tests. The results were analyzed using GraphPad Prism 7.0. All statistical tests were two-tailed, with $p < 0.05$ considered significant.

Univariate and multivariate Cox regression analyses were performed to determine the prognostic value of the risk score and various clinical characteristics. The prediction accuracy of the risk signature were tested with operating characteristic (ROC) curves.

Patients were divided into three groups with the expression of m[superscript 6]A RNA methylation regulatory factor by PCA, or patients were divided into high group and low group with the cut-off value of the median risk. Chi-square test was used to compare the distribution of fustat status of T, N, M, staging, gender, grade and age between the two risk groups.

The Kaplan–Meier method with log-rank test was used to compare the OS of the patients in the cluster subgroups or in the high- and low-risk groups. All statistical analyses were conducted using R v3.4.1 (https://www.r-project.org/).

Discussion

Urothelial carcinoma of the bladder is the fourth most common malignancy in men, with ~ 81,190 new cases and 17,240 deaths estimated in 2018 in the United States [21]. Analogous to DNA and histone, epigenetic modification to RNA species has been well documented for several decades [22].

Emerging evidence demonstrated that aberrant regulation of RNA methylation is tumorigenic. Furthermore, dysregulated expression of m[superscript 6]A writers, erasers, and readers is widespread in diversified human cancers. Similarity, Epigenetic dysregulation is essential in determining bladder cancer phenotype with regard to pathogenesis and tumor biology.

Based on the expression of m[superscript 6]A RNA methylation regulatory genes, three bladder cancer subgroups, namely cluster1, cluster 2, and cluster 3 were determined by consistent cluster analysis. We found that subgroup is not only related to clinical traits, but were also closely to the prognosis. In addition, 3 selected m[superscript 6]A RNA methylation regulatory genes were used to obtain prognostic risk scores, and the overall survival rate of patients with bladder cancer was divided into high-risk and low-risk groups.

We analyzed the expression of all m[superscript 6] A RNA methylation regulators in bladder cancer with different clinical characteristics. As the Writer of m[superscript 6]A regulator genes, METTL3 and ZC3H13 were elevated in bladder cancer. As the reader of m[superscript 6]A regulator genes, YTHDF1, YTHDF2 and HNRNPC were highly expressed in bladder cancer tissues compared with the normal tissues. Graphs from univariate Cox regression and risk models. As the expression of the YTDHC1and WTAP gene increased, the patient's risk value decreased. We concluded that YTDHC1and WTAP are low-risk genes. TFO is a high-risk gene among the m[superscript 6]A RNA methylation regulators. We found that three genes were correlated with the prognosis of bladder cancer, namely YTHDC1, FTO, WTAP. Wen's study also demonstrated that the expression of FTO mRNA in bladder urothelial carcinoma decreases significantly compared with the normal controls from both the data of real-time PCR ($p < 0.05$) and TCGA ($p < 0.01$), which is consistent with our study [23].

The discovery of proteins involved in m[superscript 6]A regulation has been among the most significant achievements in this area of study, elucidating their roles as "writers" (binding protein), "erasers" (demethylase), and "readers" (methyltransferase). METTL3 promote tumor growth in breast cancer, lung cancer and liver cancer [24–26] but as suppressor genes in Glioblastoma [27]. METTL14 performed tumor suppressor functions similar to that of METTL3 in the development of GSCs by targeting mRNA levels of ADAM19, EPHA3 and KLF4 [27]. Surprisingly, YTHDF2 promotes migration in prostate cancer in vitro, while the opposite has been investigated in the case of pancreatic cancer. It inhibits migration and invasion in pancreatic cancer cells [28, 29] and the eraser FTO is an oncogene in AML and glioma [30–32]. ALKBH5 plays an oncogene that Promotes GSCs proliferation and tumor progression by positively regulating FOXM1 in GBM. Oppositely, suppressor genes in AML [33, 34].

Emerging evidence demonstrated that m[superscript 6]A modification of mRNA is deregulated in numerous cancers, and its role in cancers has been verified by both in vitro and in vivo studies. What's more, evidence has shown that both writers and erasers can assume an oncogenic or tumor suppressor role in different tumor models. Some proteins may exert similar influence on different types of cancers, while some others may function differently in similar types of cancers.

RNA m[superscript 6]A patterns are involved in various aspects of mRNA metabolism including mRNA export, translation, and decay and perform an important function in post-transcriptional regulation of gene expression and protein translation. Similarly, the biological functions of m[superscript 6]A-related regulatory factors and related mRNAs were also revealed in our study. RNA splicing, RNA transport. Nuclear speck, chromosomal region, spliceosomal complex were related to the cellular component. Helicase activity, single-stranded DNA binding were related to molecular mechanism. These genes were enriched in RNA transport, mRNA surveillance pathway, signaling pathways regulating pluripotency of stem cells, cell cycle, basal transcription factors.

Three m[superscript 6]A-related genes related to prognosis were used to construct a prognostic risk model. We separated bladder cancer patients into high and low risk categories and found its significant statistically. Next, through the Cox regression. We found in addition to age as an independent prognostic factor, more importantly, risk score can also be an independent prognostic factor.

There are still some shortcomings in our data mining. Due to the limited amount of data, we failed to distinguish the clearly separate of the three clusters when grouping through the "ConsensusClusterPlus". We did not validate the data from the external. To exclude bias, we plan to address the functional importance of these genes in clinical experiments, which should determine whether their combinations have more predictive value than any of them alone.

In conclusion, if m[superscript 6]A level and its regulators could be potential biomarkers for prognosis of some caners is not clear, specific mechanism of m[superscript 6]A in tumorigenesis needs to be fully explored. Considering the dual role of m[superscript 6]A, additional study are required to address the cross-talk among m[superscript 6]A writers, erasers, and readers and determine its role in bladder cancer. With the thorough study of the m[superscript 6]A mechanism, it is believed that effective strategies for the diagnosis, prognosis and treatment of bladder cancer.

Abbreviations

METTL3: Methyl-transferase-Like 3; METTL14: Methyltransferase-like 14; RBM15: RNA binding motif protein 15; WTAP: Wilms Tumor 1-Associated Protein; ZC3H13: Domain-containing protein 13; HNRNPC: Heterogeneous nuclear ribonucleoprotein C; YTHDC1: YTH domain-containing 1; YTHDC2: YTH domain-containing 2; YTHDF1: YTH N6-methyl-adenosine RNA binding protein 1; YTHDF2: YTH N6-methyl-adenosine RNA binding protein 2; ALKBH5: α-Ketoglutarate-dependent dioxygenase alkB homolog 5; FTO: Obesity-associated protein; PCA: Principal component analysis; GO: Gene Ontology; TCGA : The Cancer Genome Atlas; ROC: Receiver operating characteristic; OS: Overall survival; LASSO: The least absolute shrinkage and selection operator.

Acknowledgements

Not applicable.

Authors' contributions

YZ and BZ analyzed the data and drafted the manuscript. BZ, YZ and QL contributed to the interpretation of data and revised the manuscript. YZ and BZ conceived and designed the study. All authors have reviewed and approved the final version of the manuscript.

Author details

[1]Department of Urology, Xiangyang No.1 People's Hospital, Hubei University of Medicine, Xiangyang, Hubei, People's Republic of China. [2]Department of Gynaecoogy and Obstetrics, Xiangyang No.1 People's Hospital, Hubei University of Medicine, Xiangyang, Hubei, People's Republic of China.

References

1. Pan Y, Ma P, Liu Y, Li W, Shu Y. Multiple functions of m(6)A RNA methylation in cancer. J Hematol Oncol. 2018;11:48. https://doi.org/10.1186/s13045-018-0590-8.
2. Wang S, Sun C, Li J, Zhang E, Ma Z, Xu W, Li H, Qiu M, Xu Y, Xia W, Xu L, Yin R. Roles of RNA methylation by means of N(6)-methyladenosine (m(6)A) in human cancers. Cancer Lett. 2017;408:112–20.
3. Yang Z, Li J, Feng G, et al. MicroRNA-145 modulates -methyladeno sine levels by targeting the 3'-untranslated mRNA region of the -methyladenosine binding YTH domain family 2 protein. J Biol Chem. 2017;292(9):3614–23.
4. Berulava T, Rahmann S, Rademacher K, et al. N6-adenosine methylation in MiRNAs. PLoS ONE. 2015;10(2):e0118438.
5. Yang D, Qiao J, Wang G, et al. N6-Methyladenosine modification of lincRNA 1281 is critically required for mESC differentiation potential. Nucleic Acids Res. 2018;46(8):3906–20.
6. Cozen AE, Quartley E, Holmes AD, et al. ARM-seq: AlkB-facilitated RNA methylation sequencing reveals a complex landscape of modified tRNA fragments. Nat Methods. 2015;12(9):879–84.
7. Sergiev PV, Aleksashin NA, Chugunova AA, et al. Structural and evolutionary insights into ribosomal RNA methylation. Nat Chem Biol. 2018;14(3):226–35.

8. Karijolich J, Yu Y-T. Spliceosomal snRNA modifications and their function. RNA Biol. 2014;7:192–204.
9. Dai D, Wang H, Zhu L, et al. N6-methyladenosine links RNA metabolism to cancer progression. Cell Death Dis. 2018;9:124.
10. Yang Y, Hsu PJ, Chen YS, Yang YG. Dynamic transcriptomic m[superscript 6]A decoration: writers, erasers, readers and functions in RNA metabolism. Cell Res. 2018;28:616–24.
11. Li X, Tang J, Huang W, et al. The M[SUPERSCRIPT 6]A methyltransferase METTL3: acting as a tumor suppressor in renal cell carcinoma. Oncotarget. 2017;8(56):96103–16.
12. Sun T, Wu R. The role of m[superscript 6]A RNA methylation in cancer. Biomed Pharmacother. 2019;112:108613.
13. Lobo J, Costa AL, Cantante M, et al. mA RNA modification and its writer/reader VIRMA/YTHDF3 in testicular germ cell tumors: a role in seminoma phenotype maintenance. J Transl Med. 2019;17(1):79.
14. Li Y, Zheng D, Wang F, et al. Expression of demethylase genes, FTO and ALKBH1, is associated with prognosis of gastric cancer. Dig Dis Sci. 2019;64(6):1503–13.
15. Tang C, Klukovich R, Peng H, Wang Z, Yu T, Zhang Y, Zheng H, Klungland A, Yan W. ALKBH5-dependent m[superscript 6]A demethylation controls splicing and stability of long 3′-UTR mRNAs in male germ cells. Proc Natl Acad Sci USA. 2018;115:E325–33.
16. Wang X, Li Z, Kong B, et al. Reduced mA mRNA methylation is correlated with the progression of human cervical cancer. Oncotarget. 2017;8(58):98918–30.
17. Lin S, Liu J, Jiang W, et al. METTL3 promotes the proliferation and mobility of gastric cancer cells. Open Med (Wars). 2019;14:25–31.
18. Kwok CT, Marshall AD, Rasko JE, Wong JJ. Genetic alterations of m[superscript 6]A regulators predict poorer survival in acute myeloid leukemia. J Hematol Oncol. 2017;10:39.
19. Cheng M, Sheng L, Gao Q, et al. The mA methyltransferase METTL3 promotes bladder cancer progression via AFF4/NF-κB/MYC signaling network. Oncogene. 2019;38(19):3667–80.
20. Han J, Wang JZ, Yang X, et al. METTL3 promote tumor proliferation of bladder cancer by accelerating pri-miR221/222 maturation in m[superscript 6]A-dependent manner. Mol Cancer. 2019;18:110.
21. Siegel RL, Miller KD, Jemal A. Cancer statistics, 2018. CA. 2018;68:7–30.
22. He C. Grand challenge commentary: RNA epigenetics? Nat Chem Biol. 2010;6:863–5.
23. Wen L, Pan X, Yu Y, Yang B. Down-regulation of FTO promotes proliferation and migration, and protects bladder cancer cells from cisplatin-induced cytotoxicity. BMC Urol. 2020;20(1):39.
24. Cai X, Wang X, Cao C, Gao Y, Zhang S, Yang Z, et al. HBXIP-elevated methyltransferase METTL3 promotes the progression of breast cancer via inhibiting tumor suppressor let-7g. Cancer Lett. 2018;415:11–9.
25. Lin S, Choe J, Du P, Triboulet R, Gregory RI. The m(6)A methyltransferase METTL3 promotes translation in human cancer cells. Mol Cell. 2016;62:335–45.
26. Chen M, Wei L, Law CT, Tsang FH, Shen J, Cheng CL, et al. RNA N6-methyladenosine methyltransferase METTL3 promotes liver cancer progression through YTHDF2 dependent post-transcriptional silencing of SOCS2. Hepatology. 2017;67:2254–70.
27. Cui Q, Shi H, Ye P, Li L, Qu Q, Sun G, et al. m[superscript 6]A RNA methylation regulates the self-renewal and tumorigenesis of glioblastoma stem cells. Cell Rep. 2017;18(11):2622–34.
28. Li JF, Meng S, Xu MJ, Wang S, He LJ, Xu X, et al. Downregulation of N6-methyladenosine binding YTHDF2 protein mediated by miR-493-3p suppresses prostate cancer by elevating N6-methyladenosine levels. Oncotarget. 2018;9:3752–64.
29. Chen JX, Sun YC, Xu X, Wang DW, He JB, Zhou HL, et al. YTH domain family 2 orchestrates epithelial-mesenchymal transition/proliferation dichotomy in pancreatic cancer cells. Cell Cycle. 2017;16:2259–71.
30. Su R, Dong L, Li C, Nachtergaele S, Wunderlich M, Qing Y, et al. R-2HG exhibits anti-tumor activity by targeting FTO/m[superscript 6]A/MYC/CEBPA signaling. Cell. 2018;172(1–2):90-105.e23.
31. Li Z, Weng H, Su R, Weng X, Zuo Z, Li C, et al. FTO plays an oncogenic role in acute myeloid leukemia as a N6-methyladenosine RNA demethylase. Cancer Cell. 2017;31(1):127–41.
32. Xu D, Shao W, Jiang Y, et al. FTO expression is associated with the occurrence of gastric cancer and prognosis. Oncol Rep. 2017;38(4):2285–92.
33. Zhang S, Zhao BS, Zhou A, Lin K, Zheng S, Lu Z, Chen Y, Sulman EP, Xie K, Bogler O, Majumder S, He C, Huang S. M(6)A demethylase ALKBH5 maintains tumorigenicity of glioblastoma stem-like cells by sustaining FOXM1 expression and cell proliferation program. Cancer Cell. 2017;31(4):591-606.e6.
34. Kwok CT, Marshall AD, Rasko JE, Wong JJ. Genetic alterations of m(6)A regulators predict poorer survival in acute myeloid leukemia. J Hematol Oncol. 2017;10(1):39.

17

A rare case of eosinophilic cystitis involving the inside and outside of the urinary bladder associated with an infected urachal cyst

Hyun Bin Shin[1], Hyun Sik Park[1], Joo Heon Kim[2] and Jinsung Park[1,3*]

Abstract

Background: Eosinophilic cystitis is a rare inflammatory disease of the bladder characterized by eosinophilic infiltration of the bladder wall. Most Eosinophilic cystitis cases present with mucosal lesions of the urinary bladder. We present a very rare case of large mass-forming eosinophilic cystitis, involving the inside and outside of the bladder associated with an infected urachal cyst.

Case presentation: A 59-year-old man presented with gross hematuria, fever, dysuria, and suprapubic pain. Computed tomography showed a heterogeneously enhancing mass that measured 7.6 cm × 4 cm located on the anterosuperior portion of the bladder with an internal fluid collection. Cystoscopy revealed a raspberry-like mass lesion on the bladder dome. Transurethral resection of the bladder was initially performed. The mass lesion protruding from inside the bladder was removed, and pus-like fluid was drained. The pathologic diagnosis was eosinophilic cystitis. Follow-up computed tomography showed a remnant mass outside the bladder and urachal cyst. To eliminate the remnant lesion, robot-assisted partial cystectomy was performed. The patient showed no evidence of recurrent disease on follow-up cystoscopy and computed tomography for up to 2 years.

Conclusions: Clinicians should consider the possibility of eosinophilic cystitis in patients who present with hematuria, fever, and suprapubic pain and have both intravesical and extravesical masses.

Keywords: Eosinophilic cystitis, Urachal cyst, Partial cystectomy

Background

Eosinophilic cystitis (EC) is a rare inflammatory disease of the bladder, characterized by eosinophilic infiltration of the bladder wall and associated with fibrosis with or without muscle necrosis [1]. Because of the small number of patients afflicted with EC, the etiology of EC is not well understood. But subsequent mast cell degranulation is thought to be due to antigenic stimulation that promotes IgE-mediated attraction of eosinophils throughout the bladder wall [2–5]. The most common symptoms include urinary frequency, hematuria, dysuria, urinary retention, and suprapubic pain.

Most EC cases present with mucosal lesions of the urinary bladder [6, 7], although several studies have reported mass-forming or malignancy-mimicking EC [1, 2, 6–9]. To diagnose EC, pathologic diagnosis of bladder mucosal lesions such as transmural eosinophil infiltration and absence of malignant cells by transurethral resection of the bladder (TURB) or cystoscopic biopsy, is essential [1, 2, 4, 6, 7]. To date, there is only one case report on EC associated with infected urachal remnants [8]; but the patient was a 4-year-old child diagnosed with EC at 7 months after surgical excision of the infected urachal cyst, with recurrent abscesses in the abdomen, pelvis,

*Correspondence: jspark.uro@gmail.com
[3] Department of Urology, Uijeongbu Eulji Medical Center, Eulji University School of Medicine, 712, Dongil-ro, Uijeongbu-si, Gyeonggi-do 11759, Republic of Korea
Full list of author information is available at the end of the article

and at the operation site. In our case report, we present a rare case of large mass-forming EC, involving both the inside and outside of the urinary bladder associated with an infected urachal cyst.

Case presentation

A 59-year-old man presented with gross hematuria, fever (37.9 °C), dysuria, and suprapubic pain at the Eulji University Hospital. The patient had no history of allergies or bladder injury, and had an unremarkable medical history. Laboratory tests showed elevation in c-reactive protein levels (17.31 mg/dL) but no leukocytosis (7.810×10^3/μL), elevation of erythrocyte sedimentation rate (ESR, 6 mm/h), and peripheral eosinophilia (270 cells/μL). Urinalysis revealed hematuria, but no bacterial growth was found in urine culture.

Computed tomography (CT) showed a heterogeneously enhancing mass that measured 7.6 cm × 4 cm on the anterosuperior portion of the bladder (Fig. 1). The mass had a sphere-like shape and a thickened outer wall with an internal fluid collection. Initially, an infected urachal cyst was suspected because the patient had a fever, and empirical intravenous antibiotics (third-generation cephalosporin) were initiated. Cystoscopy showed a huge raspberry-like mass lesion on the bladder dome with a definite margin, which occupied more than half of the bladder (Fig. 2A, B). Because the possibility of a tumorous condition could not be fully excluded, percutaneous drainage was not performed. After infection control with intravenous antibiotics, TURB was performed for pathologic diagnosis. During resection, a pus-like fluid was found inside the mass (Fig. 2C), and most mass lesions inside the bladder were removed (Fig. 2D). Tissue and fluid culture were performed, but no bacterial growth was observed.

Histopathological examination revealed numerous eosinophilic infiltrates in the bladder wall. These were diffusely infiltrated and gathered around vessels in the lamina propria and muscularis propria. Mild urothelial papillary hyperplasia was present. No viral inclusions were observed. Immunohistochemical staining showed patchy positive reaction on CK20 and CD 44 proteins. The tumor protein P53 showed score 1 (less than 5%) positivity. The pathologic diagnosis was EC (Fig. 3).

At 2 weeks postoperatively, follow-up CT showed shrinkage of the mass lesion, but a remnant ulcerative lesion, which was thought to be the outer part of the mass lesion, was still noted at the bladder anterior and dome side (Fig. 4A). Another 1.4-cm cystic mass, thought to be the urachal cyst, was incidentally detected above the remnant mass (Fig. 4B). Thus, the mass that was resected with a resectoscope had EC, and the infected urachal cyst existed above the mass. To eliminate the remnant EC lesion and urachal cyst,

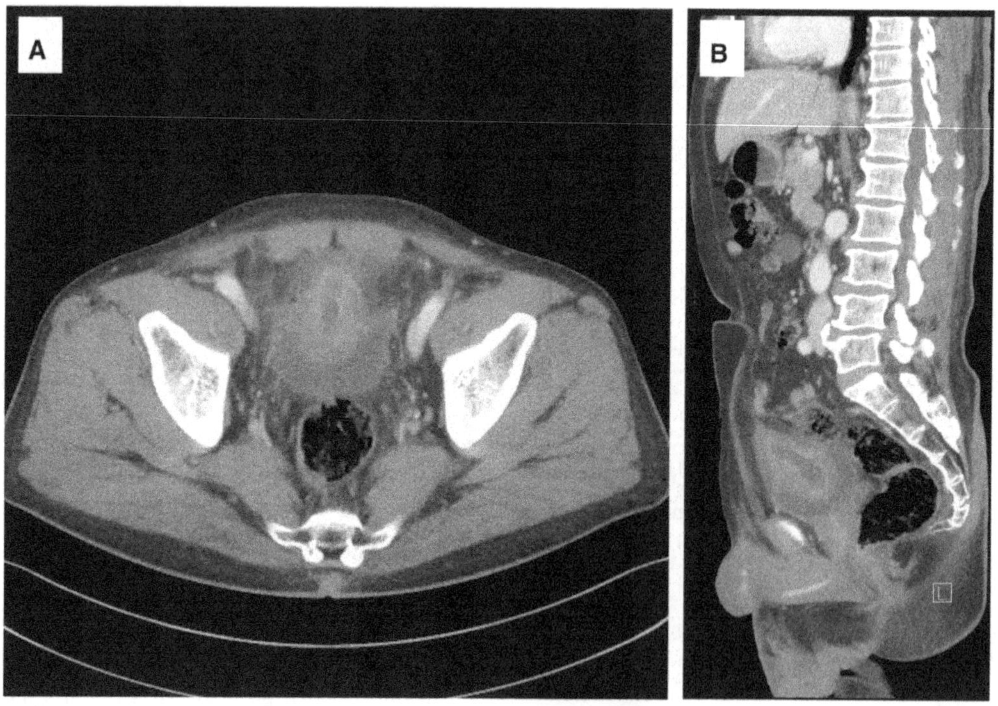

Fig. 1 Computed tomography showing a heterogeneous enhancing mass on the anterosuperior portion of the bladder. **A** Axial view, **B** sagittal view

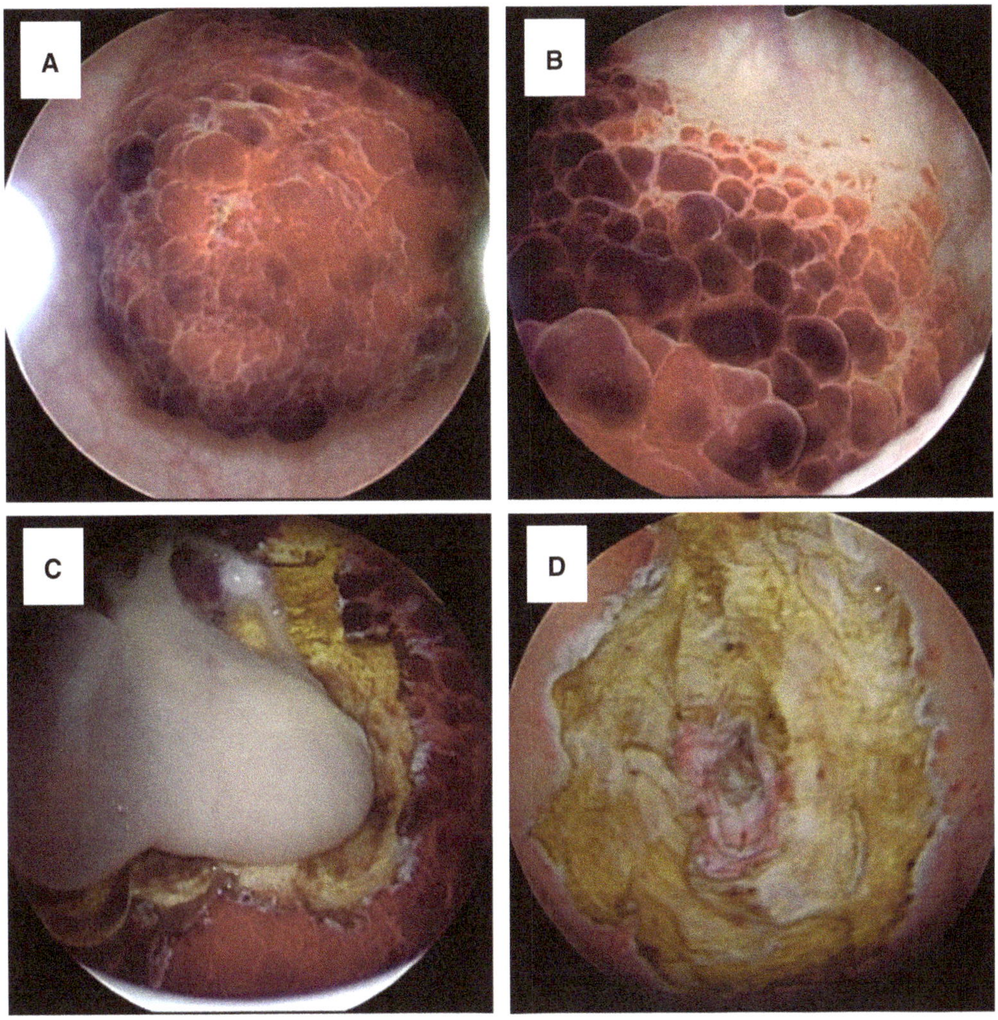

Fig. 2 Cystoscopic findings of bladder lesion. **A**, **B** Raspberry-like lesion on bladder dome. **C** At transurethral resection of the bladder, pus-like fluid is visible after resection of the mass lesion. **D** Tumor bed after mass resection. After resection of the mass lesion inside the bladder, the lesion outside the bladder is observed in the center

robot-assisted partial cystectomy was performed (Fig. 5). The urachal cyst was removed with a whole layer of the bladder wall that was, associated with the EC lesion. Similar to that seen in TURB lesions, partial cystectomy specimens showed heavy eosinophilic infiltration on the whole layers of the bladder wall, mucosal erosion, and fibrosis in the subepithelial connective tissue. An infected urachal cyst is accompanied by numerous lymphocytes, plasma cells, and histiocytic infiltrates. The benign epithelium of the urachal cyst is made up of cuboidal-type urothelium.

After partial cystectomy, the patient recovered uneventfully and was discharged on postoperative day 7. The patient was treated with antihistamine (hydroxyzine hydrochloride) for 15 months and regularly followed up. There was no evidence of recurrence in the follow-up CT and cystoscopy for up to 23 months.

Discussion and conclusion

To the best of our knowledge, this is the first report on EC that formed mass lesions involving both the inside and outside of the urinary bladder associated with infected urachal cysts. The majority of EC cases present with erythematous bladder mucosal lesions or bullous edematous lesions without a definite cause [4, 5, 7, 10, 11]. Although a few patients have been reported to present with bladder tumor-mimicking lesions [4, 5, 7, 10, 12], there is a case report of a pediatric patient who had a bladder tumor-mimicking lesion wherein the same was found after surgical excision of the infected urachal

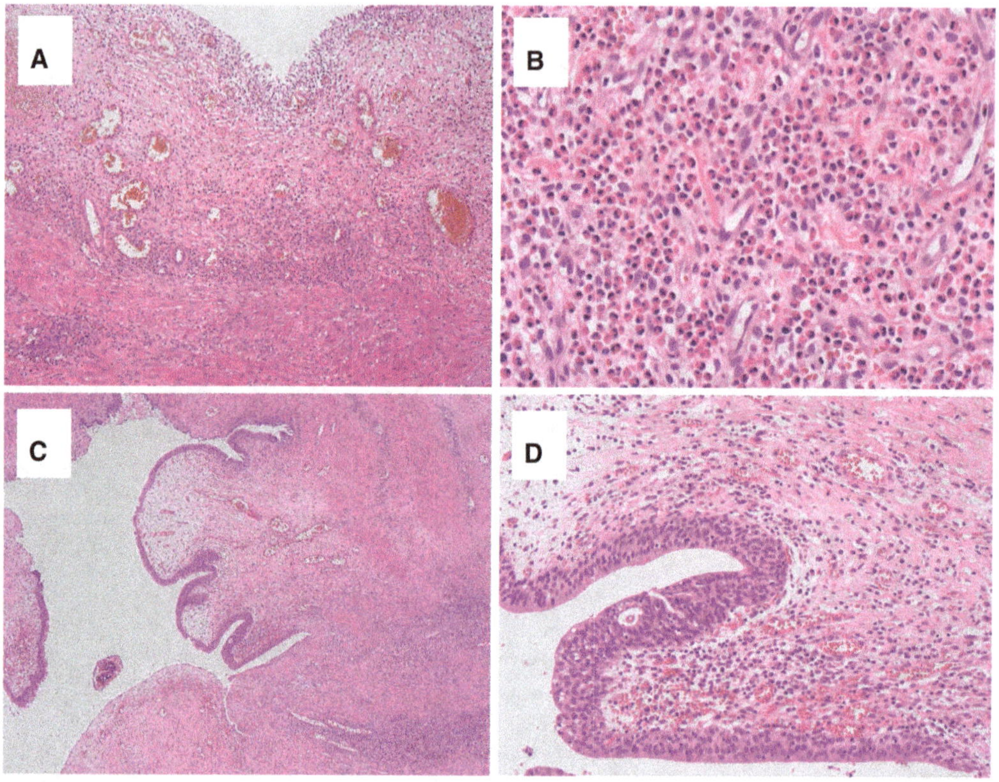

Fig. 3 Histologic findings of partial cystectomy specimen. **A** Low magnification photomicrography showing subepithelial and perivascular inflammatory cell infiltrate in the bladder (H&E. ×100). **B** Histopathology showing many eosinophils in the bladder wall (H&E. ×400). **C** The infected urachal cyst lined by urothelium and surrounded by mixed inflammatory cell infiltrate. (H&E. ×40). **D** The infected urachal cyst, histopathology showing numerous lymphocytes and plasma cells (H&E. ×200)

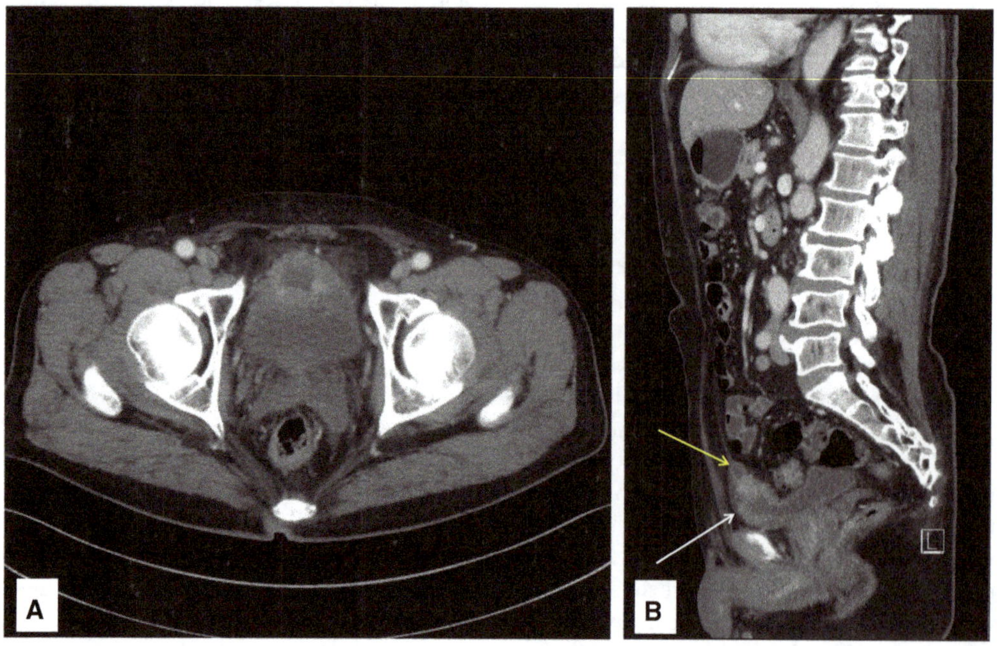

Fig. 4 Follow-up computed tomography after transurethral resection shows heterogeneous enhancing mass, reduced in size, on the anterosuperior portion of the bladder. **A** Axial view of bladder mass. **B** Sagittal view of remnant bladder mass (white arrow) with an urachal cyst (yellow arrow)

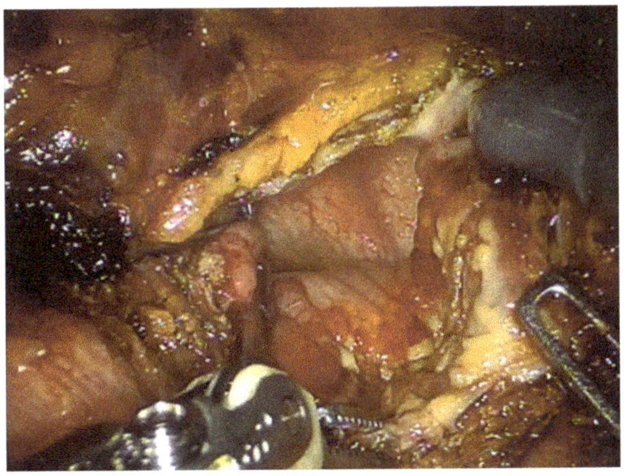

Fig. 5 Intraoperative view of robot-assisted partial cystectomy. Remnant lesion of eosinophilic cystitis after transurethral resection of the bladder (TURB) is identified at the bladder dome, i.e., remnant ulcerative, and a raspberry-like lesion is still visible. The lesion is completely removed with the infected urachal cyst, and the bladder is closed with continuous running suture

remnant [8]. In our case report, the patient presented with a sphere-like mass involving the inside and outside of the bladder as well as an infected urachal cyst. When the patient was initially presented, the bladder lesion was difficult to diagnose with EC because a huge berry-looking mass mimicking a bladder tumor was visible. To confirm the pathologic diagnosis and distinguish malignancy, TURB was performed.

Histopathological examination revealed heavy infiltration of eosinophils around vessels in the lamina propria and muscularis propria of the bladder mucosa. The diagnosis of EC can be made when many eosinophils are visible in bladder specimens [1, 2, 4, 6, 7]. There are no definite pathologic criteria for EC, but more than 25 eosinophils per high power field of view can be thought of as indicating EC, similar to eosinophilic esophagitis and gastritis [13]. In our case, heavy infiltration of eosinophils was visible around the mucosa and vessels in the lamina propria and muscularis propria, therefore diagnosis of EC could be made.

In laboratory findings, EC usually shows hematuria or proteinuria [14]. Furthermore, peripheral eosinophilia was observed in 42.5% to > 50% of the patients, and elevated ESR was observed in 7% of the patients [1, 7, 14]. In our case, the patient only showed hematopyuria without bacterial growth, and no elevation of ESR and peripheral eosinophilia was observed.

The etiology of EC is not well known because of the small number of cases. In most cases, allergies or bladder injuries are present [6]. Since EC is a result of antigen–antibody complexes [4, 5], avoiding antigens is also an effective method to treat EC. However, finding antigen is difficult in most cases, aside from using bladder instillation therapy. In our case, the patient had no allergies or history of bladder injury, but an infected urachal cyst was incidentally detected. Infected urachal cysts can act as allergens and attract eosinophils to the bladder wall. The infected urachal cyst may also have caused bladder injury due to the mass effect. Hypothetically, bladder inflammation induced by an infected urachal cyst could be the cause of EC. However, because the urachal cyst in our case was small (maximum diameter 1.7 cm) and the patient had no specific history (allergy, medical history, or bladder injury), it is not clear whether the small urachal cyst caused EC in this patient.

There is no definite curative treatment for EC, but medical treatments such as corticosteroids, antihistamines, and antibiotics can be considered as the primary treatment [3–5, 7, 14–16]. Corticosteroids can help control inflammation and symptoms, and antihistamines can help suppress the inflammatory reaction, which inhibits the formation of immune complexes. Antibiotics can be used when EC is associated with urinary tract infection. In our case, antibiotics were initially used because the mass was thought to be related to an infected cystic lesion, and antihistamines were used to prevent recurrence after partial cystectomy.

If corticosteroids or antihistamines could not resolve EC, surgical treatment is also an option [1, 5, 7, 16–18]. Surgical treatment not only has a high treatment success rate, but also a low recurrence rate [4, 7]. In our case, the reason for choosing partial cystectomy was that it required removal of the remnant urachal cyst. On CT, both urachal cysts and EC lesions were visible after TURB, and partial cystectomy was a good option to remove both lesions in one surgery.

Although the prognosis of EC is not well known, recurrences are common even after treatment. In a pooled analysis involving 135 patients, among 59 patients who received medical treatment, 10 patients (17.0%) showed recurrence of EC after medical treatment [7], whereas only 1 patient (2.6%) showed recurrence after surgery among 38 patients who were treated with surgery. However, in generalized lesions, medical treatment should be accompanied by surgical treatment [4]. Therefore, to prevent recurrence, our patient was treated with antihistamines (hydroxyzine hydrochloride) for 15 months. After 15 months, CT and cystoscopy showed no recurrence, and we decided to discontinue treatment with hydroxyzine hydrochloride and closely monitor the patient with CT. The patient was followed-up for 23 months without evidence of recurrence.

In conclusion, clinicians should consider the possibility of EC in patients presenting with hematuria, fever, and suprapubic pain with a bladder mass. Pathologic diagnosis can be made using cystoscopic biopsy or TURB, and this is essential to distinguish malignancy. In many cases, medical treatment shows successful outcomes, but partial cystectomy can be safely performed in patients with large mass-forming EC associated with urachal cyst, without any major complications.

Abbreviations

EC: Eosinophilic cystitis; TURB: Transurethral resection of the bladder tumor; CT: Computed tomography.

Acknowledgements

Not applicable.

Authors' contributions

HBS wrote the initial manuscript and substantively revised it. HSP has participated in searching the prior references. JHK performed the histologic examination of the bladder. JP, corresponding author, has made contributions to the conception of the study and revised the manuscript. All authors read and approved the final manuscript.

Author details

[1]Department of Urology, Eulji University Hospital, Eulji University School of Medicine, Daejeon, Korea. [2]Department of Pathology, Eulji University Hospital, Eulji University School of Medicine,, Daejeon, Korea. [3]Department of Urology, Uijeongbu Eulji Medical Center, Eulji University School of Medicine, 712, Dongil-ro, Uijeongbu-si, Gyeonggi-do 11759, Republic of Korea.

References

1. Kilic S, Erguvan R, Ipek D, Gokce H, Gunes A, Aydin NE, et al. Eosinophilic cystitis. A rare inflammatory pathology mimicking bladder neoplasms. Urol Int. 2003;71:285–9.
2. Thomas JC, Ross JH. Eosinophilic cystitis in a child presenting with a bladder mass. J Urol. 2004;171:1654–5.
3. Popescu OE, Landas SK, Haas GP. The spectrum of eosinophilic cystitis in males: case series and literature review. Arch Pathol Lab Med. 2009;133:289–94.
4. Teegavarapu PS, Sahai A, Chandra A, Dasgupta P, Khan MS. Eosinophilic cystitis and its management. Int J Clin Pract. 2005;59:356–60.
5. Thompson RH, Dicks D, Kramer SA. Clinical manifestations and functional outcomes in children with eosinophilic cystitis. J Urol. 2005;174:2347–9.
6. Hellstrom HR, Davis BK, Shonnard JW. Eosinophilic cystitis. A study of 16 cases. Am J Clin Pathol. 1979;72:777–84.
7. van den Ouden D. Diagnosis and management of eosinophilic cystitis: a pooled analysis of 135 cases. Eur Urol. 2000;37:386–94.
8. Goodman TR, Connolly B, Taylor G. Eosinophilic cystitis following an infected urachal remnant. Pediatr Radiol. 1999;29:487–8.
9. Devasia A, Kekre NS, Date A, Pandey AP, Gopalakrishnan G. Eosinophilic cystitis—not that uncommon! Scand J Urol Nephrol. 1999;33:396–9.
10. Itano NM, Malek RS. Eosinophilic cystitis in adults. J Urol. 2001;165:805–7.
11. Sidh SM, Smith SP, Silber SB, Young JD Jr. Eosinophilic cystitis: advanced disease requiring surgical intervention. Urology. 1980;15:23–6.
12. Oh SJ, Chi JG, Lee SE. Eosinophilic cystitis caused by vesical sparganosis: a case report. J Urol. 1993;149:581–3.
13. Zhou AG, Amin A, Yates JK, Diamond DA, Tyminski MM, Badway JA, et al. Mass forming eosinophilic cystitis in pediatric patients. Urology. 2017;101:139–41.
14. Kumar S, Sharma V, Ganesamoni R, Singh S. Eosinophilic cystitis mimicking tuberculosis: an analysis of five cases with review of literature. Urol Ann. 2013;5:50–2.
15. Park H. Eosinophilic cystitis with recurrent urinary retention: case report. Res Rep Urol. 2017;9:51–3.
16. Werbrouck C, Marrannes J, Verhamme L, Steenkiste E, Laridon E, Van Holsbeeck B. Eosinophilic cystitis mimicking bladder tumor. JBR-BTR. 2014;97:375.
17. Rossanese M, Palumbo V, Sioletic S, Crestani A, Giannarini G, Ficarra V. Surgical treatment of eosinophilic cystitis in adults: a report of two cases and a literature review. Urol Int. 2019;102:122–4.
18. Li G, Cai B, Song H, Yang Z. Clinical and radiological character of eosinophilic cystitis. Int J Clin Exp Med. 2015;8:533–9.

18

FAM83H and Nectin1 expression are related with survival and relapse of bladder urothelial carcinoma patients

Ae-Ri Ahn[1†], Sang Jae Noh[2†], Usama Khamis Hussein[1,3], Ho Sung Park[1], Myoung Ja Chung[1], Ho Lee[2], Woo Sung Moon[1], Myoung Jae Kang[1], Hyung Jin Kim[4], Na Ri Lee[5], Kyu Yun Jang[1*] and Kyoung Min Kim[1,6*]

Abstract

Background: FAM83H was originally reported to be essential for dental enamel formation. However, FAM83H has recently been implicated in tumorigenesis and tumor progression. Analysis of a publicly available gene expression database revealed a significant correlation between FAM83H and Nectin1 mRNA expression and bladder urothelial carcinoma (BUC). Therefore, we investigated the association between FAM83H and Nectin1 expression levels and the survival and recurrence of BUC in BUC patients using a tissue microarray.

Methods: We performed immunohistochemical staining of FAM83H and Nectin1 in 165 human BUC tissue sections, and analyzed the prognostic significance of FAM83H and Nectin1 expression.

Results: Both FAM83H and Nectin1 were mainly expressed in the cytoplasm, and their expression was significantly associated. FAM83H expression was significantly correlated with higher histologic grade, higher T stage, higher TNM stage, and recurrence. Nectin1 expression was significantly associated with higher histologic grade and recurrence. Univariate analysis showed FAM83H expression and Nectin1 expression were significantly associated with worse overall survival (OS) and shorter relapse-free survival (RFS) of BUC patients. In multivariate analysis, levels of FAM83H and Nectin1 were independent indicators of shorter survival of BUC patients.

Conclusions: Our results suggest that FAM83H and Nectin1 are important in the progression of BUC, and that expression patterns of these two proteins can be used as prognostic indicators of survival in BUC patients.

Introduction

Bladder cancer is a common cancer, accounting for approximately 3.0% of new cancers and 2.1% of cancer deaths worldwide [1]. The prognosis of patients with bladder cancer is relatively good, with a 5-year survival rate of approximately 70% [2]. However, the survival rate has not improved over the years. Moreover, the prognosis of patients with metastasis is poor, with a median survival of 5–7 months and a 5-year survival rate of only 15% [3, 4]. Therefore, new approaches are necessary to supplement the current platinum-based therapeutic strategy.

There are two distinct pathways for development of bladder urothelial carcinoma (BUC): a hyperplasia pathway and a dysplasia pathway [5–8]. The hyperplasia pathway is more common and accounts for 80% of BUCs [6]. Tumors that develop by activation of the hyperplasia pathway first manifest as urothelial hyperplasia with advancement to low-grade papillary urothelial carcinoma [6, 7, 9]. The hyperplasia pathway is characterized by alterations in the *FGFR3* gene, and is genetically stable [8]. Tumors that develop due to activation of this pathway

*Correspondence: kyjang@jbnu.ac.kr; kmkim@jbnu.ac.kr
†Ae-Ri Ahn and Sang Jae Noh have contributed equally to this work
[1] Department of Pathology, Jeonbuk National University Medical School, Jeonju, Republic of Korea
Full list of author information is available at the end of the article

are non-aggressive [9]. Tumors that result from activation of the dysplasia pathway initially present as dysplasia that then progresses to high-grade papillary urothelial carcinoma or urothelial carcinoma in situ and account for approximately 20% of BUC cases. These tumors are associated with a high risk of muscle invasion and metastasis [7, 8]. This pathway is genetically instable and inactivating mutations of *TP53* are the most common genetic alterations [7].

FAM83H was originally reported to be an essential molecule for dental enamel formation [10, 11]. However, FAM83H has more recently been found to be involved in tumorigenesis and tumor progression [12–15]. In colorectal cancer, FAM83H regulates the organization of the keratin cytoskeleton and formation of desmosomes and is involved in the movement of cancer cells [12]. FAM83H has also been suggested to contribute to the progression of androgen-independent prostate cancer [16]. FAM83H is transcriptionally controlled by the well-known oncogene MYC and regulates the proliferation of hepatocellular carcinoma cells [13]. In osteosarcomas, FAM83H stabilizes β-catenin and regulates Wnt signaling [14]. Expression of FAM83H was found to be associated with poor survival of renal cell carcinoma patients [17] and FAM83H expression was associated with a worse prognosis and found to be involved in PI3K-Akt-mTOR signaling in pancreatic cancer [18]. However, neither the expression nor role of FAM83H in BUC has been studied to date.

Nectin1 is a member of the Nectin family of immunoglobulin-like cell adhesion molecules. Nectins participate in various cellular activities such as cell differentiation, polarization, migration, proliferation, and survival [19, 20]. Although limited number of studies have analyzed the role of Nectin1 in tumors, most of these studies have found that Nectin1 expression is associated with cancer progression. In colorectal cancer, Nectin1 expression was associated with a worse 3-year progression-free survival rate [21]. Furthermore, Nectin1 expression in cancer-associated fibroblasts was correlated with a poor prognosis in pancreatic ductal adenocarcinoma patients [22]. However, similar to FAM83H, the role of Nectin1 in BUC has not previously been explored.

We analyzed the BUC dataset of The Cancer Genome Atlas (TCGA), Cell 2017 [23] through the cBioPortal public database (http://www.cbioportal.org), and found that Nectin1 mRNA expression was significant associated with FAM83H mRNA expression in BUCs (Additional file 1: Figure 1). Therefore, in this study, we investigated the prognostic impact of FAM83H and Nectin1 expression using immunohistochemical staining of a human BUC tissue microarray. In addition, we also evaluated FAM83H and Nectin1 expression in low-grade and high-grade non-invasive BUCs because of the considerable differences in biologic behavior and underlying genetic alterations of these BUCs.

Materials and methods

Ethical approval

This study was approved by the Institutional Review Board of Jeonbuk National University Hospital (IRB number, CUH 2020-02-007) and was performed in accordance with the principles of the Declaration of Helsinki. Signed informed consent form was obtained from all eligible participants.

Patients and follow-up

One hundred sixty-five BUC patients who underwent surgery at Jeonbuk National University Hospital between January 2008 and September 2018 were included in this study. Clinicopathologic information was obtained by reviewing medical records. Clinicopathological factors evaluated in this study were sex, age, histologic grade, T stage, N stage, M stage, TNM stage, and recurrence. Histologic slides were reviewed according to the WHO classification of tumors of the urinary system and male genital organs [24]. The 8th edition of the American Joint Committee Cancer Staging System was referenced to classify the TNM stage of BUC patients [3].

After the surgery, follow-up of the patients was carried out every 3 months in the first year. After the first year, the patients visited the hospital every 6 to 8 months period. During the follow-up, physical examination and blood and urine analysis were performed. For 3 years after the surgery, cystoscopic screening was performed in every 6 months. The survival data were most recently renewed in March 2020. The mean follow-up duration was 53.8 months.

Immunohistochemical staining and scoring

In May 2020, we established a tissue microarray from paraffin-embedded tissue blocks of surgical specimens of BUC patients to evaluate the immunohistochemical expression of FAM83H and Nectin1. Two 3.0 mm cores without necrosis or degenerative changes were obtained from the tumor for each case. Tissue sections were deparaffinized followed by antigen retrieval using a microwave oven in pH 6.0 antigen retrieval solution (DAKO, Glostrup, Denmark). Then, tissue sections were incubated with primary antibodies for FAM83H (1:100, catalogue no. A304-328A, Bethyl Laboratories, Montgomery, TX) and Nectin1 (1:50, catalogue no. sc-21722, Santa Cruz Biotechnology, Santa Cruz, CA) overnight at 4°C.

Immunohistochemical staining results were evaluated by two pathologists (KYJ and KMK) by consensus without knowledge of the patients' clinical status using a multi-viewing microscope (Nikon Eclipse 80i; Nikon, Tokyo, Japan). Both FAM83H and Nectin1 were mainly expressed in the cytoplasm. Intensity of immunohistochemical staining was scored as follows: negative, 0; weak, 1; intermediate, 2; and strong, 3. In addition, the proportion of tissue area stained was scored as follows: no staining, 0; ~ 1% staining, 1; 2–10% staining, 2; 11–33% staining, 3; 34–66% staining, 4; and 67–100% staining, 5. The staining intensity score and staining area score were added for each tissue section, and then the scores for the two tissue sections per case were added to obtain the final score for each patient. The immunohistochemical staining score therefore ranged from 0 to 16.

Statistical analysis

Patients were divided into negative and positive subgroups based on the immunohistochemical expression of FAM83H and Nectin1. The cut-off points for both FAM83H and Nectin1 were determined by receiver operating characteristic curve analysis as the highest predictive point for death [25]. We excluded non-invasive low-grade BUC cases from the survival analysis because of the significant difference in the prognosis of these cases compared to non-invasive high-grade and invasive cases. Overall survival (OS) and relapse-free survival (RFS) were evaluated through March 2020. In OS analysis, death of the patient by urothelial carcinoma was considered an event. Cases characterized by death due to other causes or being alive at the last follow-up were censored. Relapse of urothelial carcinoma or patient death by urothelial carcinoma were treated as events in the RFS analysis. Cox proportional hazards regression analysis and Kaplan–Meier survival analysis were utilized to evaluate the prognosis of urothelial carcinoma patients. Features independently associated with survival were included in multivariate analysis of Cox's proportional hazards model using the stepwise method. The relationship between immunohistochemical expression and clinicopathological factors was analyzed with Pearson's chi-square test. Pearson's method was utilized to evaluated the correlation between FAM83H and Nectin1 expression. SPSS software (IBM, version 19.0, Armonk, NY) was used throughout for statistical analysis. P values less than 0.05 were considered statistically significant.

Results

Expression of FAM83H and Nectin1 in BUC tissue sections and the correlation between expression levels of these two proteins and clinicopathologic characteristics

Typical immunohistochemical staining results for FAM83H and Nectin1 in BUC tissue sections are shown in Fig. 1. Both FAM83H and Nectin1 were expressed primarily in the cytoplasm (Fig. 1A). We performed receiver operating characteristic curve analysis according to the death of BUC patients to assign patients to FAM83H and Nectin1 negative- and positive expression groups. The cut-off points for the expression of FAM83H and Nectin1 were both eight (Fig. 1B). Using these cut-off values, 110 (66.7%) and 101 (61.2%) BUC patients were classified as belonging to the FAM83H positive-group and Nectin1 positive-group, respectively.

Positive FAM83H expression was significantly correlated with higher histologic grade ($P<0.001$), higher T stage ($P=0.004$), higher TNM stage ($P=0.008$), and recurrence ($P=0.022$) (Table 1). Positive Nectin1 expression was significantly associated with higher histologic grade ($P<0.001$), higher N stage ($P=0.031$), and recurrence ($P=0.014$) (Table 1).

Expression of FAM83H and Nectin1 in non-invasive BUCs

Because of the significant difference in prognosis and underlying molecular characteristics of low- and high-grade non-invasive BUCs, we investigated FAM83H and Nectin1 expression according to histologic grade in non-invasive BUCs (Table 2). High-grade non-invasive BUC tissue sections were significantly more likely to be positive for FAM83H and Nectin1 expression than low-grade non-invasive BUCs ($P=0.02$, $P=0.034$, respectively).

Expression of FAM83H and Nectin1 correlates with poor prognosis in BUC patients

We excluded non-invasive low-grade BUCs from the survival analysis because these tumors rarely progress to invasive carcinoma. Univariate analysis showed that histologic grade, T stage, N stage, M stage, TNM stage, FAM83H expression ($P<0.001$), and Nectin1 expression ($P=0.002$) were significantly associated with the OS of bladder urothelial carcinoma patients (Table 3). Histologic grade, T stage, N stage, TNM stage, FAM83H expression ($P<0.001$), and Nectin1 expression ($P=0.001$) were significantly correlated with the RFS of BUC patients based on univariate analysis (Table 3). FAM83H-positive patients had a 3.42-fold [95% confidence interval (95% CI); 1.75–6.7, $P<0.001$] increased risk of death and a 3.83-fold (95% CI 2.06–7.12, $P<0.001$) increased risk of relapse or death compared to FAM83H-negative patients (Table 3). Nectin1-positive patients had a 2.48-fold (95% CI 1.42–4.35, $P=0.002$) increased risk of death and a 2.48-fold (95% CI 1.47–4.17, $P=0.001$) increased risk of relapse or death compared to Nectin1-negative patients (Table 3). Kaplan–Meier survival analysis curves for OS and RFS of BUC patients according to the expression of FAM83H and Nectin1 are presented in Fig. 2.

We also performed multivariate analysis of OS and RFS in BUC patients. Factors significantly associated with OS

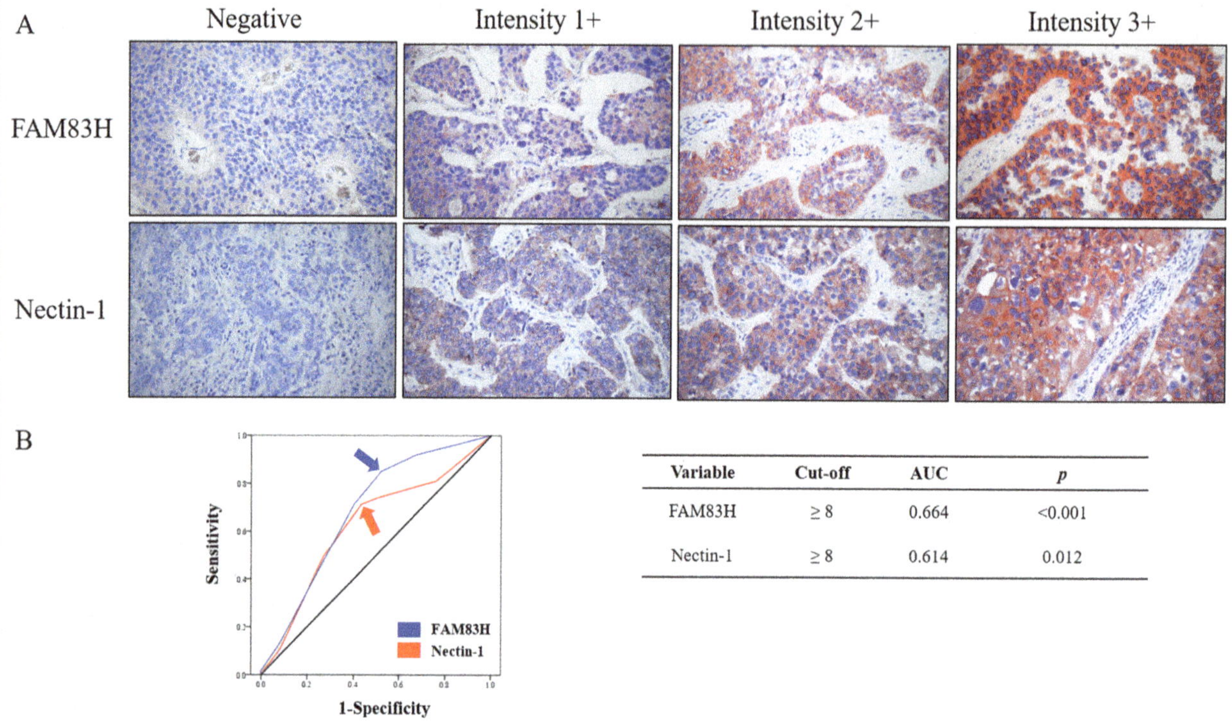

Variable	Cut-off	AUC	p
FAM83H	≥ 8	0.664	<0.001
Nectin-1	≥ 8	0.614	0.012

Fig. 1 Immunohistochemical expression of FAM83H and Nectin1 in Bladder urothelial carcinoma. **A** FAM83H and Nectin1 are expressed mainly in the cytoplasm of the cancer cells. Original magnification: × 400. **B** Receiver operating characteristic curve analysis to determine cut-off points for the expression of nuclear FAM83H (blue arrow) and cytoplasmic Nectin1 (red arrow). The cut-off points indicate the point of the highest area under the curve (AUC) to predict the death of bladder urothelial carcinoma patients

or RFS were included in the analysis. T stage, N stage, M stage, and FAM83H expression were independent prognostic factors associated with OS in BUC patients (Table 4, model 1). Positive-FAM83H expression group had a 3.14-fold (95% CI 1.59–6.22, $P=0.001$) increased risk of death comparted to the negative-FAM83H expression group (Table 4, model 1). TNM stage and FAM83H expression were independent prognostic factors of RFS based on multivariate analysis (Table 5, model 1). FAM83H-positive expression group had a 3.69-fold (95% CI 1.98–6.89, $P<0.001$) increased risk of relapse or death compared to the FAM83H-negative expression group (Table 5, model 1).

Co-expression patterns of FAM83H and Nectin1 expression and their correlations with clinicopathologic features and survival in patients with non-invasive high-grade or invasive BUC

We re-classified patients into three sub-groups (FAM83H+/Nectin1+, FAM83H+/Nectin1− or FAM83H−/Nectin1+, and FAM83H−/Nectin1−) based on FAM83H and Nectin1 expression. Co-expression of FAM83H/Nectin1 was significantly associated with histologic grade ($P<0.001$), T stage ($P=0.021$), and recurrence ($P=0.002$) (Table 1). FAM83H/Nectin1 co-expression also showed a significant correlation with histologic grade in non-invasive BUCs (Table 2). The number of FAM83H+/Nectin1+ group was highest in high-grade non-invasive BUC with FAM83H−/Nectin1− group showing lowest number in high-grade non-invasive BUC ($P=0.021$).

Univariate analysis indicated that co-expression of FAM83H/Nectin1 was significantly associated with the OS and RFS of BUC patients (Table 3). FAM83H+/Nectin1− and FAM83H−/Nectin1+ cases had a 3.89-fold (95% CI 1.42–10.62) and 3.36 (95% CI 1.39–8.11) greater risk of death and relapse or death, respectively, than FAM83H−/Nectin1− cases (Table 3). Co-expression of FAM83H+/Nectin1+ was associated with a 5.58-fold (95% CI 2.22–14.05) and 5.31 (95% CI 2.4–11.74) greater risk of death and relapse or death, respectively, compared to FAM83H−/Nectin1− cases (Table 3). Kaplan–Meier survival analysis curves for OS and RFS of BUC patients according to co-expression patterns of FAM83H and Nectin1 are presented in Fig. 2. Overall survival and relapse-free survival of BUC patients showed a stepwise decrease from the FAM83H−/Nectin1− group to the FAM83H+/Nectin1+ group. However, there was

Table 1 Clinicopathologic variables and the expression of FAM83H and Nectin1 in bladder urothelial carcinomas

Characteristics		Total	FAM83H expression		*p*	Nectin1 expression		*p*	Combined expression			*p*
			Positive	Negative		Positive	Negative		FAM83H+/Nectin1+	FAM83H+/Nectin1− or FAM83H−/Nectin1+	FAM83H−/Nectin1−	
All cases		165	110 (66.7%)	55 (33.3%)		101 (61.2%)	64 (38.8%)		86 (52.1%)	39 (23.6%)	40 (24.2%)	
Sex	Male	145	96 (66.2%)	49 (33.8%)		87 (60%)	58 (40%)		74 (51%)	35 (24.1%)	36 (24.8%)	
	Female	20	14 (70%)	6 (30%)	0.736	14 (70%)	6 (30%)	0.39	12 (60%)	4 (20%)	4 (20%)	0.753
Age (years)	≤65	44	25 (56.8%)	19 (43.2%)		25 (56.8%)	19 (43.2%)		20 (45.5%)	10 (22.7%)	14 (31.8%)	
	>65	121	85 (70.2%)	36 (29.8%)	0.106	76 (62.8%)	45 (37.2%)	0.485	66 (54.5%)	29 (24%)	26 (21.5%)	0.377
Histologic grade	Low	56	23 (41.1%)	33 (58.9%)		21 (37.5%)	35 (62.5%)		14 (25%)	16 (28.6%)	26 (46.4%)	
	High	109	87 (79.8%)	22 (20.2%)	<0.001	80 (73.4%)	29 (26.6%)	<0.001	72 (66.1%)	23 (21.1%)	14 (12.8%)	<0.001
T stage	Ta	37	18 (48.6%)	19 (51.4%)		19 (51.4%)	18 (48.6%)		12 (32.4%)	13 (35.1%)	12 (32.4%)	
	T1	77	50 (64.9%)	27 (35.1%)		46 (59.7%)	31 (40.3%)		39 (50.6%)	18 (23.4%)	20 (26%)	
	T2-4	51	42 (82.4%)	9 (17.6%)	0.004	36 (70.6%)	15 (29.4%)	0.176	35 (68.6%)	8 (15.7%)	8 (15.7%)	0.021
N stage	N0	158	104 (65.8%)	54 (34.2%)		94 (59.5%)	64 (40.5%)		80 (50.6%)	38 (24.1%)	40 (25.3%)	
	N1-3	7	6 (85.7%)	1 (14.3%)	0.275	7 (100%)	0 (0%)	0.031	6 (85.7%)	1 (14.3%)	0 (0%)	0.163
M stage	M0	160	105 (65.6%)	55 (34.4%)		97 (60.6%)	63 (39.4%)		82 (51.3%)	38 (23.8%)	40 (25%)	
	M1	5	5 (100%)	0 (0%)	0.108	4 (80%)	1 (20%)	0.381	4 (80%)	1 (20%)	0 (0%)	0.359
TNM stage	Stage 0	37	18 (48.6%)	19 (51.4%)		19 (51.4%)	18 (48.6%)		12 (32.4%)	13 (35.1%)	12 (32.4%)	
	Stage I	77	50 (64.9%)	27 (35.1%)		46 (59.7%)	31 (40.3%)		39 (50.6%)	18 (23.4%)	20 (26%)	
	Stage II, III	46	37 (80.4%)	9 (19.6%)		32 (69.6%)	14 (30.4%)		31 (67.4%)	7 (15.2%)	8 (17.4%)	
	Stage IV	5	5 (100%)	0 (0%)	0.008	4 (80%)	1 (20%)	0.298	4 (80%)	1 (20%)	0 (0%)	0.056
Recurrence	Present	49	39 (79.6%)	10 (20.4%)		37 (75.5%)	12 (24.5%)		30 (61.2%)	16 (32.7%)	3 (6.1%)	
	Absent	116	71 (61.2%)	45 (38.8%)	0.022	64 (55.2%)	52 (44.8%)	0.014	56 (48.3%)	23 (19.8%)	37 (31.9%)	0.002

Table 2 Expression of FAM83H and Nectin1 in non-invasive bladder urothelial carcinomas

Characteristics		Total	FAM83H expression		*p*	Nectin1 expression		*p*	Combined expression			*p*
			Positive	Negative		Positive	Negative		FAM83H+/ Nectin1+	FAM83H+/Nectin1− or FAM83H−/Nectin1+	FAM83H−/Nectin1−	
Histologic grade	Low	27	10 (37%)	17 (63%)		11 (40.7%)	16 (59.3%)		6 (22.2%)	9 (33.3%)	12 (44.4%)	
	High	10	8 (80%)	2 (20%)	0.02	8 (80%)	2 (20%)	0.034	6 (60%)	4 (40%)	0 (0%)	0.021

Table 3 Univariate Cox proportional hazards regression analysis for overall survival and relapse-free survival in non-invasive high-grade and invasive bladder urothelial carcinomas

Characteristics	OS		RFS	
	HR (95% CI)	*p*	HR (95% CI)	*p*
Sex, female (vs. male)	1.014 (0.503–2.042)	0.969	1.065 (0.532–2.134)	0.859
Age, y ≥ 65 (vs. < 65)	1.776 (0.953–3.309)	0.055	1.265 (0.738–2.167)	0.392
Grade, high (vs. low)	2.924 (1.398–6.117)	0.004	2.547 (1.307–4.963)	0.006
T stage, Ta	1	< 0.001	1	0.012
T1	1.372 (0.419–4.497)	0.601	0.916 (0.361–2.323)	0.854
T2–4	5.054 (1.55–16.475)	0.007	1.842 (0.717–4.729)	0.204
N stage, N1-3 (vs. N0)	5.832 (2.575–13.211)	< 0.001	3.087 (1.319–7.227)	0.009
M stage, M1 (vs. M0)	7.814 (3.038–20.096)	< 0.001	0.894 (0.123–6.48)	0.912
TNM stage, Stage 0	1	< 0.001	1	0.027
Stage I	1.374 (0.419–4.503)	0.6	0.916 (0.362–2.323)	0.916
Stage II, III	4.625 (1.41–15.177)	0.012	1.88 (0.731–4.835)	0.19
Stage IV	17.793 (4.119–76.872)	< 0.001	1.085 (0.126–9.368)	0.879
FAM83H, positive (vs. negative)	3.423 (1.748–6.704)	< 0.001	3.83 (2.06–7.121)	< 0.001
Nectin1, positive (vs. negative)	2.48 (1.415–4.346)	0.002	2.475 (1.469–4.169)	0.001
Combined expression, FAM83H−/Nectin1−	1	0.001	1	< 0.001
FAM83H−/Nectin1+ or FAM83H+/Nectin1−	3.89 (1.424–10.624)	0.008	3.36 (1.392–8.11)	0.007
FAM83H+/Nectin1+	5.579 (2.216–14.046)	< 0.001	5.309 (2.402–11.735)	< 0.001

no significant differences in survival rate between the FAM83H+/Nectin1− and FAM83H−/Nectin1+ group versus the FAM83H+/Nectin1+ group (Fig. 2).

In multivariate analysis, co-expression pattern of FAM83H and Nectin1 was an independent prognostic factor. FAM83H+/Nectin1− and FAM83H−/Nectin1+ cases had a 4.73-fold (95% CI 1.7–13.16) greater risk of death than FAM83H−/Nectin1− cases while FAM83H+/Nectin1+ cases had a 5.46-fold (95% CI 2.14–13.91) greater risk of death than FAM83H−/Nectin1− cases (Table 4, model 2). FAM83H+/Nectin1− cases and FAM83H−/Nectin1+ cases had a 3.88-fold (95% CI 1.58–9.5) greater risk of death or relapse than FAM83H−/Nectin1− cases while FAM83H+/Nectin1+ cases had a 5.27-fold (95% CI 2.38–11.69) greater risk of death or relapse than FAM83H−/Nectin1− cases (Table 5, model 2).

FAM83H and Nectin1 expression are significantly correlated

Analysis of data in the cBioPortal database revealed that mRNA levels of FAM83H and Nectin1 were significantly correlated (Supplemental Figure S1). Therefore, we analyzed the relationship between immunohistochemical expression of FAM83H and Nectin1. The χ^2 test showed significant associations between positive- and negative-expression groups of FAM83H and Nectin1 ($P < 0.001$) (Table 6). Moreover, there was a significant correlation between immunohistochemical staining scores for FAM83H and Nectin1 (both variables analyzed as continuous data, Pearson's $r = 0.502$, $P < 0.001$; Spearman's $r = 0.545$, $P < 0.001$; Fig. 3).

Discussion

In the present study, we investigated the immunohistochemical expression of FAM83H and Nectin1 in a human BUC tissue microarray. This is the first report to assess if the expression of FAM83H and Nectin1 in BUCs is correlated. We found that (1) positive expression of FAM83H and Nectin1 was correlated with unfavorable clinicopathologic characteristics; (2) FAM83H and Nectin1 expression were significantly higher in high-grade non-invasive BUCs than low-grade BUCs; (3) BUC patients whose tumors were positive for FAM83H and Nectin1 had shorter OS and RFS; (4) individual and co-expression patterns of FAM83H and Nectin1 were poor independent prognostic factors for OS and RFS; and (5) expression of FAM83H and Nectin1 were significantly positively correlated.

Although FAM83H was originally identified as important in dental enamel formation, expression of this protein has been found to be increased in stomach, pancreas, liver, ovary, colon and breast cancers [26]. FAM83H is thought to stabilize β-catenin in osteosarcomas [14] while in colon cancer, FAM83H has been reported to contribute to tumor progression via keratin cytoskeleton

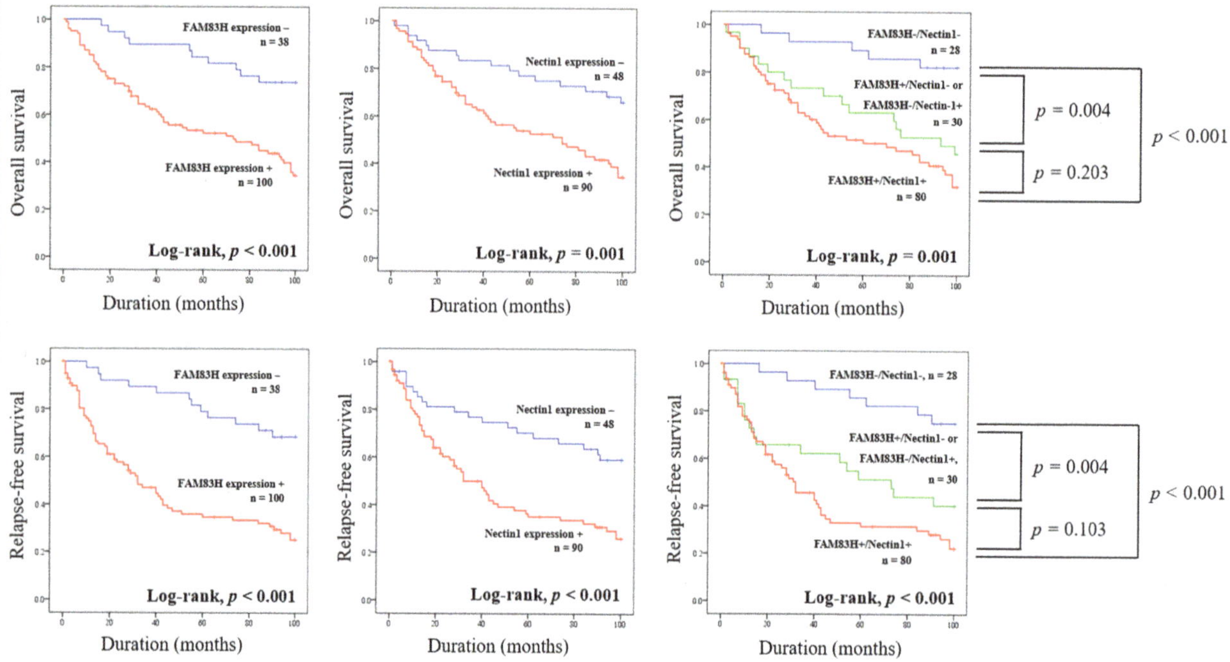

Fig. 2 Survival analysis according to expression of FAM83H and Nectin1 in bladder urothelial carcinoma patients. Kaplan–Meier survival curves for overall survival and relapse-free survival of bladder urothelial carcinoma patients according to the individual and coexpression of FAM83H, and Nectin1

disorganization [15]. Moreover, FAM83H is thought to be involved in hepatocellular carcinoma progression by controlling the transcription of MYC [13]. In addition, higher expression of FAM83H was found to be associated with shorter survival in patients with clear cell renal cell carcinoma, pancreatic cancer, or uterine cancer [17, 18, 26]. However in contrast to the majority of the reports, one study reported that FAM83H expression was associated with better disease-free survival in brain astrocytoma and oligodendroglioma patients [26]. Therefore, the role of FAM83H in tumorigenesis or tumor progression may differ according to cancer type. Consistent with the majority of reports, we found that FAM83H expression was associated with tumor progression in BUC patients. Positive expression of FAM83H was associated with higher histologic grade, higher T stage, and higher TNM stage BUCs. Moreover, patients with positive FAM83H expression had significantly shorter OS and RFS in univariate analysis. Multivariate analysis revealed that FAM83H expression was an independent factor for shorter OS and RFS in BUC patients.

Nectin proteins are Ca^{2+}-independent immunoglobulin-like cell adhesion molecules involved in cell to cell adhesion, and are involved in various cellular activities such as differentiation, proliferation, survival, and movement [19]. Nectin1 is one of the four members of the Nectin family and is expressed in many cell types, including neurons, fibroblasts, and epithelial cells [27]. In the context of cancer research, one study reported that Nectin1 expression was associated with shorter progression-free survival of colorectal cancer patients [21]. Another study reported that Nectin1 expression in cancer-associated fibroblasts of pancreatic ductal adenocarcinoma was significantly related to invasion, metastasis, and shorter OS [22]. However, absent or decreased Nectin1 expression was found in the invading edge of uterine cervical squamous cell carcinomas compared to the center of these tumors [28]. In addition, Nectin1 expression was decreased in gastric cancer compared to normal gastric tissue and was associated with better OS [29]. Therefore, similar to FAM83H, Nectin1 might play different roles in different cancer types. In the present study, positive Nectin1 expression was significantly associated with poor prognostic factors such as higher histologic grade and higher N stage. In univariate analysis, patients with BUCs that stained positive for Nectin1 had a significantly shorter OS and RFS than patients with BUCs that were negative for Nectin1 expression. In addition, positive Nectin1 expression was an independent prognostic factor for RFS survival in BUC patients in multivariate analysis.

Another interesting finding in our study is that FAM83H expression and Nectin1 expression were significantly positively correlated in BUC samples,

Table 4 Multivariate Cox regression analysis for overall survival in non-invasive high-grade and invasive bladder urothelial carcinomas

Characteristics	OS	
	HR (95% CI)	*p*
Model 1[a]		
T stage, Ta	1	< 0.001
T1	1.647 (0.501–5.411)	0.411
T2-4	4.78 (1.434–15.932)	0.011
N stage, N1-3 (vs. N0)	2.774 (1.185–6.492)	0.019
M stage, M1 (vs. M0)	3.435 (1.291–9.142)	0.013
FAM83H positive (vs. negative)	3.141 (1.587–6.215)	0.001
Model 2[b]		
T stage, Ta	1	< 0.001
T1	1.831 (0.556–6.025)	0.32
T2-4	5.76 (1.707–19.436)	0.005
N stage, N1-3 (vs. N0)	2.382 (1.016–5.586)	0.046
M stage, M1 (vs. M0)	3.428 (1.277–9.196)	0.014
Combined expression, FAM83H−/Nectin1−	1	0.002
FAM83H−/Nectin1+ or FAM83H+/Nectin1−	4.731 (1.7–13.163)	0.003
FAM83H+/Nectin1+	5.46 (2.144–13.905)	< 0.001

OS overall survival, *HR* hazard ratio, *95% CI* 95% confidence interval

[a] Variables considered in model 1 were histologic grade, T stage, N stage, M stage, TNM stage, FAM83H expression, and Nectin1 expression

[b] Variables considered in model 2 were histologic grade, T stage, N stage, M stage, TNM stage, and combined expression of FAM83H and Nectin1

Table 5 Multivariate Cox regression analysis for relapse-free survival in non-invasive high-grade and invasive bladder urothelial carcinomas

	RFS	
	HR (95% CI)	*p*
Model 1[a]		
TNM stage, Stage 0	1	0.067
Stage I	1.075 (0.423–2.729)	0.88
Stage II, III	1.983 (0.77–5.106)	0.156
Stage IV	0.906 (0.105–7.837)	0.929
FAM83H positive (vs. negative)	3.691 (1.977–6.889)	< 0.001
Model 2[b]		
TNM stage, Stage 0	1	0.037
Stage I	1.175 (0.871–3.021)	0.738
Stage II, III	2.305 (0.871–6.1)	0.093
Stage IV	1.106 (0.128–9.584)	0.927
Combined expression, FAM83H−/Nectin1−	1	< 0.001
FAM83H−/Nectin1+ or FAM83H+/Nectin1−	3.877 (1.582–9.502)	0.003
FAM83H+/Nectin1+	5.272 (2.377–11.693)	< 0.001

RFS relapse free survival, *HR* hazard ratio, *95% CI* 95% confidence interval

[a] Variables considered in model 1 were histologic grade, T stage, N stage, TNM stage, FAM83H expression, and Nectin1 expression

[b] Variables considered in model 2 were histologic grade, T stage, N stage, TNM stage, and combined expression of FAM83H and Nectin1

Table 6 Correlation between expression of FAM83H and Necin-1

Characteristics		FAM83H expression		*p*
		Positive	Negative	
Nectin1 expression	Positive	96 (58.2%)	16 (9.7%)	
	Negative	14 (8.5%)	39 (23.6%)	< 0.001

consistent with the association between the mRNA expression of FAM83H and Nectin1 in the cBioPortal public database. When we subdivided BUC patients according to co-expression patterns of FAM83H and Nectin1 (FAM83H+/Nectin1+, FAM83H+/Nectin1− or FAM83H−/Nectin1+, and FAM83H−/Nectin1−), we found that positive expression of both FAM83H and Nectin1 was significantly associated with higher T stage, higher histologic grade, and recurrence. Survival analysis revealed FAM83H+/Nectin1+ patient had the shortest OS and RFS of the three groups analyzed. Moreover, FAM83H+/Nectin1− or FAM83H−/Nectin1+ patients had a shorter OS and RFS than FAM83H−/Nectin1− patients. Multivariate survival analysis showed that combined expression of FAM83H and Nectin1 was an independent prognostic factor for OS and RFS in BUC patients. The results from this study indicate that FAM83H and Nectin1 are closely related to each other and play an important role in BUC progression. As mentioned above, Nectin1 is involved in cell adhesion and interacts with actin filaments [19, 20]. In a previous report, FAM83H was suggested to be a linker protein between CK-1α and keratin filaments and to be involved in the migration of cancer cells by reorganizing the keratin cytoskeleton [12]. Therefore, FAM83H and Nectin1 may interact to control the organization of cellular microfilaments such as keratin and actin filaments.

Our study has certain limitations. A major limitation is that this was a single center study and included a relatively small number of BUC patients. Therefore, additional studies with larger numbers of BUC patients from multiple centers are needed to confirm the association between FAM83H and Nectin1 expression and BUC progression. Furthermore, despite our findings indicating a possible oncogenic role for FAM83H and Nectin1 in BUC, the underlying mechanisms require clarification. In addition, future studies should determine the molecular mechanisms underlying the correlation in expression of FAM83H and Nectin1.

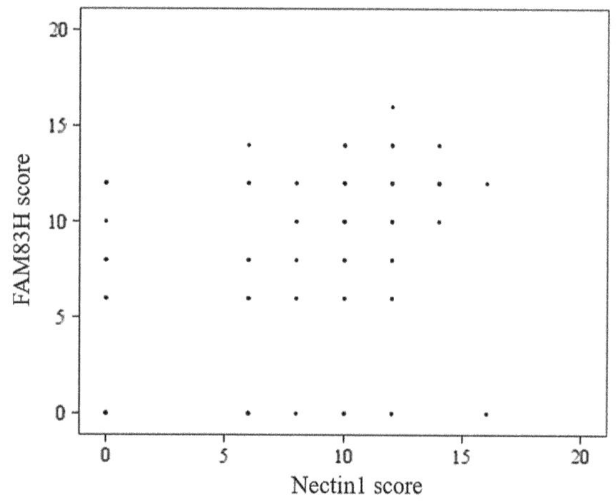

	r	p
Pearson's correlation coefficient	0.502	<0.001
Spearman's correlation coefficient	0.545	<0.001

Fig. 3 Scattergram comparing immunohistochemical score of FAM83H and Nectin1 expression in bladder urothelial carcinoma. Immunohistochemical score of FAM83H and Nectin1 showing significant positive correlation

In conclusion, we found that FAM83H and Nectin1 expression are significantly positively associated in BUCs, and that higher expression of these proteins is significantly associated with shorter OS and RFS. Therefore, FAM83H and Nectin1 may be potential therapeutic targets in BUC patients, and the co-expression pattern of FAM83H and Nectin1 could be used as a novel prognostic indicator in BUC patients.

Abbreviations

TCGA: The Cancer Genome Atlas; BUC: Bladder urothelial carcinoma; HR: Hazard ratio; OS: Overall survival; RFS: Relapse-free survival; 95% CI: 95% Confidence interval.

Supplementary Information

Additional file 1: Figure 1. Relationship between mRNA expression of FAM83H and Nectin1 in bladder urothelial carcinoma. The mRNA level of FAM83H and Nectin1 showing significant correlation in TCGA, Cell 2017 database. The dataset is selected and analyzed in cBioportal database.

Acknowledgements

The biospecimens and data used in this study were provided by the Biobank of Jeonbuk National University Hospital, a member of the Korea Biobank Network, which is supported by the Ministry of Health, Welfare and Family Affairs. All samples derived from the Korea Biobank Network were obtained with informed consent under institutional review board-approved protocols.

Authors' contributions

Conception: ARA, KYJ and KMK. Interpretation or analysis of data: ARA, SJN, UKH, KYJ, and KMK. Preparation of the manuscript: SJN, ARA, and KMK. Revision for important intellectual content: KYJ and MJC. Supervision: HSP, HL, WSM, MJC, NRL, MJK and HJK. All authors read and approved the final manuscript.

Author details

[1]Department of Pathology, Jeonbuk National University Medical School, Jeonju, Republic of Korea. [2]Department of Forensic Medicine, Jeonbuk National University Medical School, Jeonju, Republic of Korea. [3]Faculty of Science, Beni-Suef University, Beni-Suef, Egypt. [4]Department of Urology, Jeonbuk National University Medical School, Jeonju, Republic of Korea. [5]Department of Internal Medicine, Jeonbuk National University Hospital-Jeonbuk National University Medical School, Jeonju, Republic of Korea. [6]Research Institute of Clinical Medicine of Jeonbuk National University-Biomedical Research Institute of Jeonbuk National University Hospital, Jeonju, Republic of Korea.

References

1. Bray F, Ferlay J, Soerjomataram I, et al. Global cancer statistics 2018: GLOBOCAN estimates of incidence and mortality worldwide for 36 cancers in 185 countries. CA Cancer J Clin. 2018;68(6):394–424.
2. Marcos-Gragera R, Mallone S, Kiemeney LA, et al. Urinary tract cancer survival in Europe 1999–2007: results of the population-based study EUROCARE-5. Eur J Cancer. 2015;51(15):2217–30.
3. Amin M, Edge S. American Joint Committee on C. AJCC cancer staging manual Eighth edition Switzerland. New York: Springer; 2017.
4. Nadal R, Bellmunt J. Management of metastatic bladder cancer. Cancer Treat Rev. 2019;76:10–21.
5. Spruck CH, Ohneseit PF, Gonzalez-Zulueta M, et al. Two molecular pathways to transitional cell carcinoma of the bladder. Cancer Res. 1994;54(3):784–8.
6. Castillo-Martin M, Domingo-Domenech J, Karni-Schmidt O, et al. Molecular pathways of urothelial development and bladder tumorigenesis. Urol Oncol. 2010;28(4):401–8.
7. Al Hussain TO, Akhtar M. Molecular basis of urinary bladder cancer. Adv Anat Pathol. 2013;20(1):53–60.
8. Knowles MA, Hurst CD. Molecular biology of bladder cancer: new insights into pathogenesis and clinical diversity. Nat Rev Cancer. 2015;15(1):25–41.
9. Amin MB, Smith SC, Reuter VE, et al. Update for the practicing pathologist: the international consultation on urologic disease-European association of urology consultation on bladder cancer. Mod Pathol. 2015;28(5):612–30.
10. Urzúa B, Ortega-Pinto A, Morales-Bozo I, Rojas-Alcayaga G, Cifuentes V. Defining a new candidate gene for amelogenesis imperfecta: from molecular genetics to biochemistry. Biochem Genet. 2011;49(1–2):104–21.
11. Urzúa B, Martínez C, Ortega-Pinto A, et al. Novel missense mutation of the FAM83H gene causes retention of amelogenin and a mild clinical phenotype of hypocalcified enamel. Arch Oral Biol. 2015;60(9):1356–67.
12. Kuga T, Kume H, Kawasaki N, et al. A novel mechanism of keratin cytoskeleton organization through casein kinase Iα and FAM83H in colorectal cancer. J Cell Sci. 2013;126(20):4721–31.
13. Kim KM, Park SH, Bae JS, et al. FAM83H is involved in the progression of hepatocellular carcinoma and is regulated by MYC. Sci Rep. 2017;7(1):1–13.
14. Kim KM, Hussein UK, Park SH, et al. FAM83H is involved in stabilization of β-catenin and progression of osteosarcomas. J Exp Clin Cancer Res. 2019;38(1):267.
15. Kuga T, Kume H, Adachi J, et al. Casein kinase 1 is recruited to nuclear speckles by FAM83H and SON. Sci Rep. 2016;6(1):1–13.
16. Nalla AK, Williams TF, Collins CP, et al. Lentiviral vector-mediated insertional mutagenesis screen identifies genes that influence androgen independent prostate cancer progression and predict clinical outcome. Mol Carcinog. 2016;55(11):1761–71.
17. Kim KM, Hussein UK, Bae JS, et al. The expression patterns of FAM83H and PANX2 are associated with shorter survival of clear cell renal cell carcinoma patients. Front Oncol. 2019;9:14.

18. Zhuang H, Zhang C, Hou B. FAM83H overexpression predicts worse prognosis and correlates with less CD8+ T cells infiltration and Ras-PI3K Akt-mTOR signaling pathway in pancreatic cancer. Clin Transl Oncol. 2020;22(12):2244–52.
19. Takai Y, Irie K, Shimizu K, et al. Nectins and nectin-like molecules: roles in cell adhesion, migration, and polarization. Cancer Sci. 2003;94(8):655–67.
20. Takai Y, Miyoshi J, Ikeda W, et al. Nectins and nectin-like molecules: roles in contact inhibition of cell movement and proliferation. Nat Rev Mol Cell Biol. 2008;9(8):603–15.
21. Tampakis A, Tampaki EC, Nonni A, et al. Nectin-1 expression in colorectal cancer: is there a group of patients with high risk for early disease recurrence? Oncology. 2019;96(6):318–25.
22. Yamada M, Hirabayashi K, Kawanishi A, et al. Nectin-1 expression in cancer-associated fibroblasts is a predictor of poor prognosis for pancreatic ductal adenocarcinoma. Surg Today. 2018;48(5):510–6.
23. Robertson AG, Kim J, Al-Ahmadie H, et al. Comprehensive molecular characterization of muscle-invasive bladder cancer. Cell. 2017;171(3):540–56.
24. Moch H, Humphrey PA, Ulbright TM, et al. WHO classification of tumours of the urinary system and male genital organs. International Agency for Research on Cancer (IARC); 2016.
25. Park HJ, Bae JS, Kim KM, et al. The PARP inhibitor olaparib potentiates the effect of the DNA damaging agent doxorubicin in osteosarcoma. J Exp Clin Cancer Res. 2018;37(1):107.
26. Snijders AM, Lee SY, Hang B, et al. FAM83 family oncogenes are broadly involved in human cancers: an integrative multi-omics approach. Mol Oncol. 2017;11(2):167–79.
27. Takai Y, Nakanishi H. Nectin and afadin: novel organizers of intercellular junctions. J Cell Sci. 2003;116(1):17–27.
28. Guzman G, Oh S, Shukla D, et al. Nectin-1 expression in the normal and neoplastic human uterine cervix. Arch Pathol Lab Med. 2006;130(8):1193–5.
29. Takahashi Y, Yamamichi N, Ki I, et al. Nectin1 expression is frequently decreased in gastric cancers. Pathol Int. 2018;68(10):557–62.

19

Prevalence of overactive bladder symptoms and their impact on health-related quality of life of medical and dentistry students

Ramzi Shawahna[1,2*], Hatim Hijaz[3,4], Khaled Jallad[3], Mohammad Abushamma[3] and Mothana Sawafta[3]

Abstract

Background: Overactive bladder (OAB) is a popular distressing health condition that has negative impact on health-related quality of life (HRQoL) of the inflicted individuals. This multicenter study was conducted to determine the prevalence of OAB symptoms and their impact on the HRQoL of medical and dentistry students.

Methods: This study was conducted in a cross-sectional design in the 3 main universities in Palestine. In addition to the sociodemographic, health, and academic characteristics of the medical and dentistry students, the questionnaire also contained the OAB symptom bother (6-items) and HRQoL (13-items) Short-Form (OAB-q SF) scales. Kruskal–Wallis test, Mann–Whitney U test, Pearson Chi-Square/Fisher's Exact Test, Spearman's rank correlations, and a multiple linear regression model were used to analyze the data.

Results: Responses were collected from medical and dentistry students ($n = 402$). The median OAB symptom bother score was 54.1 [44.8, 81.9] and the median HRQoL score was 94.4 [88.4, 94.4]. There was a strong negative correlation between the OAB and HRQoL scores (Spearman's rho = 64.4%, p value < 0.001). OAB scores were significantly higher among dentistry students, females, who had chronic disease, and those who reported stressful life. HRQoL scores were significantly higher among medicine students, those who reported less stressful life, and those who reported satisfaction with their social life. Dentistry students, female, and those who self-reported high stress were 1.94-fold (95% CI 1.05, 3.56), 1.91-fold (95% CI 1.16, 3.14), and 1.88-fold (95% CI 1.21, 2.91) more likely to report less than optimal HRQoL compared to medicine students, male, and those who self-reported low stress, respectively.

Conclusions: Our findings suggested that OAB symptoms were prevalent among medical and dentistry students across Palestinian universities. Decision makers in academia, healthcare authorities, and advocacy groups might need to design appropriate interventions to address health and wellbeing issues of medical and dentistry students. Using appropriate diagnostic procedures, reducing stress, and improving the social life might help in reducing the burden on OAB and improve the HRQoL of medical and dentistry students. More investigations should be conducted to investigate if such interventions are effective in reducing OAB symptoms and improving HRQoL.

Keywords: Overactive bladder, Medical students, Dentistry students, Health-related quality of life, Palestine

*Correspondence: ramzi_shawahna@hotmail.com
[1] Department of Physiology, Pharmacology and Toxicology, Faculty of Medicine and Health Sciences, An-Najah National University, New Campus, Building: 19, Office: 1340, P.O. Box 7, Nablus, Palestine
Full list of author information is available at the end of the article

Background

Overactive bladder (OAB) is a popular and distressing condition that has negative impact on health-related quality of life (HRQoL) of the inflicted individuals [1].

According to the International Continence Society, OAB is symptomatic health condition characterized by abnormal urinary urgency that is often accompanied by nocturia and/or daytime frequency that could be with or without urgent urinary incontinence in the absence of any obvious urinary tract infections and/or any other underlying pathologies [2, 3]. Previous epidemiological studies have reported variable prevalence rates of OAB among the general public that ranged from 3 to 43% [4–7]. Previous studies also reported that OAB was largely underestimated and undertreated among the general public [7, 8].

Previous studies have reported negative impact of OAB on the HRQoL that can be translated as negative effects on the physical, social, and psychological well-being [9]. OAB can also have negative interference with the daily activities of the affected individuals [9, 10]. Additionally, OAB affects the patients' relationships with spouse/partner, family, and friends. As a result, anxiety, depression, embarrassment, and difficulties in sleep and sexual relationships were previously reported as common among individuals with OAB [11].

Previous studies have identified different factors that could promote urinary incontinence and OAB like occupational stress, delayed voiding, consumption of tea, carbonated drinks, and smoking [8, 12–14]. The literature reported little on the prevalence of OAB symptoms among young adults and its impact of their HRQoL [8, 13, 14]. Additionally, little was reported on the factors associated with OAB symptoms among young adults [13]. Reisch et al. reported that OAB symptoms were prevalent among 21.7% of female health profession students in a university in the Pacific Northwest [13]. OAB symptoms was more prevalent among participants who consumed caffeine and carbonated drinks compared to those who did not consume caffeine and carbonated drinks. The study also reported lower HRQoL among students with OAB symptoms compared to those without OAB symptoms. Özgür Yeniel et al. OAB symptoms were prevalent among 35.4% of Turkish midwifery students [8]. Turkish midwifery students with OAB symptoms also reported lower HRQoL compared to those without OAB symptoms. Similarly, Hagovska et al. reported lower HRQoL among overweight female university students with OAB symptoms compared to students without OAB symptoms [14].

Studying medicine and dentistry can be highly stressful. Throughout their medical school, medical and dentistry students face multiple highly demanding tasks [15]. As a result, medical and dentistry students often reported lower HRQoL compared to their age-matched peers and students of other disciplines [16–18]. Additionally, previous studies have reported higher prevalence of anxiety and depression symptoms among medical and dentistry students when compared to their age-matched groups of students in other non-medical disciplines [19–21].

Recently, there has been many calls to improve the HRQoL of medical and dentistry students [18, 22, 23]. As OAB symptoms are common and distressing, they could also worsen the HRQoL of medical and dentistry students. Little was reported on the prevalence of OAB symptoms among medical and dentistry students. Additionally, little was reported on the factors that could be associated with prevalence of OAB symptoms and the HRQoL of medical and dentistry students. Associations between sociodemographic, health, and academic variables with OAB symptoms and HRQoL were not investigated. Therefore, this study was conducted to determine the prevalence of OAB symptoms among the medical and dentistry students in Palestine. The study also aimed to investigate the associations between the sociodemographic, health, and academic characteristics of the medical and dentistry students with the prevalence of OAB symptoms and their HRQoL.

Methods

Study settings/context

This study was conducted in the 3 major universities in Palestine. The Doctor of Medicine (MD) program in Palestinian universities consists of 265 credited hours of basic and clinical courses/training and the dentistry program consists of 210 credited hours. The students often complete one of the programs in 6 academic years. Graduates are the future physicians and dentists in primary, secondary, and tertiary healthcare centers in Palestine. The study was conducted in the context of improving the HRQoL of the medical and dentistry students in Palestine.

Study design and the study tool

This study was conducted in a cross-sectional design among medical and dentistry students in Palestine using a questionnaire as the study tool. The study was conducted and reported in compliance with the Strengthening the Reporting of Observational Studies in Epidemiology (STROBE) Statement [24]. Compliance with the STROBE statement is shown in Additional file 1: Table S1. Because the study was conducted during the ongoing COVID-19 pandemic, an online version was used to collect the data in this study.

The questionnaire contained two parts. The first part collected sociodemographic, health, and academic characteristics of the medical and dentistry students like age, gender, height, body weight, smoking habits, employment status, presence of chronic disease, history of surgery, history of trauma, the university where the student was enrolled, academic discipline, academic year, number of study hours, self-rated satisfaction with the academic achievement, self-rated degree of stress, self-rated satisfaction with the financial status, and self-rated satisfaction with the social life. The second part contained the Overactive Bladder Symptom and Health-Related Quality of Life Short-Form (OAB-q SF) [25]. The OAB symptom bother scale contained 6-items and the HRQoL Scale contained 13-items. The Scales were abridged from the 33-items OAB-q Scale [26]. The OAB-q SF measures three HRQoL domains: coping, sleep, and emotional/ social interactions. Higher OAB symptom bother scores and lower HRQoL indicate greater effect [25, 26]. The scales were developed and assessed for subscale structure and psychometric performance [25]. The scales were shown to have excellent model fit and internal consistency. The convergent validity, discriminant validity, and internal reliability of the scales were good. Scores of the scales were reproducible and responsive to change.

Pilot testing of the questionnaire

The questionnaire was pilot tested among 18 medical students who did not take part in the larger study. The students were asked to evaluate the questionnaire for readability and comprehensibility. Based on the feedback of the students in the pilot testing, some items were revised for clarity. To ensure the stability of scores over a short period of time, the test–retest method was used. The students were asked to respond to the questionnaire. After a short time period (30 min to 2 h), the same students who participated in the pilot testing were asked to respond to the questionnaire once again. The scores obtained in both rounds were correlated using Pearson's correlations. It was decided a priori that a Pearson's correlation coefficient of $\geq 80\%$ would be considered acceptable to indicate stability of the scores over a short time period. The Cronbach's alpha statistics were used to assess the relatedness of the items (internal consistency of the study tool). It was decided a priori that a Cronbach's alpha of $\geq 70\%$ would be considered acceptable to indicate internal consistency of the questionnaire.

Study population, sample size, and sampling

The study population in this study was medical and dentistry students in Palestine. We used an online sample size calculator to calculate the sample size needed for this study. Assuming a population of approximately 9000 medical and dentistry students in the different Palestinian universities, the sample size calculated at a 95% confidence interval (CI) and accepting a 5% margin of error. The sample size needed for this study was 369 students. Medical and dentistry students in the 3 major universities in Palestine were invited to take part in the study using their formal mailing groups. A convenience sampling technique was used and the data collection was terminated when 402 responses were obtained.

Data analysis

The data collected were entered into SPSS for Windows v.21.0. Sociodemographic, health, and academic data were grouped into categories. The OAB-q SF consisted of 2 domains: OAB symptom bother (6-items) and HRQoL (13-items). The students could rate each of the OAB symptom bother items on a Likert scale of 1–6 (1 = not at all, 6 = a very great deal). The possible raw scores of the OAB symptom bother items could range from 6 to 36 (possible raw score range = 30). Similarly, the students could rate each of the HRQoL items on a Likert scale of 1–6 (1 = none of the time, 6 = all of the time). The lowest and highest possible raw scores of the HRQoL items could range from 13 to 78 (possible raw score range = 65) [25].

Scores of the OAB symptom bother (6-items) were transformed as in the Eq. (1):

$$\text{Transformed Score} = \frac{(\text{Actual raw score} - \text{lowest possible raw score})}{\text{Possible raw score range}} \times 100\% \tag{1}$$

Scores of the QoL scores were transformed as in the Eq. (2):

$$\text{Transformed Score} = \frac{(\text{Highest possible score} - \text{Actual raw score})}{\text{Possible raw score range}} \times 100\% \tag{2}$$

The transformed scores of the OAB symptom bother and HRQoL items were assessed for normal distribution using Kolmogorov–Smirnov test of normality. As the distribution of the data was not normal, nonparametric tests were used. The data are presented as median [lower quartile (Q1), upper quartile (Q3)]. Categories were compared using Kruskal–Wallis test or Mann–Whitney *U* test, as appropriate. Associations between sociodemographic, health, and academic variables of the medical and dentistry students and presence of OAB symptoms and less than optimal HRQoL were investigated using Pearson Chi-Square (χ^2)/Fisher's Exact Test (FET). Correlations were investigated using Spearman's rank correlations. To control potential confounding factors, a multiple linear regression model was used to investigate predictors of higher scores. Then variables with statistically significant differences in the Mann–Whitney U test were retained in the regression model. The goodness of fit of the model was indicated by an R^2 value of 0.30. The variance inflation factor (VIF) and tolerance were assessed using collinearity statistics. Tolerance values were > 1.02 and the VIF values were less than 1.50 which indicated absence of multicollinearity issues. Presence of OAB symptom bother was indicated by a sum transformed score of > 35.6 on the 6-item OAB symptom bother Scale and less than optimal HRQoL was indicated by a sum transformed score of < 94.4 on the 13-item HRQoL Scale. A multivariate logistic regression model was used to determine which variables were predictors of presence of any OAB symptom bother and less than optimal HRQoL. Odds ratios (OR) with their 95% CI were calculated. Statistical significance was considered when the p-value was < 0.05.

Ethics approval and consent to participate

The study was conducted in compliance with local and international ethical guidelines including those followed at An-Najah National University and Declaration of Helsinki. Because this study was conducted in the context of improving the HRQoL of the medical and dentistry students in Palestine and in view of the no/minimal risk to the study participants, this study fell within the "Exempt" review category. The Institutional Review Board (IRB) of An-Najah National University approved this exemption. All students provided written informed consent to participate in the study.

Results

Reliability of the study tool

When the scores of the students in the pilot testing were correlated, the Pearson's correlation coefficient (r) was 93.0%. This indicated an excellent stability of scores over the short period of time. The Cronbach's alpha of all items (6 OAB symptom bother and 13 HRQoL items) was 93.3% (95% CI of 92.4% to 94.3%). For the 6 OAB symptom bother items, the Cronbach's alpha was 81.1% (95% CI of 78.1% to 83.8%). For the 13 HRQoL items, the Cronbach's alpha was 93.3% (95% CI of 92.3% to 94.2%). This indicated that the items in each domain as well as in the questionnaire as a whole were internally consistent.

Sociodemographic, health, and academic characteristics of the medical and dentistry students

Responses ($n = 402$) were collected from medical and dentistry students who were enrolled in the 3 major universities in Palestine. Of the students, 276 (68.7%) were female, 205 (51.0%) were in their clinical stage (3rd to 6th year), 228 (56.7%) were 21 years and older, 131 (32.6%) were overweight or obese, 24 (6.0%) had chronic disease, 78 (19.4%) had a history of surgery, 8 (2.0%) had a history of trauma, 14 (3.5%) had a side/part-time job, 65 (16.2%) were smokers, 320 (79.6%) were satisfied with their academic achievement, 147 (36.6%) rated their life as stressful, 225 (56.0%) studied for 5 or more hours per day, 253 (62.9%) were satisfied with their financial status as high, and 277 (68.9%) were satisfied with their social life. Medical and dentistry students were similar with regard to their sociodemographic, health, and academic characteristics except for smoking habits and number of study hours/day. Dentistry students smoked more than medical students (Pearson Chi-Square/Fisher's Exact Test = 5.10, p value = 0.028). On the other hand, medical students studied more than dentistry students (Pearson Chi-Square/Fisher's Exact Test = 5.59, p value = 0.024). Comparison between the sociodemographic, health, and academic characteristics of the medical and dentistry students is shown in Additional file 1: Table S2. Detailed sociodemographic, health, and academic characteristics of the medical and dentistry students are shown in Table 1.

Prevalence of OAB symptom bother among medical and dentistry students

The median transformed OAB symptom bother among medical and dentistry students was 54.1 [44.8, 81.9]. The students reported some OAB symptom bother relevant to an uncomfortable urge to urinate (60.4%), a sudden urge to urinate with little or no warning (36.3%), accidental loss of small amounts of urine (20.1%), nighttime urination (28.1%), waking up at night because you had to urinate (43.8%), and urine loss associated with a strong desire to urinate, respectively (16.9%). Distribution of the rating of the medical and dentistry students on the 6 OAB symptom bother items is shown in Table 2.

Health related quality of life scores

The median transformed HRQoL scores was 94.4 [88.4, 94.4]. The students reported less than optimal HRQoL scores relevant to the domains: coping, sleep, and emotional/social interactions. The detailed responses of the medical and dentistry students on the 13 HRQoL items are shown in Table 3.

Table 1 Sociodemographic, health, and academic characteristics of the students who participated in the study ($n=402$)

Variable	n	%
University*		
University 1	250	62.2
University 2	114	28.4
University 3	38	9.5
Discipline		
Medicine	350	87.1
Dentistry	52	12.9
Academic stage		
Basic stage (1st–3rd year)	197	49.0
Clinical stage (4th–6th year)	205	51.0
Gender		
Male	126	31.3
Female	276	68.7
Age (years)		
<21	174	43.3
≥21	228	56.7
Body mass index		
<24.9	271	67.4
≥24.9	131	32.6
Presence of chronic disease		
No	378	94.0
Yes	24	6.0
History of surgery		
Yes	78	19.4
No	324	80.6
History of trauma		
Yes	8	2.0
No	394	98.0
Employment		
Yes	14	3.5
No	388	96.5
Smoking		
Yes	65	16.2
No	337	83.8
Self-rated satisfaction with academic achievement		
Not satisfied	82	20.4
Satisfied	320	79.6
Self-rated stress		
Low stress	255	63.4
High stress	147	36.6
Number of study hours/day		
<5	177	44.0
≥5	225	56.0
Self-rated satisfaction with the financial status		
Not satisfied	149	37.1
Satisfied	253	62.9
Self-rated satisfaction with the social life		
Not satisfied	125	31.1
Satisfied	277	68.9

*1, 2, and 3 denotes the largest universities in Palestine in terms of number of students

Association of the sociodemographic, health, and academic characteristics with the OAB Bother Symptom and health related quality of life scores

There was a strong negative correlation between the transformed OAB symptom bother and HRQoL scores obtained in this study (Spearman's rho = 64.4%, p value < 0.001).

The OAB symptom bother scores were significantly higher for students who studied dentistry, were of female gender, had chronic diseases, reported high stressful life, and were not satisfied with their social life compared to students who studied medicine, were male in gender, did not have chronic disease, reported less stressful life, and were satisfied with their social life. Comparison of the median and interquartile range of the OAB symptom bother scores is shown in Table 4. On the other hand, the HRQoL scores were significantly higher for students who studied medicine, were male in gender, reported low stressful life, studies less than 5 h, and were satisfied with their social life. Comparison of the median and interquartile range of the HRQoL scores is shown in Table 4.

The multiple linear regression model showed that OAB symptom bother scores were significantly higher for dentistry students, those of female gender, had chronic disease, and those reported stressful life. On the other hand, the model showed that HRQoL scores were significantly higher for medicine students, those who reported less stressful life, and those reported satisfaction with their social life. Details of the multiple linear analysis are shown in Table 5.

Presence of any OAB symptom bother were associated with female gender (Pearson Chi-Square/Fisher's Exact Test = 5.20, p value = 0.027) and high self-reported stress (Pearson Chi-Square/Fisher's Exact Test = 4.91, p value = 0.032). Less than optimal HRQoL was associated with studying dentistry (Pearson Chi-Square/Fisher's Exact Test = 5.63, p value = 0.020), female gender (Pearson Chi-Square/Fisher's Exact Test = 12.17, p value < 0.001), high self-reported stress (Pearson Chi-Square/Fisher's Exact Test = 10.67, p value = 0.001), and studying ≥ 5 h/day (Pearson Chi-Square/Fisher's Exact Test = 4.89, p value = 0.028). Details of associations between presence of any OAB symptom bother and less than optimal HRQoL with sociodemographic, health, and academic variables of the students are shown in Table 6.

Multivariate logistic regression showed that dentistry students were 1.94-fold (95% CI 1.05, 3.56) more likely to report less than optimal HRQoL compared to medicine students, female students were 1.91-fold (95% CI 1.16, 3.14) more likely to report less than optimal HRQoL compared to male students, and students who self-reported high stress were 1.88-fold (95% CI 1.21, 2.91) more likely to report less than optimal HRQoL compared

Table 2 Distribution of the responses of the medical and dentistry students on the 6 overactive bladder symptom bother items ($n=402$)

#	Item	Not at all		A little bit		Some-what		Quite a bit		A great deal		A very great deal	
		n	%	n	%	n	%	n	%	n	%	n	%
1	An uncomfortable urge to urinate	159	39.6	118	29.4	46	11.4	48	11.9	23	5.7	8	2.0
2	A sudden urge to urinate with little or no warning	256	63.7	75	18.7	29	7.2	31	7.7	8	2.0	3	0.7
3	Accidental loss of small amounts of urine	321	79.9	48	11.9	12	3.0	15	3.7	5	1.2	1	0.2
4	Nighttime urination	289	71.9	71	17.7	14	3.5	16	4.0	8	2.0	4	1.0
5	Waking up at night because you had to urinate	226	56.2	120	29.9	20	5.0	19	4.7	14	3.5	3	0.7
6	Urine loss associated with a strong desire to urinate	334	83.1	37	9.2	16	4.0	7	1.7	8	2.0	0	0.0

to the students who self-reported low stress. Details of the multivariate logistic regression model are shown in Table 7.

Discussion

During their training, medical and dentistry students could be exposed to a huge amount of stress that deteriorates their HRQoL [15]. Identifying and addressing stressors are prerequisite steps in improving the HRQoL of medical and dentistry students. In this multicenter study, prevalence of OAB symptom bother among medical and dentistry students, the associated sociodemographic, health, and academic factors, and their impact on the HRQoL were identified. To the best of our knowledge, this is the first study to investigate prevalence of OAB symptom bother and HRQoL among medical and dentistry students. A considerable percentage of the students were bothered with OAB symptom bother which affected their HRQoL. The study showed strong negative association between OAB symptom bother and HRQoL scores. OAB symptom bother and HRQoL scores were associated with discipline and stressful life. Findings of this study could be informative to decision makers in academia, health regulatory authorities, and advocacy groups who could be interested in improving the HRQoL of medical and dentistry students.

Findings of this study showed considerable percentage of medical and dentistry students reporting some degree of OAB symptom bother which affected their HRQoL. Findings of this study were consistent with those reported among university students including those in healthcare disciplines like midwifery in the US, Turkey, and Slovak Republic [8, 13, 14]. Together, these findings might indicate higher prevalence of OAB symptom bother among students of stressful disciplines like dentistry and medicine and lower HRQoL compared to their age-matched peers in other disciplines. Several previous studies have reported high prevalence of anxiety and depressive symptoms among students in healthcare disciplines including medical students in Palestine [15, 18, 19, 22, 23]. Findings of this study showed that OAB symptom bother scores were higher among female students compared to male students. Although some studies reported that prevalence of OAB symptom bother among male and female patients was similar, the majority of the studies have reported higher prevalence of OAB symptom bother among females compared to males [7, 27]. Results of this study were consistent with those reported in the previous studies on the higher prevalence of OAB symptoms among female students compared to male students in Korea, Turkey, Slovak Republic, and Japan [7, 8, 14, 27–30]. Presence of chronic diseases was also associated with higher OAB symptom bother. Previous studies have shown that chronic diseases like diabetes, irritable bowel syndrome, asthma, heart disease, depression, arthritis, and neurological conditions like multiple sclerosis and cerebral palsy [31–34]. In a study among 1025 patients with type 2 diabetes, 14% reported OAB symptoms [35]. Matsumoto et al. reported that among patients with irritable bowel syndrome, about 33% reported concurrent OAB symptoms [36]. The study population in this study were young medical students in their twenties. However, chronic diseases were prevalent in a small percentage (6%) of them. Findings of this study might add to the ability of the OAB symptom bother scale used in this study to differentiate between patient populations [25]. Students who rated their life as stressful reported higher OAB symptoms and lower HRQoL scores compared to others who reported less stressful life. Findings of this study were consistent with those reported in previous studies in which perceive stress was significantly correlated with OAB symptoms and HRQoL [37–40]. Lai et al. showed that severity of OAB symptoms were associated with higher perceived psychological stress [38]. In another study among nurses, Zhang et al. showed that OAB symptoms were associated with occupational stress

Table 3 Distribution of the responses of the medical and dentistry students on the 13 health-related quality of life items ($n = 402$)

#	Item	None of the time		A little of the time		Some of the time		A good bit of the time		Most of the time		All of the time	
		n	%	n	%	n	%	n	%	n	%	n	%
1	Caused you to plan "escape routes" to restrooms in public places	315	78.4	42	10.4	18	4.5	15	3.7	8	2.0	4	1.0
2	Made you feel like there is something wrong with you	327	81.3	37	9.2	9	2.2	14	3.5	9	2.2	6	1.5
3	Interfered with your ability to get a good night's rest	352	87.6	25	6.2	4	1.0	12	3.0	6	1.5	3	0.7
4	Made you frustrated or annoyed about the amount of time you spend in the restroom	355	88.3	28	7.0	6	1.5	4	1.0	4	1.0	5	1.2
5	Made you avoid activities away from restrooms (i.e., walks, running, hiking)	364	90.5	0	0.0	21	5.2	12	3.0	2	0.5	3	0.7
6	Awakened you during sleep	316	78.6	52	12.9	9	2.2	11	2.7	9	2.2	5	1.2
7	Caused you to decrease your physical activities (exercising, sports, etc.)	368	91.5	19	4.7	4	1.0	7	1.7	3	0.7	1	0.2
8	Caused you to have problems with your partner or spouse	396	98.5	5	1.2	0	0.0	1	0.2	0	0.0	0	0.0
9	Made you uncomfortable while traveling with others because of needing to stop for a restroom	348	86.6	27	6.7	9	2.2	9	2.2	3	0.7	6	1.5
10	Affected your relationships with family and friends	383	95.3	11	2.7	7	1.7	1	0.2	0	0.0	0	0.0
11	Interfered with getting the amount of sleep you needed	361	89.8	26	6.5	4	1.0	8	2.0	2	0.5	1	0.2
12	Caused you embarrassment	344	85.6	27	6.7	11	2.7	12	3.0	6	1.5	2	0.5
13	Caused you to locate the closest restroom as soon as you arrive at a place you have never been	344	85.6	28	7.0	11	2.7	7	1.7	6	1.5	6	1.5

Table 4 Comparison of the median and interquartile range of the overactive bladder symptom bother and health-related quality of life scores

Variable	n	%	OAB scores		HRQoL scores	
			Median [Q1, Q3]	*p* value	Median [Q1, Q3]	*p* value
University*						
University 1	250	62.2	54.1 [44.8, 81.9]	0.181	94.4 [90.4, 94.4]	0.362
University 2	114	28.4	54.1 [44.8, 91.1]		94.4 [86.5, 94.4]	
University 3	38	9.5	63.3 [44.8, 91.1]		94.4 [80.6, 94.4]	
Discipline						
Medicine	350	87.1	54.1 [44.8, 81.9]	0.003	94.4 [90.4, 94.4]	0.003
Dentistry	52	12.9	72.6 [44.8, 116.6]		93.4 [73.6, 94.4]	
Academic stage						
Basic stage (1st–3rd year)	197	49.0	54.1 [44.8, 81.9]	0.195	94.4 [88.4, 94.4]	0.329
Clinical stage (4th–6th year)	205	51.0	54.1 [35.6, 81.9]		94.4 [90.4, 94.4]	
Gender						
Male	126	31.3	54.1 [35.6, 72.6]	0.009	94.4 [94.4, 94.4]	0.001
Female	276	68.7	54.1 [44.8, 91.1]		94.4 [88.4, 94.4]	
Age (years)						
<21	174	43.3	54.1 [44.8, 84.2]	0.213	94.4 [88.4, 94.4]	0.494
≥21	228	56.7	54.1 [44.8, 81.9]		94.4 [90.4, 94.4]	
Body mass index						
<24.9	271	67.4	54.1 [44.8, 81.9]	0.994	94.4 [90.4, 94.4]	0.995
≥24.9	131	32.6	54.1 [44.8, 81.9]		94.4 [88.4, 94.4]	
Presence of chronic disease						
No	378	94.0	54.1 [44.8, 81.9]	0.018	94.4 [90.4, 94.4]	0.067
Yes	24	6.0	81.9 [44.8, 135.1]		94.4 [66.3, 94.4]	
History of surgery						
Yes	78	19.4	54.1 [44.8, 91.1]	0.531	94.4 [88.4, 94.4]	0.832
No	324	80.6	54.1 [44.8, 81.9]		94.4 [90.4, 94.4]	
History of trauma						
Yes	8	2.0	63.3 [44.8, 93.4]	0.666	92.4 [71.7, 94.4]	0.328
No	394	98.0	54.1 [44.8, 81.9]		94.4 [89.9, 94.4]	
Employment						
Yes	14	3.5	44.8 [35.6, 56.4]	0.092	94.4 [93.4, 94.4]	0.291
No	388	96.5	54.1 [44.8, 81.9]		94.4 [88.4, 94.4]	
Smoking						
Yes	65	16.2	63.3 [44.8, 91.1]	0.494	94.4 [88.4, 94.4]	0.758
No	337	83.8	54.1 [44.8, 81.9]		94.4 [89.4, 94.4]	
Self-rated satisfaction with academic achievement						
Not satisfied	82	20.4	54.1 [44.8, 81.9]	0.704	94.4 [89.9, 94.4]	0.866
Satisfied	320	79.6	54.1 [44.8, 81.9]		94.4 [88.4, 94.4]	
Self-rated stress						
Low stress	255	63.4	54.1 [35.6, 72.6]	0.003	94.4 [92.4, 94.4]	0.001
High stress	147	36.6	63.3 [44.8, 100.4]		94.4 [84.5, 94.4]	
Number of study hours/day						
<5	177	44.0	54.1 [40.2, 81.9]	0.056	94.4 [92.4, 94.4]	0.028
≥5	225	56.0	54.1 [44.8, 91.1]		94.4 [88.4, 94.4]	
Self-rated satisfaction with the financial status						
Not satisfied	149	37.1	54.1 [44.8, 86.5]	0.259	94.4 [86.5, 94.4]	0.099
Satisfied	253	62.9	54.1 [44.8, 81.9]		94.4 [90.4, 94.4]	
Self-rated satisfaction with the social life						
Not satisfied	125	31.1	63.3 [44.8, 91.1]	0.009	94.4 [86.5, 94.4]	0.038
Satisfied	277	68.9	54.1 [44.8, 81.9]		94.4 [90.4, 94.4]	

*1, 2, and 3 denotes the largest universities in Palestine in terms of number of students, HRQoL: Health-related quality of life, Q1: Lower quartile, Q3: Upper quartile, OAB: Overactive bladder

Table 5 Multiple linear regression between sociodemographic, health, and academic variables of the students with overactive bladder Symptom Bother health related quality of life scores

Variable	Unstandardized coefficients	SE	Standardized coefficients	t	*p* value
OAB symptom bother scores					
Discipline	16.35	6.05	0.13	2.70	0.007
Gender	8.88	4.41	0.10	2.01	0.045
Presence of chronic disease	18.92	8.55	0.11	2.21	0.028
Self-rated stress	11.50	4.26	0.13	2.70	0.007
Self-rated satisfaction with the social life	− 8.18	4.35	− 0.09	− 1.88	0.061
HRQoL scores					
Discipline	17.39	6.06	0.14	2.87	0.004
Gender	7.16	4.48	0.08	1.60	0.111
Self-rated stress	11.95	4.27	0.14	2.80	0.005
Number of study hours	4.88	4.14	0.06	1.18	0.240
Self-rated satisfaction with the social life	− 8.77	4.36	− 0.10	− 2.01	0.045

HRQoL: Health-related quality of life, OAB: Overactive bladder, SE: Standard error, t: t-statistics

[39]. Findings of this study were not surprising as in our previous study, depressive and anxiety symptoms were highly prevalent among medical students in Palestine [19].

In all healthcare systems, medical and dentistry students are the future workforce of physicians and dentists in primary, secondary, and tertiary healthcare centers. Therefore, addressing their health issues and improving their well-being and HRQoL could be crucial for optimal delivery of healthcare services and sustainability of the healthcare system [41, 42]. Decision makers in academia, health regulatory authorities, and advocacy groups might need to address health issues among medical and dentistry students. Improving care of chronic diseases that might comorbid with OAB symptoms, reducing stress through implementation of mindfulness and/or lifestyle programs, and providing support to female students might reduce OAB symptoms and improve HRQoL among medical and dentistry students [41, 43, 44].

Strengths and limitations

Findings of this study should be interpreted after considering a number of strengths and limitations. First, in this multicenter study, data were collected from the major universities in Palestine. This should have improved the external validity of the study. Second, although the scales used were previously validated, appropriate diagnostic tests were also used in this study to ensure test–retest reliability and internal consistency of the study tool. Third, the number of students included in this study was larger than the sample size needed. Additionally, the participants were diversified in terms of sociodemographic, health, and academic variables. The sample included participants from both genders, who rated their social and financial status differently. This should have added depth and width to the results obtained in this study. Fourth, associations between the OAB symptom bother and HRQoL scores with the sociodemographic, health, and academic variables of the students were investigated using powerful statistical tests.

This study had a number of limitations. First, the study was conducted among medical and dentistry students only. We did not compare the prevalence of OAB symptom bother among university students in nonmedical disciplines. It could have been interesting to compare findings of the medical and dentistry students with those in nonmedical disciplines. Future studies would be conducted to compare prevalence of OAB symptom bother and HRQoL among university students in different health and non-health related disciplines. Second, the study was conducted in a cross-sectional design. Findings of cross-sectional studies are limited to the time period in which the study was conducted. A longitudinal study could have shown more interesting results and might have allowed detecting and investigating changes in OAB and/or HRQoL scores. Third, the items in the study tool were in both English and Arabic. Forward and backward translations were used to ensure accuracy [45, 46]. The items originally in English were translated into Arabic which were then translated back into English. Previous Arabic tools used to measure OAB symptoms were also reviewed [47, 48]. It is noteworthy mentioning that English is the language of instructions and teaching in Palestinian medical and dentistry schools. Additionally, Test of English as a Foreign Language (TOEFL) is a prerequisite for medical education in Palestinian universities. Fourth,

Table 6 Associations between presence of any overactive bladder symptom bother and less than optimal health-related quality of life with sociodemographic, health, and academic variables of the students

Variable	OAB symptoms						HRQoL					
	Absent		Present		χ^2/FET	*p* value	Less than optimal		Optimal		χ^2/FET	*p* value
	n	%	n	%			n	%	n	%		
University*												
University 1	58	14.4	192	47.8	1.27	0.553	88	21.9	162	40.3	1.89	0.388
University 2	23	5.7	91	22.6			37	9.2	77	19.2		
University 3	6	1.5	32	8.0			17	4.2	21	5.2		
Discipline												
Medicine	80	19.9	270	67.2	2.36	0.150	116	28.9	234	58.2	5.63	0.020
Dentistry	7	1.7	45	11.2			26	6.5	26	6.5		
Academic stage												
Basic stage (1st–3rd year)	35	8.7	162	40.3	3.42	0.070	76	18.9	121	30.1	1.79	0.210
Clinical stage (4th–6th year)	52	12.9	153	38.1			66	16.4	139	34.6		
Gender												
Male	36	9.0	90	22.4	5.20	0.027	29	7.2	97	24.1	12.17	<0.001
Female	51	12.7	225	56.0			113	28.1	163	40.5		
Age (years)												
<21	31	7.7	143	35.6	2.65	0.113	67	16.7	107	26.6	1.36	0.249
≥21	56	13.9	172	42.8			75	18.7	153	38.1		
Body mass index												
<24.9	56	13.9	215	53.5	0.47	0.519	96	23.9	175	43.5	0.00	1.000
≥24.9	31	7.7	100	24.9			46	11.4	85	21.1		
Presence of chronic disease												
No	84	20.9	294	73.1	1.26	0.318	131	32.6	247	61.4	1.23	0.277
Yes	3	0.7	21	5.2			11	2.7	13	3.2		
History of surgery												
Yes	14	3.5	64	15.9	0.78	0.445	28	7.0	50	12.4	0.01	1.000
No	73	18.2	251	62.4			114	28.4	210	52.2		
History of trauma												
Yes	1	0.2	7	1.7	0.40	0.693	4	1.0	4	1.0	0.77	0.461
No	86	21.4	308	76.6			138	34.3	256	63.7		
Employment												
Yes	4	1.0	10	2.5	0.41	0.743	3	0.7	11	2.7	1.22	0.395
No	83	20.6	305	75.9			139	34.6	249	61.9		
Smoking												
Yes	15	3.7	50	12.4	0.09	0.869	21	5.2	44	10.9	0.31	0.671
No	72	17.9	265	65.9			121	30.1	216	53.7		
Self-rated satisfaction with academic achievement												
Not satisfied	19	4.7	63	15.7	0.14	0.764	29	7.2	53	13.2	0.00	1.000
Satisfied	68	16.9	252	62.7			113	28.1	207	51.5		
Self-rated stress												
Low stress	64	15.9	191	47.5	4.91	0.032	75	18.7	180	44.8	10.67	0.001
High stress	23	5.7	124	30.8			67	16.7	80	19.9		
Number of study hours/day												
<5	44	10.9	133	33.1	1.93	0.181	52	12.9	125	31.1	4.89	0.028
≥5	43	10.7	182	45.3			90	22.4	135	33.6		
Self-rated satisfaction with the financial status												
Not satisfied	27	6.7	122	30.3	1.73	0.211	59	14.7	90	22.4	1.89	0.195
Satisfied	60	14.9	193	48.0			83	20.6	170	42.3		

Table 6 (continued)

Variable	OAB symptoms						HRQoL					
	Absent		Present		χ^2/FET	*p* value	Less than optimal		Optimal		χ^2/FET	*p* value
	n	%	n	%			n	%	n	%		
Self-rated satisfaction with the social life												
Not satisfied	21	5.2	104	25.9	2.51	0.119	52	12.9	73	18.2	3.13	0.091
Satisfied	66	16.4	211	52.5			90	22.4	187	46.5		

HRQoL: Health-related quality of life, OAB: Overactive bladder, χ^2/FET: Pearson Chi-Square/Fisher's Exact Test

Table 7 Multivariate regression analysis of association between overactive bladder symptom bother and health-related quality of life with sociodemographic, health, and academic variables of the students

Domain	Variable	β	SE	Wald	*p* value	OR	95% CI for OR	
							Lower	Upper
OAB symptom bother	Gender							
	Male	Reference						
	Female	−0.49	0.25	3.66	0.056	0.61	0.37	1.01
	Self-rated stress							
	Low stress	Reference						
	High stress	−0.51	0.27	3.52	0.061	0.60	0.35	1.02
	Constant	1.80	0.24	57.40	0.000	6.06		
HRQoL	Discipline							
	Medicine	Reference						
	Dentistry	0.66	0.31	4.50	0.034	1.94	1.05	3.56
	Gender							
	Male	Reference						
	Female	0.65	0.25	6.49	0.011	1.91	1.16	3.14
	Self-rated stress							
	Low stress	Reference						
	High stress	0.63	0.22	8.02	0.005	1.88	1.21	2.91
	Number of study hours/day							
	<5	Reference						
	≥5	0.28	0.22	1.52	0.218	1.32	0.85	2.04
	Constant	−0.65	0.33	3.89	0.048	0.52		

CI: Confidence interval, OR: Odds ratio, SE: Standard error

this study was an observational study using a questionnaire and the results obtained were self-reported. A clinical assessment supported by laboratory findings of the students who participated in the study should have permitted collecting more meaningful data. Comparing the scores obtained in this study with more objective data such as bladder diary should have allowed better interpretation of the findings. Fifth, we did not correlate OAB symptom bother and HRQoL scores with anxiety/stress scores that could have been measured using a validated tool. Investigating correlations between OAB symptom bother, HRQoL scores, and anxiety/stress scores could have provided more meaningful data. Finally, a convenience sampling technique was followed in this study to recruit the study participants. As the study was conducted during the ongoing COVID-19 pandemic, this sampling technique allowed collecting the number of participants needed for this study respecting the stay-at-home orders and keeping social distancing.

Conclusions

Our findings suggest that OAB symptom bother were prevalent among medical and dentistry students across Palestinian universities. There was a strong negative association between OAB symptom bother and HRQoL scores. Decision makers in academia, healthcare authorities, and advocacy groups might need to design appropriate interventions to address health and wellbeing issues of medical and dentistry students. Using appropriate diagnostic procedures, reducing stress, and improving the social life might help in reducing the burden on OAB and improve the HRQoL of medical and dentistry students. More investigations should be conducted to investigate if such interventions are effective in reducing OAB symptoms and improving HRQoL of medical and dentistry students.

Abbreviations

CI: Confidence interval; HRQoL: Health-related quality of life; IRB: Institutional Review Board; MD: Doctor of Medicine; OAB: Overactive bladder; OAB-q SF: OAB symptom bother and health-related quality of life Short-Form; Q1: Lower quartile; Q3: Upper quartile; VIF: Variance inflation factor.

Supplementary Information

Additional file 1. **Supplementary Table S1**. Adherence to STROBE Statement for reporting cross-sectional studies [1]. **Supplementary Table S2** Comparison between the sociodemographic, health, and academic characteristics of the medical and dentistry students.

Acknowledgements

Author would like to thank the students who participated in the study. An-Najah National University is acknowledged for making this study possible.

Authors' contributions

RS and HH were involved in the conception and design of the work, analysis and interpretation of data, drafting and final approval the manuscript. KJ, MA, and MS collected data and participated in drafting the manuscript. All authors read and approved the final manuscript.

Author details

[1]Department of Physiology, Pharmacology and Toxicology, Faculty of Medicine and Health Sciences, An-Najah National University, New Campus, Building: 19, Office: 1340, P.O. Box 7, Nablus, Palestine. [2]An-Najah BioSciences Unit, Centre for Poison Control, Chemical and Biological Analysis, An-Najah National University, Nablus, Palestine. [3]Department of Medicine, Faculty of Medicine and Health Sciences, An-Najah National University, Nablus, Palestine. [4]An-Najah National University Hospital, An-Najah National University, Nablus, Palestine.

References

1. Foley S, Choudhury N, Huang M, Stari A, Nazir J, Freeman R. Quality of life in patients aged 65 years and older with overactive bladder treated with mirabegron across eight European countries: secondary analysis of BELIEVE. Int J Urol. 2019;26(9):890–6.
2. Haylen BT, de Ridder D, Freeman RM, Swift SE, Berghmans B, Lee J, Monga A, Petri E, Rizk DE, Sand PK, et al. An International Urogynecological Association (IUGA)/International Continence Society (ICS) joint report on the terminology for female pelvic floor dysfunction. Int Urogynecol J. 2010;21(1):5–26.
3. Coyne KS, Sexton CC, Vats V, Thompson C, Kopp ZS, Milsom I. National community prevalence of overactive bladder in the United States stratified by sex and age. Urology. 2011;77(5):1081–7.
4. Irwin DE, Milsom I, Hunskaar S, Reilly K, Kopp Z, Herschorn S, Coyne K, Kelleher C, Hampel C, Artibani W, et al. Population-based survey of urinary incontinence, overactive bladder, and other lower urinary tract symptoms in five countries: results of the EPIC study. Eur Urol. 2006;50(6):1306–14 (**discussion 1314–1305**).
5. Stewart W, Van Rooyen J, Cundiff G, Abrams P, Herzog A, Corey R, Hunt T, Wein A. Prevalence and burden of overactive bladder in the United States. World J Urol. 2003;20(6):327–36.
6. Milsom I, Stewart W, Thüroff J. The prevalence of overactive bladder. Am J Manag Care. 2000;6(11 Suppl):S565-573.
7. Eapen RS, Radomski SB. Review of the epidemiology of overactive bladder. Res Rep Urol. 2016;8:71–6.
8. Özgür Yeniel A, Mete Ergenoglu A, Meseri R, Hadimli A, Askar N, Mete Itil I. The prevalence of probable overactive bladder, associated risk factors and its effect on quality of life among Turkish midwifery students. Eur J Obstet Gynecol Reprod Biol. 2012;164(1):105–9.
9. Coyne KS, Payne C, Bhattacharyya SK, Revicki DA, Thompson C, Corey R, Hunt TL. The impact of urinary urgency and frequency on health-related quality of life in overactive bladder: results from a national community survey. Value Health. 2004;7(4):455–63.
10. Ahmad QT, Saffarini JH, Samara AM, Jabri DS, Saffarini ZH, Banijaber YM, Jaradat A, Abushamma F, Zyoud SeH. The impact of lower urinary tract symptoms on the quality of life during pregnancy: a cross-sectional study from Palestine. BMC Urol. 2020;20(1):191.
11. Balzarro M, Rubilotta E, Mancini V, Trabacchin N, Oppezzi L, Li Marzi V, Fusco F, Serati M. Impact of overactive bladder-wet syndrome on female sexual function: a systematic review and meta-analysis. Sex Med Rev. 2019;7(4):565–74.
12. Xu D, Zhu S, Li H, Gao J, Mou H, Wang K. Relationships among occupational stress, toileting behaviors, and overactive bladder in nurses: a multiple mediator model. J Adv Nurs. 2019;75(6):1263–71.
13. Reisch R, Rutt R, Dockter M, Sanders S. Overactive bladder symptoms in female health profession students: bladder diary characteristics and impact of symptoms on health-related quality of life. J Women's Health (2002). 2018;27(2):156–61.
14. Hagovska M, Švihra J, Buková A, Horbacz A, Dračková D, Švihrová V. Comparison of body composition and overactive bladder symptoms in overweight female university students. Eur J Obstet Gynecol Reprod Biol. 2019;237:18–22.
15. Kötter T, Wagner J, Brüheim L, Voltmer E. Perceived Medical School stress of undergraduate medical students predicts academic performance: an observational study. BMC Med Educ. 2017;17(1):256.
16. Angkurawaranon C, Jiraporncharoen W, Sachdev A, Wisetborisut A, Jangiam W, Uaphanthasath R. Predictors of quality of life of medical students and a comparison with quality of life of adult health care workers in Thailand. Springerplus. 2016;5(1):584.
17. Pagnin D, de Queiroz V. Comparison of quality of life between medical students and young general populations. Educ Health (Abingdon). 2015;28(3):209–12.
18. Malibary H, Zagzoog MM, Banjari MA, Bamashmous RO, Omer AR. Quality of Life (QoL) among medical students in Saudi Arabia: a study using the WHOQOL-BREF instrument. BMC Med Educ. 2019;19(1):344.
19. Shawahna R, Hattab S, Al-Shafei R. Tab'ouni M: Prevalence and factors associated with depressive and anxiety symptoms among Palestinian medical students. BMC Psychiatry. 2020;20(1):244.
20. Brenneisen Mayer F, Souza Santos I, Silveira PS, Itaqui Lopes MH, de Souza AR, Campos EP, de Abreu BA, Hoffman Ii I, Magalhães CR, Lima MC, et al. Factors associated to depression and anxiety in medical students: a multicenter study. BMC Med Educ. 2016;16(1):282.
21. Bacchi S, Licinio J. Qualitative Literature Review of the Prevalence of Depression in Medical Students Compared to Students in Non-medical Degrees. Acad Psychiatry. 2015;39(3):293–9.
22. Ribeiro ÍJS, Pereira R, Freire IV, de Oliveira BG, Casotti CA, Boery EN. Stress and quality of life among university students: a systematic literature review. Health Prof Educ. 2018;4(2):70–7.
23. Almalki SA, Almojali AI, Alothman AS, Masuadi EM, Alaqeel MK. Burnout and its association with extracurricular activities among medical students in Saudi Arabia. Int J Med Educ. 2017;8:144–50.
24. Vandenbroucke JP, von Elm E, Altman DG, Gøtzsche PC, Mulrow CD, Pocock SJ, Poole C, Schlesselman JJ, Egger M. Strengthening the reporting of observational studies in epidemiology (STROBE): explanation and elaboration. PLoS Med. 2007;4(10):e297.

25. Coyne KS, Thompson CL, Lai JS, Sexton CC. An overactive bladder symptom and health-related quality of life short-form: validation of the OAB-q SF. Neurourol Urodyn. 2015;34(3):255–63.
26. Coyne K, Revicki D, Hunt T, Corey R, Stewart W, Bentkover J, Kurth H, Abrams P. Psychometric validation of an overactive bladder symptom and health-related quality of life questionnaire: the OAB-q. Qual Life Res. 2002;11(6):563–74.
27. Sekido N, Hinotsu S, Kawai K, Shimazui T, Akaza H. How many uncomplicated male and female overactive bladder patients reveal detrusor overactivity during urodynamic study? Int J Urol. 2006;13(10):1276–9.
28. Ural ÜM, Gücük S, Ekici A, Topçuoğlu A. Urinary incontinence in female university students. Int Urogynecol J. 2021;32(2):367–73.
29. Kajiwara M, Inoue K, Mutaguchi K, Usui T. The prevalence of overactive bladder and nocturnal enuresis in Japanese early adolescents: a questionnaire survey. Hinyokika kiyo Acta urologica Japonica. 2006;52(2):107–11.
30. Shin DG, Kim HW, Lee JZ. Effect of the amount of hours spent studying on the prevalence of overactive bladder in college women. Lower Urin Tract Symptoms. 2010;2(2):113–8.
31. Liu R-T, Chung M-S, Lee W-C, Chang S-W, Huang S-T, Yang KD, Chancellor MB, Chuang Y-C. Prevalence of overactive bladder and associated risk factors in 1359 patients with type 2 diabetes. Urology. 2011;78(5):1040–5.
32. Khavari R, Elias SN, Pande R, Wu KM, Boone TB, Karmonik C. Higher neural correlates in patients with multiple sclerosis and neurogenic overactive bladder following treatment with intradetrusor injection of onabotulinumtoxinA. J Urol. 2019;201(1):135–40.
33. Chen L-C, Kuo H-C. Pathophysiology of refractory overactive bladder. LUTS Lower Urin Tract Symptoms. 2019;11(4):177–81.
34. Kim KS, Kim H-J, Lee SH, Cho ST, Moon HS. Association between irritable bowel syndrome and overactive bladder: a research survey. Urology. 2017;109:88–93.
35. Xu D, Cheng R, Ma A, Zhao M, Wang K. Toileting behaviors and overactive bladder in patients with type 2 diabetes: a cross-sectional study in China. BMC Urol. 2017;17(1):42.
36. Matsumoto S, Hashizume K, Wada N, Hori J, Tamaki G, Kita M, Iwata T, Kakizaki H. Relationship between overactive bladder and irritable bowel syndrome: a large-scale internet survey in Japan using the overactive bladder symptom score and Rome III criteria. BJU Int. 2013;111(4):647–52.
37. Ge TJ, Vetter J, Lai HH. Sleep disturbance and fatigue are associated with more severe urinary incontinence and overactive bladder symptoms. Urology. 2017;109:67–73.
38. Lai H, Gardner V, Vetter J, Andriole GL. Correlation between psychological stress levels and the severity of overactive bladder symptoms. BMC Urol. 2015;15(1):14.
39. Zhang C, Hai T, Yu L, Liu S, Li Q, Zhang X, Xu T, Wang X. Association between occupational stress and risk of overactive bladder and other lower urinary tract symptoms: a cross-sectional study of female nurses in China. Neurourol Urodyn. 2013;32(3):254–60.
40. Chen G-D, Lin T-L, Hu S-W, Chen Y-C, Lin L-Y. Prevalence and correlation of urinary incontinence and overactive bladder in Taiwanese women. Neurourol Urodyn. 2003;22(2):109–17.
41. Hassed C, de Lisle S, Sullivan G, Pier C. Enhancing the health of medical students: outcomes of an integrated mindfulness and lifestyle program. Adv Health Sci Educ. 2009;14(3):387–98.
42. Henning MA, Krägeloh CU, Hawken SJ, Zhao Y, Doherty I. The quality of life of medical students studying in New Zealand: a comparison with nonmedical students and a general population reference group. Teach Learn Med. 2012;24(4):334–40.
43. Dyrbye L, Shanafelt T. A narrative review on burnout experienced by medical students and residents. Med Educ. 2016;50(1):132–49.
44. Moir F, Henning M, Hassed C, Moyes SA, Elley CR. A peer-support and mindfulness program to improve the mental health of medical students. Teach Learn Med. 2016;28(3):293–302.
45. Tsang S, Royse CF, Terkawi AS. Guidelines for developing, translating, and validating a questionnaire in perioperative and pain medicine. Saudi J Anaesth. 2017;11(Suppl 1):S80–9.
46. Boparai JK, Singh S, Kathuria P. How to design and validate a questionnaire: a guide. Curr Clin Pharmacol. 2018;13(4):210–5.
47. Al-Shaiji TF, Alkabbani M. Validation of the Arabic linguistic version of the 8-item overactive bladder questionnaire (OAB-V8). Int Urogynecol J. 2019;30(12):2153–6.
48. Elbaset MA, Hashem A, Taha D-E, Zahran MH, El-Hefnawy AS. Validation of the arabic linguistic version of the overactive bladder symptoms score questionnaire. Arab J Urol. 2019;17(4):265–9.

20

Possible role of intravenous administration of mesenchymal stem cells to alleviate interstitial cystitis/bladder pain syndrome in a Toll-like receptor-7 agonist-induced experimental animal model in rat

Hidetoshi Tabata[1], Masanori Sasaki[2,3,4*], Yuko Kataoka-Sasaki[2], Nobuo Shinkai[1], Koji Ichihara[1], Naoya Masumori[1], Jeffery D. Kocsis[3,4] and Osamu Honmou[2,3,4]

Abstract

Background: Interstitial cystitis/bladder pain syndrome (IC/BPS) categorized with and without Hunner lesions is a condition that displays chronic pelvic pain related to the bladder with no efficacious treatment options. There are strong associations suggested between Hunner-type IC and autoimmune diseases. Recently, we established an animal model of Hunner-type IC using a Toll-like receptor-7 (TLR7) agonist. Intravenous infusion of mesenchymal stem cells (MSCs) can be used to treat injury via multimodal and orchestrated therapeutic mechanisms including anti-inflammatory effects. Here, we investigated whether infused MSCs elicit therapeutic efficacy associated with the TLR7-related anti-inflammatory pathway in our Hunner-type IC model.

Methods: Voiding behaviors were monitored 24 h prior to the Loxoribine (LX), which is a TLR7 agonist instillation in order to establish a Hunner-type IC model (from − 24 to 0 h) in female Sprague–Dawley rats. LX was instilled transurethrally into the bladder. At 0 h, the initial freezing behavior test confirmed that no freezing behavior was observed in any of the animals. The LX-instilled animals were randomized. Randomized LX-instilled rats were intravenously infused with MSCs or with vehicle through the right external jugular vein. Sampling tissue for green fluorescent protein (GFP)-positive MSCs were carried out at 48 h. Second voiding behavior tests were monitored from 72 to 96 h. After the final evaluation of the freezing behavior test at 96 h after LX instillation (72 h after MSC or vehicle infusion), histological evaluation with H&E staining and quantitative real-time polymerase chain reaction (RT-PCR) to analyze the mRNA expression levels of inflammatory cytokines were performed.

Results: Freezing behavior was reduced in the MSC group, and voiding behavior in the MSC group did not deteriorate. Hematoxylin–eosin staining showed that mucosal edema, leukocyte infiltration, and hemorrhage were suppressed in the MSC group. The relative expression of interferon-β mRNA in the bladder of the MSC group was

*Correspondence: msasaki@sapmed.ac.jp
[2] Department of Neural Regenerative Medicine, Research Institute for Frontier Medicine, Sapporo Medical University School of Medicine, Sapporo, Hokkaido 060-8556, Japan
Full list of author information is available at the end of the article

inhibited. Numerous GFP-positive MSCs were distributed mainly in the submucosal and mucosal layers of the inflammatory bladder wall.

Conclusion: Intravenous infusion of MSCs may have therapeutic efficacy in a LX-instilled Hunner-type IC rat model via a TLR7-related anti-inflammatory pathway.

Keywords: Intravenous, Mesenchymal stem cell, Hunner-type interstitial cystitis

Background

Interstitial cystitis/bladder pain syndrome (IC/BPS) is a condition that causes chronic pelvic pain related to the bladder with no efficacious treatment options [1]. The complete picture of IC/BPS remains unclear; however, IC/BPS can be categorized into IC/BPS with and without Hunner lesions [2]. Hunner-type IC is characterized by the cystoscopic finding known as Hunner lesions, reddish mucosal lesions accompanied by abnormal capillary structures. Hunner-type IC has a proven bladder histology that manifests epithelial denudation and chronic inflammatory changes, such as lymphoplasmacytic and mast cell infiltration, stromal fibrosis, and edema [3].

Recently, we established an animal model of Hunner-type IC using a Toll-like receptor 7 (TLR7) agonist [4]. Strong associations occur between Hunner-type IC and autoimmune diseases [5]. Toll-like receptors (TLRs) are key players in the innate immune system and in biological defense mechanisms against external pathogens [6]. Among TLRs, TLR7 is associated with the development and maintenance of inflammation and pain and is considered to contribute to the development of several autoimmune diseases [5]. As we identified an increase in the number of TLR7 immunoreactive cells and in TLR7 mRNA expression in the bladder of Hunner-type IC patients, loxoribine (LX) (a TLR7 agonist) was applied to the bladder of C57BL/6N female mice to induce edema, congestion and inflammation and was associated with significantly increased TLR7-mRNA expression (4). The animals instilled with LX demonstrated increased licking behavior, voiding frequency, and afferent nerve activities associated with increased single-voided volume and intercontraction interval of micturition per cystometry measurements [4].

Cellular therapy for IC/BPS, using mesenchymal stem cells (MSCs) derived from multiple sources, has been reported to provide therapeutic efficacy. The proposed mechanisms by which transplanted MSCs restrain IC/BPS symptoms include regeneration of damaged bladder tissue through the Wnt pathway [7, 8], anti-tissue fibrosis [9], anti-apoptosis via the AKT/mTOR pathway [10], antioxidant [11, 12], and anti-inflammatory effects including mast cell infiltration and inhibition of inflammatory cytokines [13, 14]. However, specific pathways inhibiting inflammation in MSCs have not been identified.

Here, we investigated whether intravenous infusion of MSCs elicits therapeutic efficacy to reduce inflammation in our established Hunner-type IC model with a TLR7 agonist. Bladder pain-like behavior and voiding behaviors were monitored. In addition, histopathological gene expression analyses was carried out to identify a TLR7-related anti-inflammatory pathway, with the intent of utilizing these data to develop approaches to reduce the symptoms in this experimental Hunner-type IC model.

Materials and methods

Preparation of MSCs from bone marrow

MSCs were cultured as described in our previous studies [15, 16]. Briefly, the bone marrow was collected from the femoral bones of adult wild-type Sprague–Dawley (SD) rats and GFP-expressing rats [W-Tg (CAG-GFP)184Ys], diluted to 25 ml with Dulbecco's modified Eagle's medium (DMEM) (Sigma, St. Louis, MO, USA), supplemented with 10% heat-inactivated fetal bovine serum (FBS) (Thermo Fisher Scientific Inc., Waltham, MA, USA), 2 mM l-glutamine (Sigma), 100 U/ml penicillin, and 0.1 mg/ml streptomycin (Thermo Fisher Scientific Inc.), and incubated for 3 days (5% CO_2, 37 °C). When the cultures almost reached confluence (over 95%), adherent cells were detached using trypsin–EDTA solution (Sigma) and subcultured on a 150 mm^2 tissue culture dish (1030–150: IWAKI, Tokyo, Japan; surface area: 148 cm^2) at 5×10^5 cells/ml in 14 ml culture medium; thus, the plating density was approximately $3.4 \times 10^3/cm^2$. The surface antigen phenotype of MSCs was as follows: $CD45^-$, $CD73^+$, $CD90^+$, and $CD106^-$ [17, 18]. The cultured MSCs were used for infusion after three passages. For infusion, the supernatants discarded and MSCs (1.0×10^6 cells) were resuspended in fresh 1 ml DMEM and injected.

Hunner-type IC model

Sixty-two female SD rats, aged 8 weeks, were used. The animals were housed under standard laboratory conditions with a 12:12 h light: dark cycle and free access to food and water. Under anesthesia with ketamine and xylazine (75 and 10 mg/kg, respectively; i.p.), a polyethylene catheter (PE-50) was atraumatically inserted into the bladder of rats, transurethrally. After urine was drained, 200 μl of 4.5 mM Loxoribine (LX) (AdipoGen Life Sciences, Liestal, Switzerland) (n = 36), a selective TLR7agonist [or distilled water (DW) for sham (n = 14)], was instilled slowly. The catheter was kept for 60 min, after which the instilled liquid was drained, and the animals were allowed to recover from anesthesia.

Experimental protocol

The experimental protocol is illustrated in Fig. 1. Voiding behaviors (1) were monitored 24 h prior to LX or DW instillation, to establish a Hunner-type IC model (from − 24 to 0 h). At 0 h, the initial freezing behavior (1) test confirmed that no freezing behavior was observed in any of the animals (Fig. 2a). LX was instilled into 48 rats, and DW was instilled into 14 rats. After the second freezing behavior (2) test following LX or DW instillation at 24 h, the 12 LX-instilled rats that displayed no freezing behavior were excluded. Thus, we included 36 LX-instilled rats and 14 DW-instilled rats for this study. Eight of the 36 LX-instilled rats were used for the detection of GFP-expressing MSCs (GFP-MSCs). GFP-MSCs were infused into LX-instilled animals (n = 4), and MSCs derived from wild-type animals were infused into LX-instilled animals (n = 4), at 48 h (24 h after MSC or vehicle infusion). The remaining LX-instilled animals (n = 28) were randomized. Randomized LX-instilled rats were intravenously infused with MSCs (MSC group: 1.0×10^6 cells in 1 ml fresh DMEM) or with vehicle (Vehicle group: 1 ml fresh DMEM), and the DW-instilled rats were infused with vehicle only (Sham group) through the right external jugular vein [15]. Second voiding behavior [2] tests were

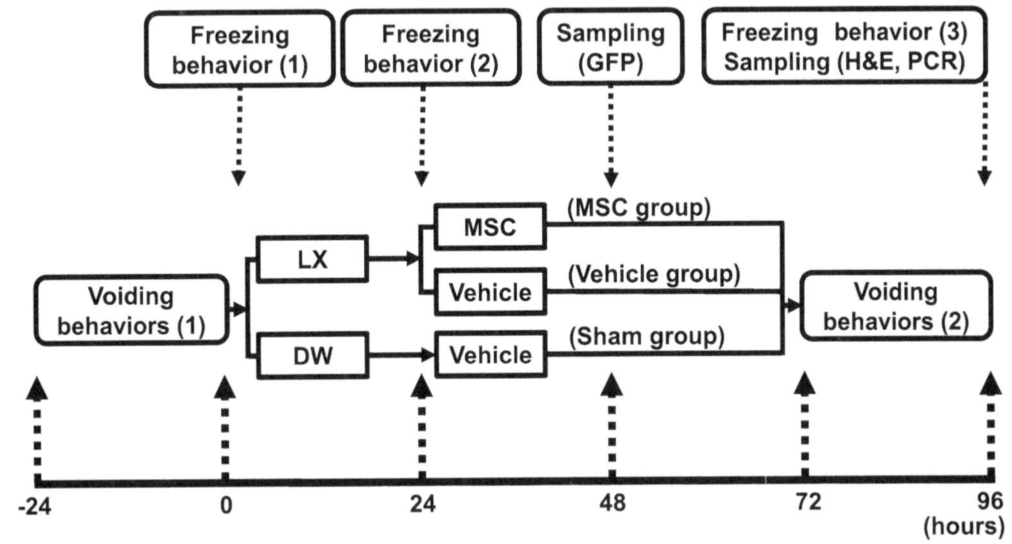

Fig. 1 Experimental protocol

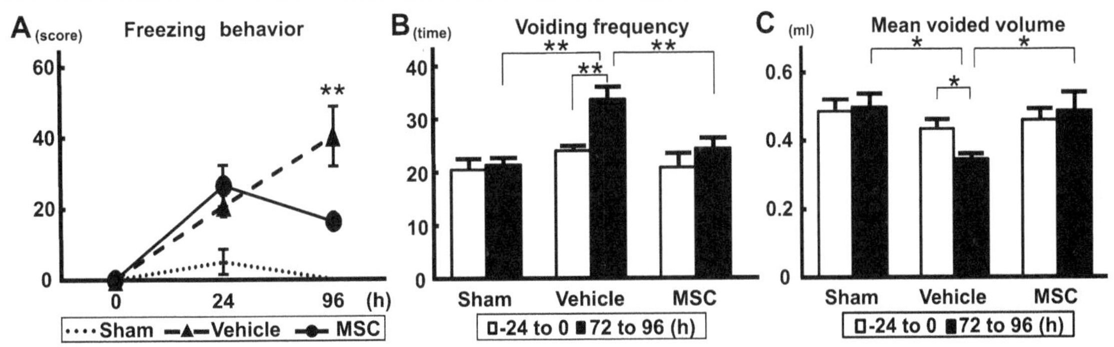

Fig. 2 Urological evaluations. **a** Bladder pain-like behavior; **b** voiding frequency; **c** mean voided volume. n = 6/group. ANOVA with the Tukey–Kramer post hoc test. $*p < 0.05$, $**p < 0.01$. *h* "hour"

monitored from 72 to 96 h. After the final evaluation of the freezing behavior [3] test at 96 h after LX instillation (72 h after MSC or vehicle infusion), histologic evaluations and quantitative real-time polymerase chain reaction (RT-PCR) were performed.

Transplantation procedure

The rats used in this study were anesthetized with an intraperitoneal (IP) injection of ketamine and xylazine (90/4 mg/kg) and received intravenous infusion of MSCs (1.0×10^6) in 1.0 ml total fluid volume (DMEM) or vehicle (1.0 ml fresh DMEM alone) via right external jugular vein. All rats were injected subcutaneously daily with cyclosporine A (10 mg/kg).

Freezing behavior

Freezing behavior was defined as bladder pain-like behavior of rats, indicated by cessation of movement and pointing of the nose toward the lower abdomen without licking. If the freezing behavior occurred within a 5-s interval, it was scored as one positive event. The number of positive events of the respective behaviors was counted for 30 min [19].

Voiding behavior

Voiding behaviors (voiding frequency and measurement of voided volume) were recorded for 24 h using a metabolic cage (Urination Monitor-100, Melquest Ltd., Toyama, Japan), after 24 h of adaptation to the environment [4]. The voiding frequency was recorded for 24 h; after a 5-min interval, it was defined as the next voiding. The cutoff for voided volume in this experiment was defined as 0.03 ml. These settings were applied according to the findings from our pilot study. During recording, the rats were allowed free access to water and food.

Histopathological analyses

Rats were deeply anesthetized with an intraperitoneal injection of ketamine (50 mg/kg) and xylazine (10 mg/kg), perfused with phosphate-buffered saline (PBS) and 4% paraformaldehyde (PFA) in 0.1 M phosphate-buffer (PB), 96 h after LX instillation (72 h after MSC or vehicle infusion). Then, the bladders were isolated from each group and opened at the dorsal side of the bladder neck, along the midline towards the dome. After macroscopic evaluation, bladders were placed in 4% formaldehyde and embedded in paraffin for microscopic evaluation via hematoxylin–eosin (H&E) staining. For H&E staining, paraffin-embedded sections were cut (3 μm) using a Leica RM2265 microtome (Leica Microsystems, Wetzlar, Hesse-Darmstadt, Germany). The deparaffinized sections were stained with hematoxylin for 5 min at room temperature, followed by staining with eosin solution (1% eosin + 95% ethanol + acetate) for 3 min at room temperature and then photographed (BZ-9000; Keyence, Osaka, Japan). During histological evaluation, ten fields of each slide were scored for mucosal edema, leukocyte infiltration, hemorrhage, and mucosal abrasion [20]. Edema was evaluated at × 200 magnification. No edema was scored as 0, minimal edema (no change in connective tissue thickness) as 1, moderate edema (connective tissue thickness increased by < twofold) as 2, and severe edema (connective tissue thickness increased by > twofold) as 3. Leukocyte infiltration was evaluated in the mucosa at × 400 magnification. No extravascular leukocytes were scored as 0, > 20 leukocytes as 1, 20–45 leukocytes as 2, and > 45 leukocytes as 3. Mucosal hemorrhage and mucosal abrasion were evaluated at × 100 magnification. The presence of hemorrhage and mucosal abrasion was scored as 1, and no change was scored as 0. The total score of all fields of view for mucosal edema, leukocyte infiltration, mucosal hemorrhage, and mucosal abrasion was divided by the maximum possible score and then multiplied by 100 [20].

RT-PCR

Quantitative RT-PCR was performed as previously described [15]. After 96 h of LX instillation (72 h after MSC or vehicle infusion), the animals were anesthetized with an intraperitoneal injection of ketamine (50 mg/kg) and xylazine (10 mg/kg), and bladders from each group were collected using a dissecting microscope. Total RNA was extracted using an RNeasy Plus Mini kit (#74134, Qiagen, Valencia, CA, USA) according to the manufacturer's instructions. The RNA concentration was quantified by determining the optical density at 260 nm. RNA (1 μg) was reverse transcribed into cDNA using SuperScript III reverse transcriptase (Qiagen) and oligo-dT. Real-time PCR for each sample was performed in triplicate with TaqMan Universal Master Mix II with no UNG (Thermo Fisher Scientific Inc.). The following sets of specific primers and TaqMan probes were purchased from Thermo Fisher Scientific Inc.: glyceraldehyde-3-phosphate dehydrogenase (GAPDH) (TaqMan rodent GAPDH control reagents, Rn01775763-g1) as an endogenous control, and TLR7 (Rn01771083) and interferon (*IFN*)-β (Rn00569434) as target genes. The reactions were run on an ABI-StepOne real-time PCR system (Thermo Fisher Scientific Inc.) using a 48-well plate format. The cycling conditions included an initial denaturation phase at 95 °C for 3 min, followed by 40 cycles of 95 °C for 15 s and 55 °C for 60 s. Relative quantification of target gene expression was performed using the comparative threshold cycle method, according to the manufacturer's guidelines.

Detection of GFP expressing MSCs

Detection of GFP expressing MSCs was performed as previously described [15]. One day after injection of GFP-MSCs from GFP-expressing rats and non-GFP-MSCs from wild-type SD rats, transcardial perfusion (4% PFA) under anesthesia with an intraperitoneal injection of ketamine (50 mg/kg) and xylazine (10 mg/kg) was performed to dissect out the bladder. After dissection, the bladders were fixed in 4% PFA for 1 h at 4 °C. Then, the frozen embedded bladder was cut into 12-μm thick sections with a cryostat and mounted on glass slides. Slides were washed thrice in PBS with Tween 20 (0.1%) (PBST) and blocked in normal goat serum (10%) and Triton X (0.3%) in PBS at room temperature for 30 min. The sections were then incubated overnight at 4 °C with the primary antibody (chicken anti-GFP antibody, 1:1000; ab13970, Abcam, Cambridge, MA, USA), diluted with normal goat serum (5%), Triton X (0.3%), and PBS. After four washes in PBST, the sections were incubated with the secondary antibody (1:2000; AF 488-conjugated goat anti-chicken immunoglobulin Y, Abcam, 150,173) for 1 h and counterstained with DAPI. The sections were then examined using a confocal microscope (Ex/Em, 405/488: LSM780 ELYRA system; Carl Zeiss, Oberkochen, Germany).

Statistical analysis

All statistical analyses were performed using SPSS 18 (SPSS Inc., Chicago, IL, USA). Comparisons were performed using one-way analysis of variance with the Tukey–Kramer post hoc test.

Results

The freezing behavior score was decreased following MSC infusion

There were no significant differences among the three experimental groups (MSC, vehicle, and sham) in the initial freezing behavior (1) test at 0 h. At 24 h after LX or DW instillation (prior to MSC or vehicle infusion), the scores of the second freezing behavior (2) test were increased in the LX-instilled groups (both vehicle and MSC groups). At 96 h, the freezing behavior score was further increased in the vehicle group; however, the score in the MSC group decreased ($p<0.01$) (Fig. 2a).

The intravenous infusion of MSCs suppressed pelvic pain evaluated with voiding behaviors

There were no significant differences among the three groups in terms of voiding frequency (Fig. 2b) and mean voided volume (Fig. 2c) from −24 to 0 h ($p=0.55$). It was difficult to measure stable voiding behaviors prior to MSC or vehicle infusion, possibly because of the effects of anesthesia and intravesical activity of catheter implantation for instillation of LX into the bladder. In addition, a 24 h period is required to measure voiding behaviors (see Materials and Methods). The voiding frequency in the vehicle group at 96 h (from 72 to 96 h) was elevated compared with that in the MSC and sham groups ($p<0.01$); there was no difference between the sham and MSC-infused groups. The voiding frequency at 96 h was also higher than that at 0 h (from −24 to 0 h) in the vehicle group, although there were no differences between the sham and MSC-infused groups. The mean voided volume in the vehicle group at 96 h (from 72 to 96 h) was lower than that in the MSC and sham groups ($p<0.05$), and there was no difference between the sham and MSC-infused groups. The mean voided volume at 96 h was lower than that at 0 h (from −24 to 0 h) in the vehicle group, although there was no difference between the sham and MSC-infused groups. These results suggest that intravenous infusion of MSCs suppressed pelvic pain following LX instillation in the bladder, indicating the therapeutic efficacy of infused MSCs for experimental IC.

Intravenous infusion of MSCs inhibited histopathological damage

Macroscopic observation revealed that the bladder wall in the vehicle group (Fig. 3b) was thicker than that in the sham group (Fig. 3a), and the bladder wall in the MSC group (Fig. 3c) was thinner than that in the vehicle group. Histopathological evaluation using H&E staining in the vehicle group revealed mucosal edema (Fig. 3e), mucosal ablation (Fig. 3e, red arrows), hemorrhage (Fig. 3h, green arrow), and leukocyte infiltration (Fig. 3h, blue arrows), although H&E staining in the sham group (Fig. 3d, g) showed no thickening and edema in the mucosal and submucosal layers, as well as no inflammatory features such as hemorrhage or leukocyte infiltration. In the vehicle group, these inflammatory features were less observed compared to the MSC group (Fig. 3f, i). Mucosal edema (Fig. 4a, $p<0.01$), leukocyte infiltration (Fig. 4b: $p<0.05$), and hemorrhage (Fig. 4c, $p<0.05$) were evident in the vehicle group after LX instillation compared with the sham group. These changes were suppressed in the MSC-treated group. Although a trend was observed, there were no significant differences among the three groups in mucosal ablation (Fig. 4d, $p=0.16$). These results indicate that intravenous infusion of MSCs inhibited histopathological damage following LX instillation in the bladder.

Infused MSCs reduced the expression of IFN-β in the TLR7 expressed bladder wall following LX instillation

The relative expression of TLR7-mRNA in the bladder wall in both vehicle and MSC groups was elevated following LX instillation compared with the sham group (Fig. 5a: $p<0.01$), and there was no significant difference

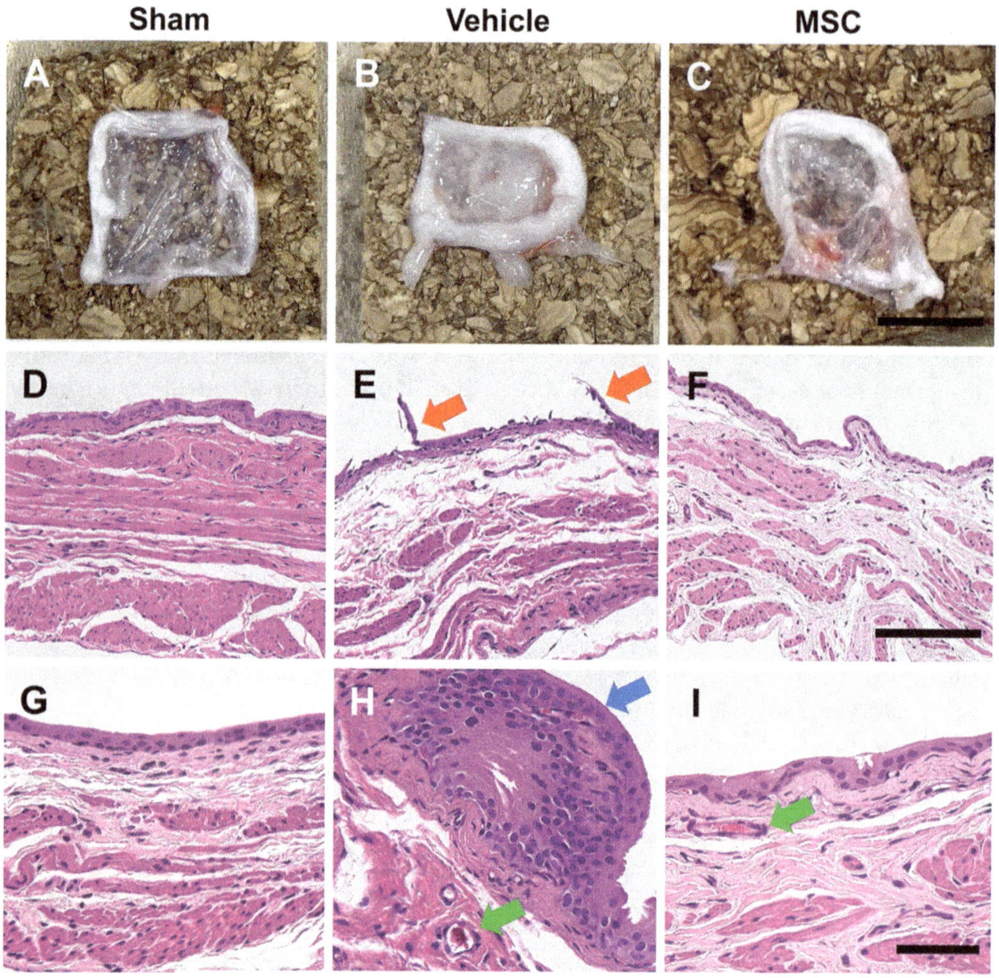

Fig. 3 Representative macroscopic and histological images of bladder at 96 h following intravenous infusion of MSCs or vehicle in a LX-instilled rat model of Hunner-type IC. (**a, d, g**) Sham, (**b, e, h**) vehicle, and (**c, f, i**) MSC groups. Red arrows indicate mucosal ablation. Blue arrows indicate leukocyte infiltration. Green arrows indicate hemorrhage. Scale bars = 1 cm (**a–c**), 150 μm (**d–f**), and 50 μm (**g–i**)

between the MSC and vehicle groups. The relative expression of *IFN-β* mRNA in the bladder wall in the vehicle group was elevated following LX instillation compared with that in the MSC and sham groups (Fig. 5b, $p<0.05$). Even though TLR7 levels were elevated in the MSC group after LX instillation, *IFN-β* mRNA levels were not.

Accumulated MSCs in the inflammatory bladder wall

GFP-MSCs were identified in the inflammatory bladder wall via observation of green fluorescence (Fig. 6a). Numerous infused GFP-MSCs were more extensively distributed in the submucosal and mucosal layers and few GFP-MSCs were present in the muscle layer (Fig. 6a). The accumulation of the infused GFP-MSCs demonstrated a homing effect in the LX-instilled bladder, suggesting that GFP-MSCs might accumulate at the inflammation lesion site in the bladder, where we observed leukocyte infiltration in the vehicle group (Fig. 3h). To confirm whether the infused MSCs showed autofluorescence at the wavelengths used to study GFP fluorescence, we examined sections of samples from animals infused with non-GFP-MSCs derived from wild-type SD rats. No GFP^+ cells were observed in these rats (Fig. 6b).

Discussion

We found that intravenous infusion of MSCs reduced the symptoms of IC/BPS in our newly established animal model of Hunner-type IC using a TLR7 agonist. The IC/BPS related freezing behavior was improved (reduced), and the voiding behaviors scored as voiding frequency and mean voided volume did not deteriorate following infusion of MSCs compared with the vehicle group. Macroscopic observation and histological analysis using H&E staining demonstrated that preservation of the bladder wall structure was clearly observed in the MSC

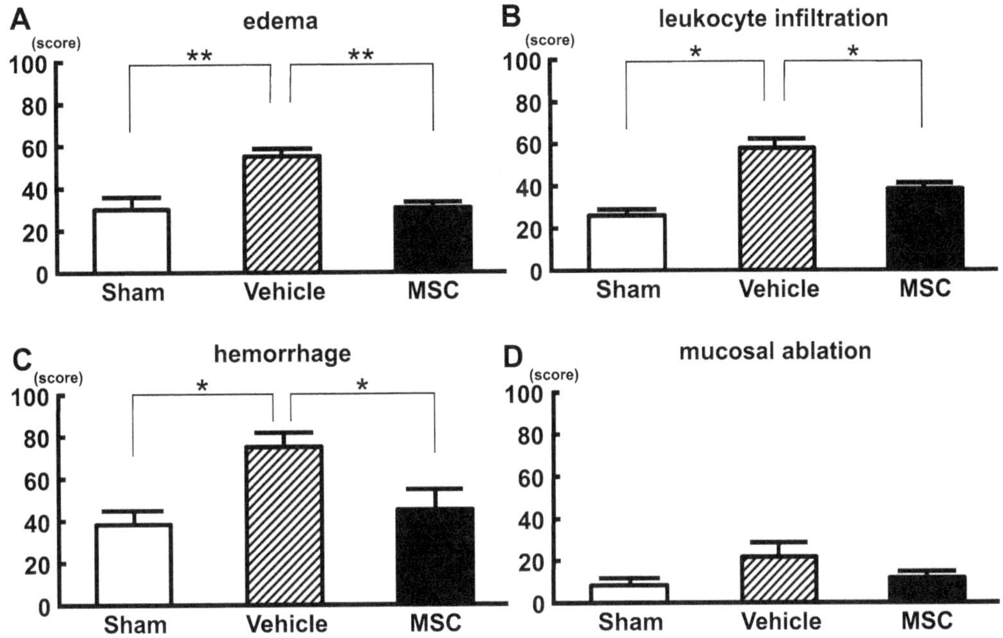

Fig. 4 Histological evaluation. **a** Edema, **b** leukocyte infiltration, **c** hemorrhage, and **d** mucosal ablation. n = 6/group. ANOVA with the Tukey–Kramer post hoc test. $^{*}p < 0.05$, $^{**}p < 0.01$

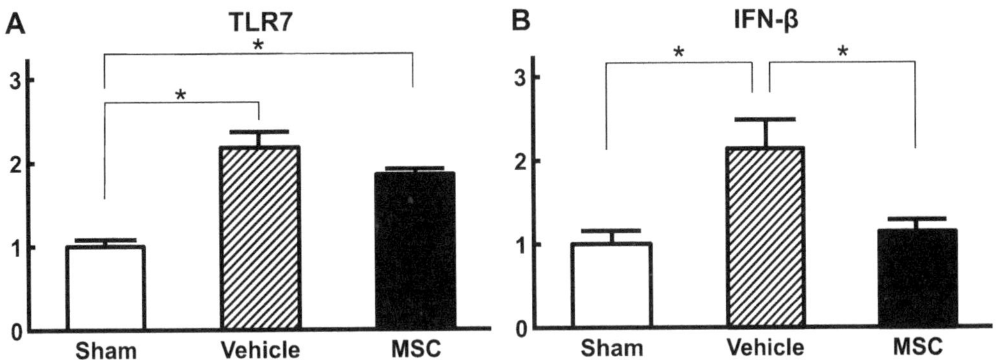

Fig. 5 mRNA expression of TLR7 (**a**) and IFN-β (**b**) in the bladder wall at 96 h following infusion of MSCs or vehicle in a LX-instilled rat model of Hunner-type IC. n = 8/group. ANOVA with the Tukey–Kramer post hoc test. $^{*}p < 0.05$.

group. The bladder wall thickness in the MSC group was thinner than that in the vehicle group, and several pathological features, including hemorrhage, edema, and leukocyte infiltration, showed improvement in bladder wall pathology. We observed a significantly higher expression of TLR7 mRNA in the bladder wall in our IC/BPS model. However, the expression of *IFN-β* mRNA in the MSC group was significantly reduced compared to that in the vehicle group. Accumulated GFP-MSCs were found mainly in the submucosal and mucosal layers in the inflammatory bladder wall after intravenous infusion of GFP-MSCs. These data suggest that MSCs might contribute to the downregulation of *IFN-β* and thus reduction in inflammation.

Although the etiology and pathophysiology of IC/BPS are uncertain, autoimmune disorders are common comorbidities of IC/BPS [21]. Thus, autoimmunity could be among the possible causes of IC/BPS [22]. In the animal model of Hunner-type IC induced by a TLR7 agonist used here [4], we elucidated that intravenous infusion of MSCs provides therapeutic efficacy for the Hunner-type IC model by downregulating the expression of *IFN-β* in a TLR7-induced rat model. Previous studies indicated that TLR7-myeloid differentiation primary response 88

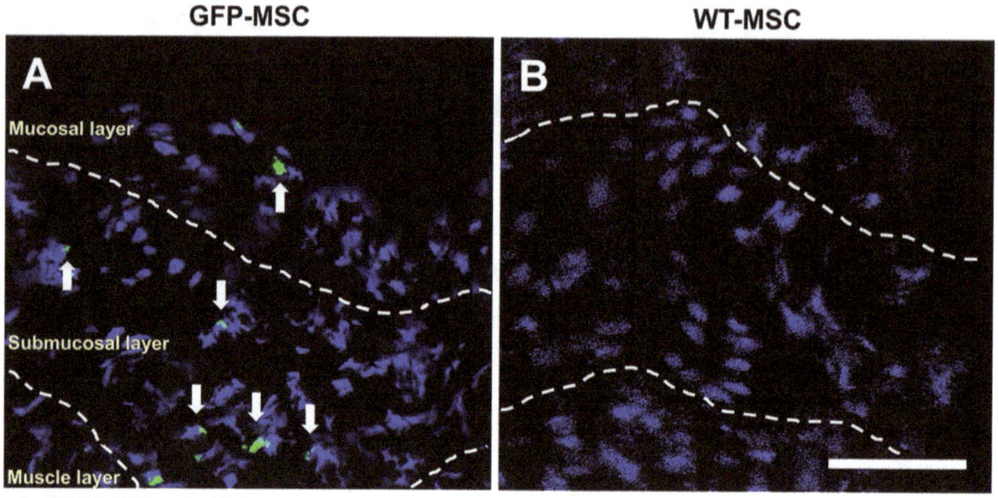

Fig. 6 Distribution of GFP-MSCs in the bladder wall at 48 h following infusion of MSCs or vehicle in a LX-instilled rat model of Hunner-type IC. **a** GFP-MSCs; **b** MSCs derived from wild type rats. Dashed lines indicate the borders of mucosal, submucosal and muscle layers. Arrows indicate GFP-MSCs. Scale bar = 50 μm

(MyD88) signaling, which activates interferon regulatory factor 7 (IRF-7), results in robust induction of *IFN-β* [23, 24]. It has been reported that MSCs secrete transforming growth factor beta *(TGF-β)* [25] and they can stimulate macrophages to secrete *TGF-β* in sites of inflammation [26]. Infused MSCs accumulated in the mucosal and submucosal layers of the bladder wall and might contribute to increased levels of *TGF-β* [25]. *TGF-β* inhibits the phosphorylation of IRF-7, reduces the protein level of MyD88 [27], and downregulates the production of *IFN-β* [28]. The expression level of TLR7 was not significantly reduced in our model system, although *IFN-β* was downregulated following intravenous infusion of MSCs. Therefore, it is conceivable that infused MSCs might play an important role in reducing the expression of *IFN-β* (Fig. 7), thereby promoting the reduction of inflammation in the bladder wall. Thus, a novel finding of this study is that the intravenous infusion of MSCs has therapeutic effects on Hunner-type IC by downregulating the expression of IFN-β in this TLR7-induced Hunner-type IC model. Therefore, using this unique model, a novel pathway for inhibiting the inflammation induced by infused MSCs has been proposed.

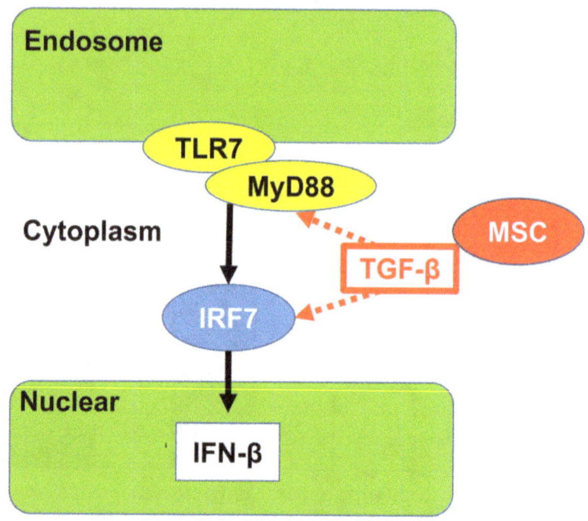

Fig. 7 Possible therapeutic mechanism of infused MSCs. TLR7: Toll like receptor 7, MyD88: myeloid differentiation primary response 88, TGF-β: transforming growth factor beta, IRF7: interferon regulatory factor 7, IFN-β: interferon beta

It is important to contextualize that Ichihara et al. used mice to develop this Hunner-type IC model with TLR7; however, we used rats because most cellular transplantation studies with Hunner-type IC models have used rats [7–10, 13, 14, 29]. We used the same concentration of LX as that in the mouse model (4.5 mM, 100 μm) [4], but we increased the volume of LX (4.5 mM, 200 μm) in the current study after considering the bladder volume of rats [30]. A potential strength of this study is the use of a TLR7-induced Hunner-type IC rat model system compared with other commonly used IC/BPS model systems induced with cyclophosphamide [31, 32], lipopolysaccharide [33], hydrochloric acid (HCl) [7, 13], uroplakin [14, 29] and ketamine [9].

We propose that the TLR7-related anti-inflammatory pathway is associated with restraining IC/BPS pathology. This study provides additional insights into the anti-inflammatory mechanism of infused MSCs, in addition to the infiltration of mast cells and reduction of inflammatory cytokines [13, 14].

A limitation of this study is that as mentioned above, that we employed the methods used in the original paper by Ichihara et al. [4]. The study period by Ichihara et al. was 96 h which we used in this study. We also would like to stress that our preliminary study with our established Hunner-type IC model with TLR7 agonist demonstrated that the bladder pain-like behavior and voiding behaviors did not last more than a week. Thus, we focused on acute therapeutic effects of infused MSCs in this study. We also realize that elucidation of the precise molecular mechanism underlying the MSC therapy is important and future studies should be performed to establish a more appropriate model for longer term study and study of corresponding pathways and proteins using western blot and ELISA.

Conclusions

Intravenous infusion of MSCs may have an impact on the mitigation of IC/BPS symptoms via *IFN-β* downregulation in a TLR7-induced rat model of Hunner-type IC model system.

Acknowledgements

We thank the National BioResource Project—Rat (http://www.anim.med.kyoto-u.ac.jp/NBR/) for providing the strain of rats used in the current study [W-Tg (CAG-GFP) 184Ys].

Authors' contributions

HT: Protocol development, data collection, data analysis. MS: Project development, data analysis and management, and manuscript writing. YKS: Project development, data analysis. NS: Protocol development. KI: Protocol development, manuscript editing. NM: Project development, data analysis, manuscript editing. JDK: Data analysis, manuscript writing. OH: Project development, data analysis, management, manuscript writing. All authors read and approved the final manuscript.

Author details

[1]Department of Urology, Sapporo Medical University School of Medicine, Sapporo 060-8556, Japan. [2]Department of Neural Regenerative Medicine, Research Institute for Frontier Medicine, Sapporo Medical University School of Medicine, Sapporo, Hokkaido 060-8556, Japan. [3]Department of Neurology, Yale University School of Medicine, New Haven, CT 06510, USA. [4]Center for Neuroscience and Regeneration Research, VA Connecticut Healthcare System, West Haven, CT 06516, USA.

References

1. Ko KJ, Cho WJ, Lee YS, Choi J, Byun HJ, Lee KS. Comparison of the efficacy between transurethral coagulation and transurethral resection of hunner lesion in interstitial cystitis/bladder pain syndrome patients: a prospective randomized controlled trial. Eur Urol. 2020;77(5):644–51.
2. van de Merwe JP, Nordling J, Bouchelouche P, Bouchelouche K, Cervigni M, Daha LK, et al. Diagnostic criteria, classification, and nomenclature for painful bladder syndrome/interstitial cystitis: an ESSIC proposal. Eur Urol. 2008;53(1):60–7.
3. Akiyama Y, Luo Y, Hanno PM, Maeda D, Homma Y. Interstitial cystitis/bladder pain syndrome: the evolving landscape, animal models and future perspectives. Int J Urol. 2020;27(6):491–503.
4. Ichihara K, Aizawa N, Akiyama Y, Kamei J, Masumori N, Andersson KE, et al. Toll-like receptor 7 is overexpressed in the bladder of Hunner-type interstitial cystitis, and its activation in the mouse bladder can induce cystitis and bladder pain. Pain. 2017;158(8):1538–45.
5. Andersson KE, Birder L. Current pharmacologic approaches in painful bladder research: an update. Int Neurourol J. 2017;21(4):235–42.
6. Iwasaki A, Medzhitov R. Regulation of adaptive immunity by the innate immune system. Science. 2010;327(5963):291–5.
7. Song M, Lim J, Yu HY, Park J, Chun JY, Jeong J, et al. Mesenchymal stem cell therapy alleviates interstitial cystitis by activating wnt signaling pathway. Stem Cells Dev. 2015;24(14):1648–57.
8. Ryu CM, Yu HY, Lee HY, Shin JH, Lee S, Ju H, et al. Longitudinal intravital imaging of transplanted mesenchymal stem cells elucidates their functional integration and therapeutic potency in an animal model of interstitial cystitis/bladder pain syndrome. Theranostics. 2018;8(20):5610–24.
9. Kim A, Yu HY, Heo J, Song M, Shin JH, Lim J, et al. Mesenchymal stem cells protect against the tissue fibrosis of ketamine-induced cystitis in rat bladder. Sci Rep. 2016;6:30881.
10. Xie J, Liu B, Chen J, Xu Y, Zhan H, Yang F, et al. Umbilical cord-derived mesenchymal stem cells alleviated inflammation and inhibited apoptosis in interstitial cystitis via AKT/mTOR signaling pathway. Biochem Biophys Res Commun. 2018;495(1):546–52.
11. Chen YT, Chiang HJ, Chen CH, Sung PH, Lee FY, Tsai TH, et al. Melatonin treatment further improves adipose-derived mesenchymal stem cell therapy for acute interstitial cystitis in rat. J Pineal Res. 2014;57(3):248–61.
12. Shin JH, Ryu CM, Ju H, Yu HY, Song S, Shin DM, et al. Synergistic effects of N-acetylcysteine and mesenchymal stem cell in a lipopolysaccharide-induced interstitial cystitis rat model. Cells. 2019;9(1):86.
13. Furuta A, Yamamoto T, Igarashi T, Suzuki Y, Egawa S, Yoshimura N. Bladder wall injection of mesenchymal stem cells ameliorates bladder inflammation, overactivity, and nociception in a chemically induced interstitial cystitis-like rat model. Int Urogynecol J. 2018;29(11):1615–22.
14. Chung JW, Chun SY, Lee EH, Ha YS, Lee JN, Song PH, et al. Verification of mesenchymal stem cell injection therapy for interstitial cystitis in a rat model. PLoS ONE. 2019;14(12):e0226390.
15. Matsuda Y, Sasaki M, Kataoka-Sasaki Y, Takayanagi A, Kobayashi K, Oka S, et al. Intravenous infusion of bone marrow-derived mesenchymal stem cells reduces erectile dysfunction following cavernous nerve injury in rats. Sex Med. 2017.
16. Takemura M, Sasaki M, Kataoka-Sasaki Y, Kiyose R, Nagahama H, Oka S, et al. Repeated intravenous infusion of mesenchymal stem cells provides enhanced functional recovery in a rat model of chronic cerebral ischemia. J Neurosurg. **(in press)**.
17. Kim S, Honmou O, Kato K, Nonaka T, Houkin K, Hamada H, et al. Neural differentiation potential of peripheral blood- and bone-marrow-derived precursor cells. Brain Res. 2006;1123(1):27–33.
18. Ukai R, Honmou O, Harada K, Houkin K, Hamada H, Kocsis J. Mesenchymal stem cells derived from peripheral blood protects against ischemia. J Neurotrauma. 2007;24(3):508–20.
19. Saitoh C, Chancellor MB, de Groat WC, Yoshimura N. Effects of intravesical instillation of resiniferatoxin on bladder function and nociceptive behavior in freely moving, conscious rats. J Urol. 2008;179(1):359–64.
20. Dönmez M, İnci K, Zeybek ND, Doğan HS, Ergen A. The Early histological effects of intravesical instillation of platelet-rich plasma in cystitis models. Int Neurourol J. 2016;20(3):188–96.
21. Homma Y, Akiyama Y, Tomoe H, Furuta A, Ueda T, Maeda D, et al. Clinical guidelines for interstitial cystitis/bladder pain syndrome. Int J Urol. 2020;27(7):578–89.
22. Bosch PC. A randomized, double-blind, placebo-controlled trial of certolizumab pegol in women with refractory interstitial cystitis/bladder pain syndrome. Eur Urol. 2018;74(5):623–30.
23. Kawai T, Sato S, Ishii KJ, Coban C, Hemmi H, Yamamoto M, et al. Interferon-alpha induction through Toll-like receptors involves a direct interaction of IRF7 with MyD88 and TRAF6. Nat Immunol. 2004;5(10):1061–8.
24. Honda K, Yanai H, Mizutani T, Negishi H, Shimada N, Suzuki N, et al. Role of a transductional-transcriptional processor complex involving MyD88 and IRF-7 in Toll-like receptor signaling. Proc Natl Acad Sci USA. 2004;101(43):15416–21.

25. Nakazaki M, Oka S, Sasaki M, Kataoka-Sasaki Y, Onodera R, Komatsu K, et al. Prevention of neointimal hyperplasia induced by an endovascular stent via intravenous infusion of mesenchymal stem cells. J Neurosurg. 2019;6:1–13.
26. Nakazaki M, Morita T, Lankford KL, Askenase PW, Kocsis JD. Small extracellular vesicles released by infused mesenchymal stromal cells target M2 macrophages and promote TGF-β upregulation, microvascular stabilization and functional recovery in a rodent model of severe spinal cord injury. J Extracell Vesicles. 2021;10(11):e12137.
27. Naiki Y, Michelsen KS, Zhang W, Chen S, Doherty TM, Arditi M. Transforming growth factor-beta differentially inhibits MyD88-dependent, but not TRAM- and TRIF-dependent, lipopolysaccharide-induced TLR4 signaling. J Biol Chem. 2005;280(7):5491–5.
28. Naiki Y, Komatsu T, Koide N, Dagvadorj J, Yoshida T, Arditi M, et al. TGF-β1 inhibits the production of IFN in response to CpG DNA via ubiquitination of TNF receptor-associated factor (TRAF) 6. Innate Immun. 2015;21(7):770–7.
29. Kim BS, Chun SY, Lee EH, Chung JW, Lee JN, Ha YS, et al. Efficacy of combination therapy with pentosan polysulfate sodium and adipose tissue-derived stem cells for the management of interstitial cystitis in a rat model. Stem Cell Res. 2020;45:101801.
30. Ito Y, Kashiwabara M, Yoshida A, Hikiyama E, Onoue S, Yamada S. Muscarinic receptor binding in rat bladder urothelium and detrusor muscle by intravesical solifenacin. Biol Pharm Bull. 2016;39(7):1167–71.
31. Taidi Z, Mansfield KJ, Bates L, Sana-Ur-Rehman H, Liu L. Purinergic P2X7 receptors as therapeutic targets in interstitial cystitis/bladder pain syndrome; key role of ATP signaling in inflammation. Bladder (San Franc). 2019;6(1):e38.
32. Augé C, Gamé X, Vergnolle N, Lluel P, Chabot S. Characterization and validation of a chronic model of cyclophosphamide-induced interstitial cystitis/bladder pain syndrome in rats. Front Pharmacol. 2020;11:1305.
33. Kogan P, Xu S, Wang Y, O'Donnell MA, Lutgendorf SK, Bradley CS, et al. Sub-noxious intravesical lipopolysaccharide triggers bladder inflammation and symptom onset in a transgenic autoimmune cystitis model: a MAPP network animal study. Sci Rep. 2018;8(1):6573.

21

Development and validation of a prognostic nomogram for predicting overall survival in patients with primary bladder sarcoma: A SEER-based retrospective study

Shijie Li, Xuefeng Liu and Xiaonan Chen*

Abstract

Background: Primary bladder sarcoma (PBS) is a rare malignant tumor of the bladder with a poor prognosis, and its disease course is inadequately understood. Therefore, our study aimed to establish a prognostic model to determine individualized prognosis of patients with PBS.

Patients and Methods: Data of 866 patients with PBS, registered from 1973 to 2015, were extracted from the surveillance, epidemiology, and end result (SEER) database. The patients included were randomly split into a training (n = 608) and a validation set (n = 258). Univariate and multivariate Cox regression analyses were employed to identify the important independent prognostic factors. A nomogram was then established to predict overall survival (OS). Using calibration curves, receiver operating characteristic curves, concordance index (C-index), decision curve analysis (DCA), net reclassification improvement (NRI) and integrated discrimination improvement (IDI), the performance of the nomogram was internally validated. We compared the nomogram with the TNM staging system. The application of the risk stratification system was tested using Kaplan–Meier survival analysis.

Results: Age at diagnosis, T-stage, N-stage, M-stage, and tumor size were identified as independent predictors of OS. C-index of the training cohort were 0.675, 0.670, 0.671 for 1-, 3- and 5-year OS, respectively. And that in the validation cohort were 0.701, 0.684, 0.679, respectively. Calibration curves also showed great prediction accuracy. In comparison with TNM staging system, improved net benefits in DCA, evaluated NRI and IDI were obtained. The risk stratification system can significantly distinguish the patients with different survival risk.

Conclusion: A prognostic nomogram was developed and validated in the present study to predict the prognosis of the PBS patients. It may assist clinicians in evaluating the risk factors of patients and formulating an optimal individualized treatment strategy.

Keywords: Primary bladder sarcoma, Nomogram, Prognosis, Survival analysis

Introduction

Primary bladder sarcoma (PBS) is a very rare malignant tumor, accounting for less than 0.5% of all bladder tumors. The 5-year survival rate is 10–35% [1]. Some subtypes of PBS show a high tendency toward distant metastasis and are associated with a shorter survival [2]. Published studies on PBS are scarce all over the world,

*Correspondence: chenxn@cmu.edu.cn
Department of Urology, Shengjing Hospital of China Medical University, 36 Sanhao Street, Shenyang 110004, Liaoning, People's Republic of China

and most of the cases are reported in the form of case reports for a certain subtype of PBS [3–5].

In view of the scarcity of PBS, the natural history of this disease is not well known. Nevertheless, its relationship with schistosomiasis [6], cyclophosphamide therapy [7, 8], and radiotherapy [9] has been documented. Leiomyosarcoma is the most common type of bladder sarcoma in adults and it is reported that the incidence rate of bladder leiomyosarcoma may increase due to an increase in the number of patients undergoing chemo or radiotherapy [10].

Insufficient understanding makes the diagnosis and treatment of PBS challenging in daily practice. Due to the low incidence rate, the treatment of PBS is largely empirical. Radical cystectomy remains the mainstay of treatment for non-metastatic PBS, and bilateral pelvic lymph node dissection is recommended because of the high risk of metastasis to the pelvic lymph nodes [11]. Transurethral resection alone is generally not recommended, except for very small lesions [3]. Chemo and radiotherapy are viable treatment options as well, and are usually used in the comprehensive treatment of rhabdomyosarcoma or high-grade metastatic leiomyosarcoma [12, 13]. Radiotherapy is also chosen in case of positive surgical margins or suspicion of residual tumor [14].

For rare tumors such as PBS, single center studies often have poor predictive power due to the small number of patients. Therefore, using a population-based cancer database to assess the clinical characteristics and prognosis is a reasonable way to acquire better understanding of this rare disease. In this study, we used the Surveillance, Epidemiology, and End Results (SEER) database (https://seer.cancer.gov/) to identify the prognostic factors and construct a nomogram for PBS patients. To the best of our knowledge, this is the first study using the SEER database to examine the clinical features of PBS. This study aimed to establish a predictive model to better understand the survival outcomes of PBS at a population level.

Material and methods

Patients

Data of the patients diagnosed with bladder sarcoma were extracted based on the International Classification of Tumor Diseases Third Edition (ICD-O-3). Inclusion criteria were as follows: (1) age at diagnosis > 18 years old; (2) histologically diagnosed as the first malignant tumor; (3) availability of complete demographic and sociological information, follow-up date, duration of survival (in months), and cause of death; (4) histological diagnosis of bladder sarcoma (ICD-O-3 Code: C67.0–C67.9); (5) adequate data regarding the patients' clinical stage, pathological grade, and other variables. After screening, 866 eligible PBS patients were finally included in the cohort. The process of data selection was shown in Fig. 1. The patients were randomly divided into two sets (training set, n = 608 and validation set, n = 258). Since SEER is a

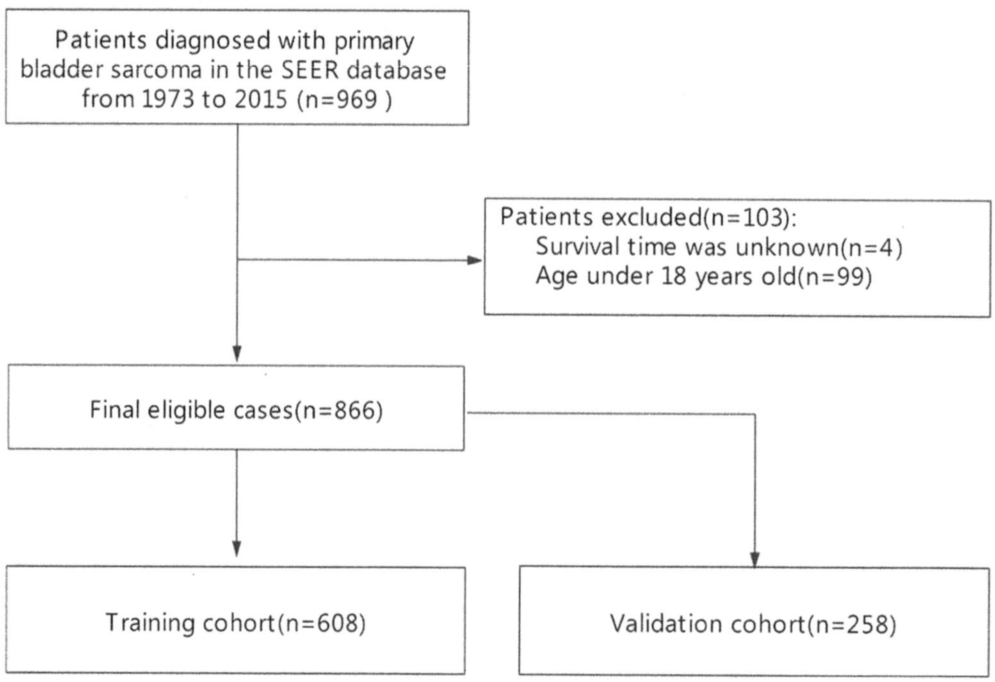

Fig. 1 Flowchart showing the selection of patients

publicly available database, studies using the SEER database do not require ethical board approval and patient consent.

Data collection

Variables in the present study included age, sex, race, marital status, histological grade, pathological classification, pathological stage (TNM stage according to the American Joint Committee on Cancer staging system, third and sixth edition), tumor size, type of intervention such as radiation, chemotherapy and/or surgery, vital status, and duration of survival. As is shown in Fig. 2B, C, tumor size was divided into three categories by X-tile software version 3.6.1 (Rimm Lab, Yale School of Medicine, New Haven, CT, USA), which is a useful tool for finding optimal cutoff points of continuous data [15]. Overall survival (OS) was the primary endpoint. Duration of survival was calculated from the date of diagnosis to the date of last follow-up or until the date of death.

Statistical analysis

Continuous variables were reported as median with range, and categorical variables as frequencies and proportions. The optimal cutoff values for age and tumor size were evaluated using the X-tile software. Univariate Cox regression analysis was performed to identify the significant prognostic factors. Afterwards, we incorporated them into the multivariable Cox proportional hazards regression models to further determine each variable's independent association with survival outcomes. A nomogram for predicting the 1-, 3- and 5-year OS was constructed using the factors which remained significant in the multivariate Cox regression model. The predictive accuracy and discriminative ability of the nomogram were determined by the receiver operating characteristics (ROC) curves, the area under the curve (AUC), and Harrell's concordance index (C-index). Calibration plots were generated to explore the performance characteristics of the nomogram at 1-, 3- and 5-year survival time. In addition, decision curve analysis (DCA), net reclassification improvement (NRI) and integrated discrimination improvement (IDI) were used to evaluate the clinical utility of the nomogram and to assess whether the model was more accurate than AJCC TNM staging system or not.

In addition, we calculated the total score of each patient based on the nomogram and constructed a risk stratification model accordingly, dividing the cohort into

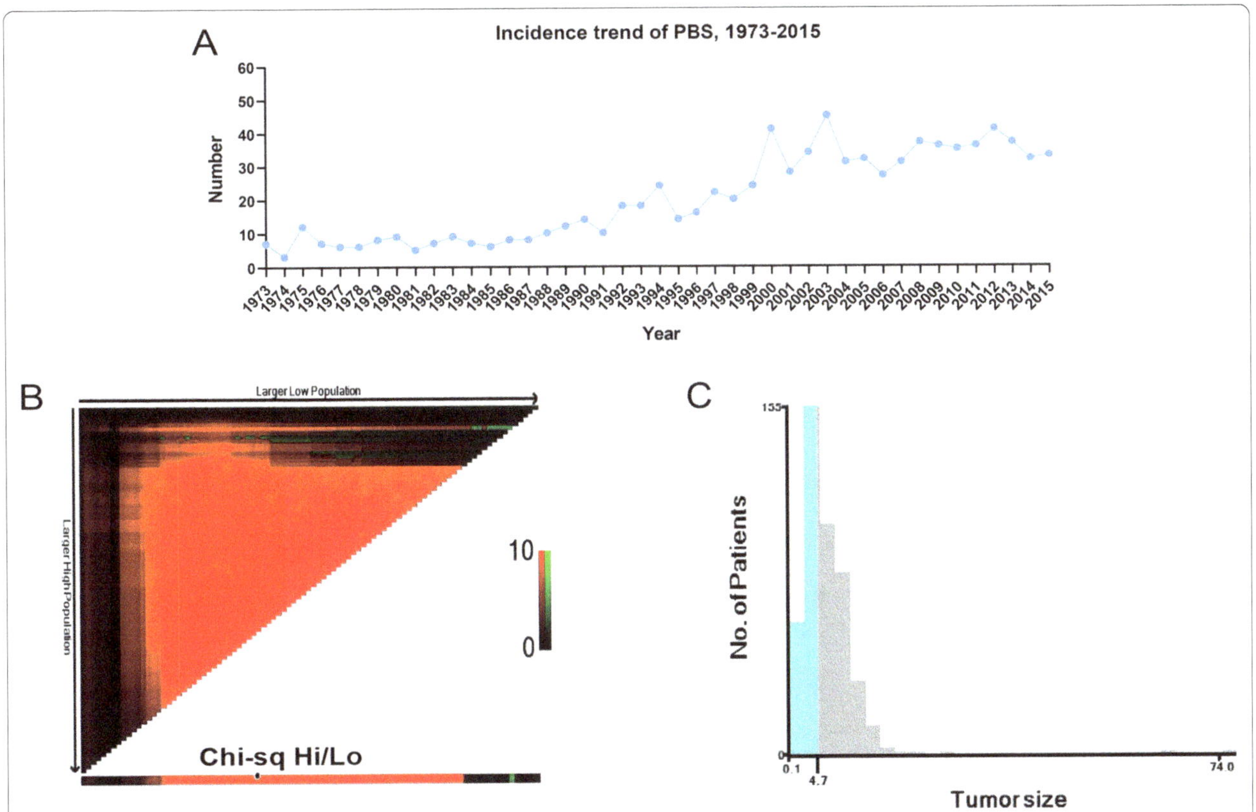

Fig. 2 (**A**) An increase in the incidence of primary bladder sarcoma over the years. (**B**) X-tile analysis to determine the best cutoff value for tumor size in the entire cohort (**C**) The distributions of the number of patients based on x-tile analysis. OS, overall survival

Table 1 Baseline demographic and clinical characteristics of patients with primary bladder sarcoma in the training cohort and validation cohort

Characteristics	Total cohort (n = 866)	Training cohort (n = 608)	Validation cohort (n = 258)	*P*-value
Total	866	608	258	
Age (IQR)	73.0 (60.2, 81.0)	73.0 (60.8, 81.0)	73.0 (60.2, 81.8)	0.963
Age, n (%)				0.517
18–29	27 (3.1)	21 (3.5)	6 (2.3)	
30–39	28 (3.2)	22 (3.6)	6 (2.3)	
40–49	56 (6.5)	33 (5.4)	23 (8.9)	
50–59	94 (10.9)	67 (11)	27 (10.5)	
60–69	156 (18.0)	109 (17.9)	47 (18.2)	
70–79	248 (28.6)	176 (28.9)	72 (27.9)	
≥ 80	257 (29.7)	180 (29.6)	77 (29.8)	
Sex, n (%)				1.000
Female	337 (38.9)	237 (39)	100 (38.8)	
Male	529 (61.1)	371 (61)	158 (61.2)	
Race, n (%)				0.189
White	743 (85.8)	530 (87.2)	213 (82.6)	
Black	90 (10.4)	58 (9.5)	32 (12.4)	
Other	33 (3.8)	20 (3.3)	13 (5)	
Marital status, n (%)				0.381
Married	484 (55.9)	342 (56.2)	142 (55)	
Single	353 (40.8)	249 (41)	104 (40.3)	
Unknown	29 (3.3)	17 (2.8)	12 (4.7)	
Pathological classification, n (%)			0.633	
Carcinosarcoma	408 (47.1)	296 (48.7)	112 (43.4)	
Leiomyosarcoma	207 (23.9)	141 (23.2)	66 (25.6)	
Sarcoma	84 (9.7)	59 (9.7)	25 (9.7)	
Spindle cell sarcoma	31 (3.6)	22 (3.6)	9 (3.5)	
Other	136 (15.7)	90 (14.8)	46 (17.8)	
Histological grade, n (%)				0.166
Well differentiated	22 (2.5)	16 (2.6)	6 (2.3)	
Moderately differentiated	38 (4.4)	29 (4.8)	9 (3.5)	
Poorly differentiated	202 (23.3)	151 (24.8)	51 (19.8)	
Undifferentiated	283 (32.7)	184 (30.3)	99 (38.4)	
Unknown	321 (37.1)	228 (37.5)	93 (36)	
T-stage, n (%)				0.124
Ta	68 (7.9)	55 (9)	13 (5)	
Tis	1 (0.1)	1 (0.2)	0 (0)	
T1	68 (7.9)	45 (7.4)	23 (8.9)	
T2	94 (10.9)	63 (10.4)	31 (12)	
T3	92 (10.6)	72 (11.8)	20 (7.8)	
T4	54 (6.2)	40 (6.6)	14 (5.4)	
Unknown	489 (56.5)	332 (54.6)	157 (60.9)	
N-stage, n (%)				0.286
No	476 (55.0)	329 (54.1)	147 (57)	
Yes	175 (20.2)	119 (19.6)	56 (21.7)	
Unknown	215 (24.8)	160 (26.3)	55 (21.3)	
M-stage, n (%)				0.326
No	593 (68.5)	407 (66.9)	186 (72.1)	
Yes	97 (11.2)	71 (11.7)	26 (10.1)	

Table 1 (continued)

Characteristics	Total cohort (n = 866)	Training cohort (n = 608)	Validation cohort (n = 258)	*P*-value
Unknown	176 (20.3)	130 (21.4)	46 (17.8)	
Tumor size, n (%)				0.622
<4.8	161 (18.6)	117 (19.2)	44 (17.1)	
≥4.8	291 (33.6)	199 (32.7)	92 (35.7)	
Unknown	414 (47.8)	292 (48)	122 (47.3)	
Surgical treatment, n (%)				0.023*
No	54 (6.2)	38 (6.2)	16 (6.2)	
Yes	537 (62.0)	360 (59.2)	177 (68.6)	
Unknown	275 (31.8)	210 (34.5)	65 (25.2)	
Radiation				0.360
No/Unknown, n (%)	754 (87.1)	534 (87.8)	220 (85.3)	
Yes	112 (12.9)	74 (12.2)	38 (14.7)	
Chemotherapy, n (%)				0.864
No/Unknown	734 (84.8)	514 (84.5)	220 (85.3)	
Yes	132 (15.2)	94 (15.5)	38 (14.7)	

**P* < 0.05 indicating statistical significance

two different risk groups (low-risk group and high-risk group). The optimal cutoff value was analyzed by X-tile software. Kaplan–Meier survival analysis and Chi-square test were used to assess the significance of the difference in survival between the low- and high-risk groups.

All the analyses were performed with the statistical software package R 4.0.2 (http://www.R-project.org, The R Foundation, Vienna, Austria). Two-sided *P* values of less than 0.05 were considered statistically significant. All procedures performed in this study involving human participants conformed to the ethical standards described in the 1964 Helsinki declaration and its subsequent amendments.

Results

Patients' baseline characteristics

Eight hundred and sixty-six patients with PBS in the SEER database met the study criteria and were included in this study. Figure 2A clearly showed an increase in the incidence of PBS over the years. Cohort demographics and tumor-related characteristics were described in Table 1. Most patients were male (529, 61.1%), white (743, 85.8%), and more than 80 years old (257, 29.7%). With regard to therapy, a majority of the patients underwent surgery (537, 62.0%), while fewer patients received radiation (112, 12.9%) or chemotherapy (132, 15.2%). Overall, the 1-, 3- and 5-year OS rates were 48.2%, 34.5% and 29.4%, respectively. Except for surgical treatment, there was no significant difference between the training and validation set ($P > 0.05$).

There were 709 events (deaths) in the cohort and the mean follow-up period was 42.1 months (median, 9.0 months; range 0–447 months).

Screening for prognostic factors of OS

We conducted a univariable and multivariable Cox proportional hazards regression analysis to demonstrate the association between selected characteristics and oncological outcomes. Univariable Cox regression analysis identified seven variables (age, pathological classification, T-stage, N-stage, M-stage, tumor size, and radiation) as factors associated with a shorter OS. Multivariable Cox regression analysis indicated that statistically significant risk factors associated with a shorter OS included age, T-stage, N-stage, M-stage, and tumor size (Table 2). For example, patients with a tumor of a higher T stage or distant metastases may have a poor prognosis and worse cancer outcomes. Similarly, patients with a large tumor (≥ 4.8 cm) were more likely to have poor prognosis. Median OS in the training cohort was 11 months, with 1-, 3- and 5-year survival rates of 51.3%, 36.2%, and 30.8%, respectively. Kaplan–Meier analysis intuitively showed the different survival outcomes stratified according to the variables listed in Table 1 (Fig. 3A–M). Log-rank test showed significant differences in OS among subgroups in terms of pathological classification, T-stage, N-stage, M-stage, tumor size and radiotherapy ($P < 0.05$).

Table 2 Univariate and multivariate Cox regression analysis of included variables for OS in training cohort

Characteristics	Univariate analysis		Multivariate analysis	
	HR (95% CI)	*P*-value	HR (95% CI)	*P*-value
Age				
18–29	Reference		Reference	
30–39	0.53 (0.27, 1.03)	0.06	0.48 (0.24, 0.96)	0.039*
40–49	0.56 (0.31, 1.03)	0.062	0.43 (0.23, 0.80)	0.008*
50–59	0.71 (0.41, 1.2)	0.202	0.74 (0.42, 1.27)	0.274
60–69	0.58 (0.35, 0.97)	0.039*	0.55 (0.32, 0.94)	0.030*
70–79	0.65 (0.4, 1.06)	0.081	0.62 (0.37, 1.03)	0.063
≥ 80	0.66 (0.4, 1.07)	0.094	0.61 (0.37, 1.03)	0.063
Sex				
Female	Reference			
Male	1.1 (0.92, 1.32)	0.308		
Race				
White	Reference			
Black	1.07 (0.79, 1.46)	0.657		
Other	1.11 (0.68, 1.8)	0.681		
Marital status				
Married	Reference			
Single	0.9 (0.75, 1.08)	0.275		
Unknown	1.07 (0.61, 1.87)	0.806		
Pathological classification				
Carcinosarcoma	Reference		Reference	
Leiomyosarcoma	0.99 (0.79, 1.25)	0.927	0.79 (0.61, 1.03)	0.086
Sarcoma	1.55 (1.16, 2.07)	0.003*	1.36 (0.99, 1.88)	0.060
Spindle cell sarcoma	1.14 (0.7, 1.84)	0.602	0.94 (0.56, 1.60)	0.829
Other	1.3 (1, 1.69)	0.051	1.10 (0.83, 1.46)	0.510
Histological grade				
Well differentiated	Reference			
Moderately differentiated	1.35 (0.71, 2.57)	0.355		
Poorly differentiated	1.19 (0.69, 2.07)	0.534		
Undifferentiated	1.28 (0.74, 2.21)	0.381		
Unknown	1.25 (0.72, 2.15)	0.426		
T-stage				
Ta	Reference		Reference	
Tis	15.53 (2.11, 114.23)	0.007*	40.68 (5.17, 319.99)	< 0.001*
T1	2.08 (1.35, 3.21)	< 0.001*	2.20 (1.29, 3.75)	0.004*
T2	2.18 (1.48, 3.22)	< 0.001*	2.07 (1.33, 3.23)	0.001*
T3	1.0051 (0.65, 1.57)	0.982	1.15 (0.68, 1.96)	0.595
T4	1.02 (0.64, 1.62)	0.926	1.17 (0.67, 2.06)	0.574
Unknown	1.86 (1.36, 2.56)	< 0.001*	2.17 (1.45, 3.25)	< 0.001*
N-stage				
No	Reference		Reference	
Yes	0.62 (0.48, 0.8)	< 0.001*	0.74 (0.56, 0.97)	0.028*
Unknown	0.83 (0.68, 1.02)	0.084	1.03 (0.71, 1.50)	0.869
M-stage				
No	Reference		Reference	
Yes	2.7 (2.05, 3.55)	< 0.001*	2.74 (2.00, 3.75)	< 0.001*
Unknown	0.87 (0.69, 1.08)	0.205	0.85 (0.62, 1.19)	0.360

Table 2 (continued)

Characteristics	Univariate analysis		Multivariate analysis	
	HR (95% CI)	*P*-value	HR (95% CI)	*P*-value
Tumor size				
<4.8	Reference		Reference	
≥4.8	2 (1.51, 2.63)	<0.001*	2.02 (1.52, 2.69)	<0.001*
Unknown	1.86 (1.44, 2.41)	<0.001*	2.11 (1.59, 2.81)	<0.001*
Surgical treatment				
No	Reference			
Yes	0.84 (0.57, 1.23)	0.364		
Unknown	0.84 (0.56, 1.25)	0.396		
Radiation				
No/Unknown	Reference			
Yes	1.39 (1.06, 1.81)	0.017*	1.26 (0.94, 1.70)	0.118
Chemotherapy				
No/Unknown	Reference			
Yes	0.97 (0.75, 1.26)	0.842		

*$P<0.05$ indicating statistical significance

Prognostic nomogram construction for OS

A nomogram was established based on the aforementioned significant prognostic factors for 1-, 3- and 5-year OS (Fig. 4), and then was validated internally. Each variable was given a score based on the hazard ratio. The total scores for each variable were added up and placed on the total subscale to obtain the probabilities of 1-, 3- and 5-year OS. As shown in Additional file 1: Figure S1, using the nomogram, it could be concluded that a 70-year-old patient with T2N0M0 and a tumor size of 5 cm would score 47.5 points, which means that the patient has about 57.5%, 42%, and 34.5% survival probability 1, 3, and 5 years after the diagnosis, respectively.

Calibration and validation of the nomogram

On the training cohort, the C-index of the nomogram for 1-, 3- and 5-year OS prediction were 0.675 [95% confidence interval (CI): 0.648–0.702], 0.670 (95% CI: 0.642–0.697) and 0.671 (95% CI: 0.643–0.698), respectively. On the validation cohort, the C-indexes at 1-, 3-, and 5-year were 0.701 (95% CI 0.674–0.728), 0.684 (95% CI 0.657–0.711), and 0.679 (95% CI 0.651–0.706), respectively. The data indicated brilliant discrimination ability of the nomogram.

Meanwhile, the calibration plots of the training cohort for 1-, 3- and 5-year OS displayed consistency between the observed and predicted results (Fig. 5A–C). Similarly, the calibration plots of the 1-, 3- and 5-year OS were well calibrated in the validation cohort (Fig. 5D–F).

Comparison of the nomogram and AJCC TNM staging system

ROC curves analysis showed that the AUCs of the nomogram for 1-, 3- and 5-year OS were better than those of TNM stage both in the training (Fig. 6A–C) and validation cohort (Fig. 6D–F).

DCA analysis showed that compared with the AJCC TNM staging system, the net benefit of the new nomogram is significantly increased and has a wide range of threshold probabilities both in the training (Fig. 7A–C) and validation cohort (Fig. 7D–F). This indicated that the nomogram can be more beneficial in the clinical application of predicting individual survival outcomes than TNM staging system.

In the NRI and IDI analyses, the nomogram performed better than TNM staging system (Table 3). In the training cohort, the 1-, 3- and 5-year NRI of the nomogram compared to TNM staging system was 15.3% ($p<0.01$), 21.0% ($p<0.01$) and 21.2% ($p<0.01$), respectively. And the 1-, 3- and 5-year IDI of the nomogram compared to TNM staging system was 3.3% ($p<0.01$), 4.6% ($p<0.01$) and 4.4% ($p<0.01$), respectively. In the validation cohort, the 1-, 3- and 5-year NRI of the nomogram compared to TNM staging system was 19.8% ($p<0.01$), 16.5% ($p=0.02$) and 17.9% ($p=0.01$), respectively. And the 1-, 3- and 5-year IDI of the nomogram compared to TNM staging system was 7.9% ($p<0.01$), 7.9% ($p<0.01$) and 8.6% ($p<0.01$), respectively.

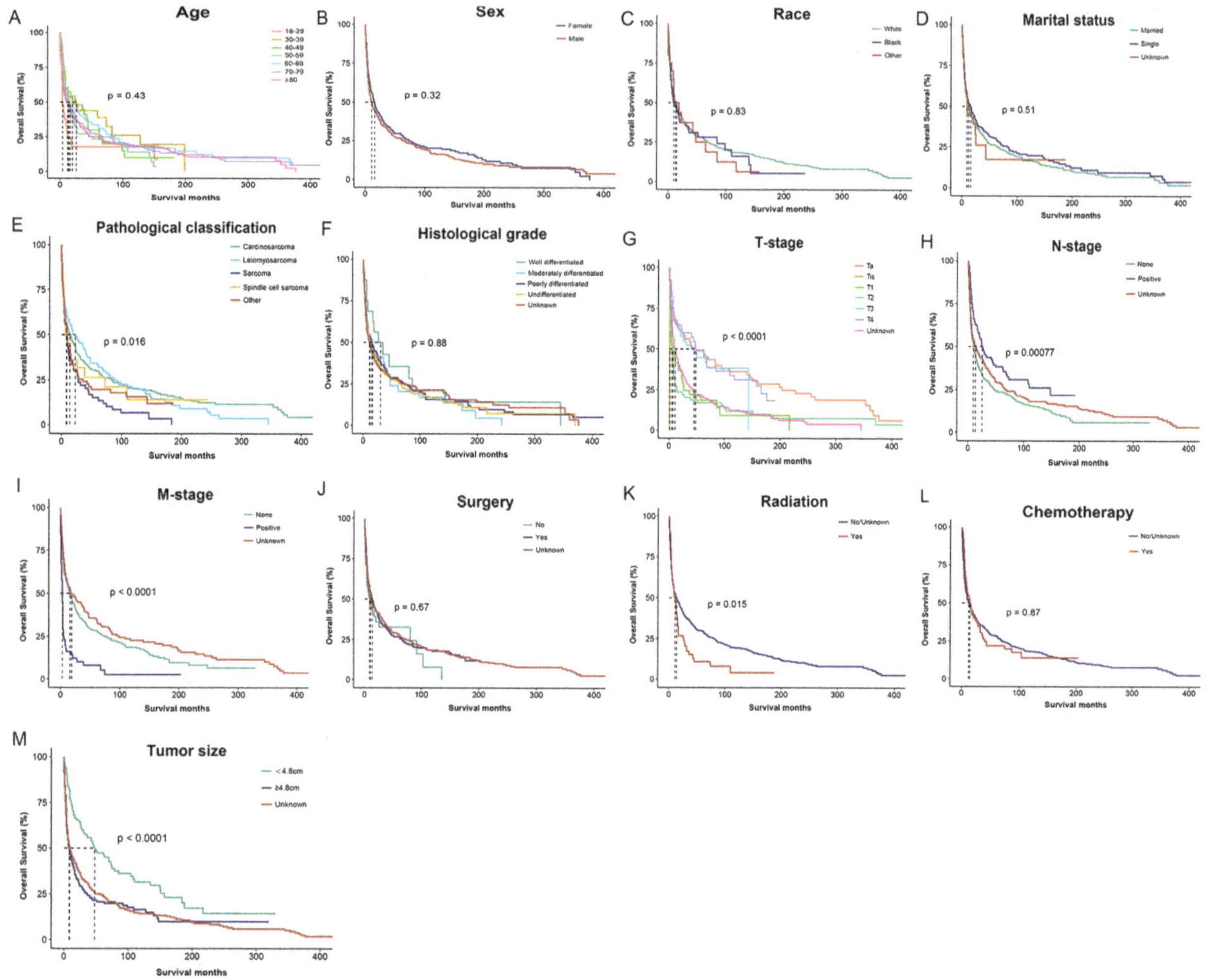

Fig. 3 Kaplan–Meier curves of overall survival in patients with primary bladder sarcoma stratified by age (**A**), sex (**B**), race (**C**), marital status (**D**), pathological classification (**E**), histological grade (**F**), T-stage (**G**), N-stage (**H**), M-stage (**I**), tumor size (**J**), surgical treatment (**K**), radiation (**L**), and chemotherapy (**M**)

Ability of nomogram to stratify patient risk

The cut-off point between the high-risk and low-risk cohorts was determined as 47 by X-tile analysis, and the 608 patients in the training cohort were divided into a high-risk group (total score > 47) and a low-risk group (total score ≤ 47) based on this cut-off value. By Kaplan–Meier analysis (Fig. 8A), 367 high-risk patients had significantly more severe OS than 241 low-risk patients ($p < 0.0001$). Application of this cutoff value also significantly distinguished the high-risk and low-risk groups in the validation cohort ($p = 0.041$) (Fig. 8B).

Discussion

Around 430,000 new cases of bladder cancer are diagnosed worldwide each year, and this cancer is associated with high morbidity and mortality [16]. As a rare subtype of bladder cancer, the incidence rate of PBS is very low, due to which tumor progression is not well-understood. The clinical significance and biologic behavior of this subtype of bladder cancer warrant additional investigation. In the present study, vast amount of data collected by the SEER program was utilized to examine the largest series of PBS cases reported to date. This study was the first attempt to date to use the SEER database to build a predictive model for better understanding the survival outcomes of PBS at a population level.

Several unique features of PBS distinguish it from urothelial bladder cancer, and are worth mentioning. PBS has multiple types, and leiomyosarcoma and rhabdomyosarcoma account for 50% and 20% of PBS cases, respectively [17]. Other histological types of PBS include osteosarcoma, angiosarcoma, myxoid liposarcoma, fibrosarcoma, malignant fibroblastic tumor, carcinosarcoma, and plexiform sarcoma [18]. Besides, previous studies

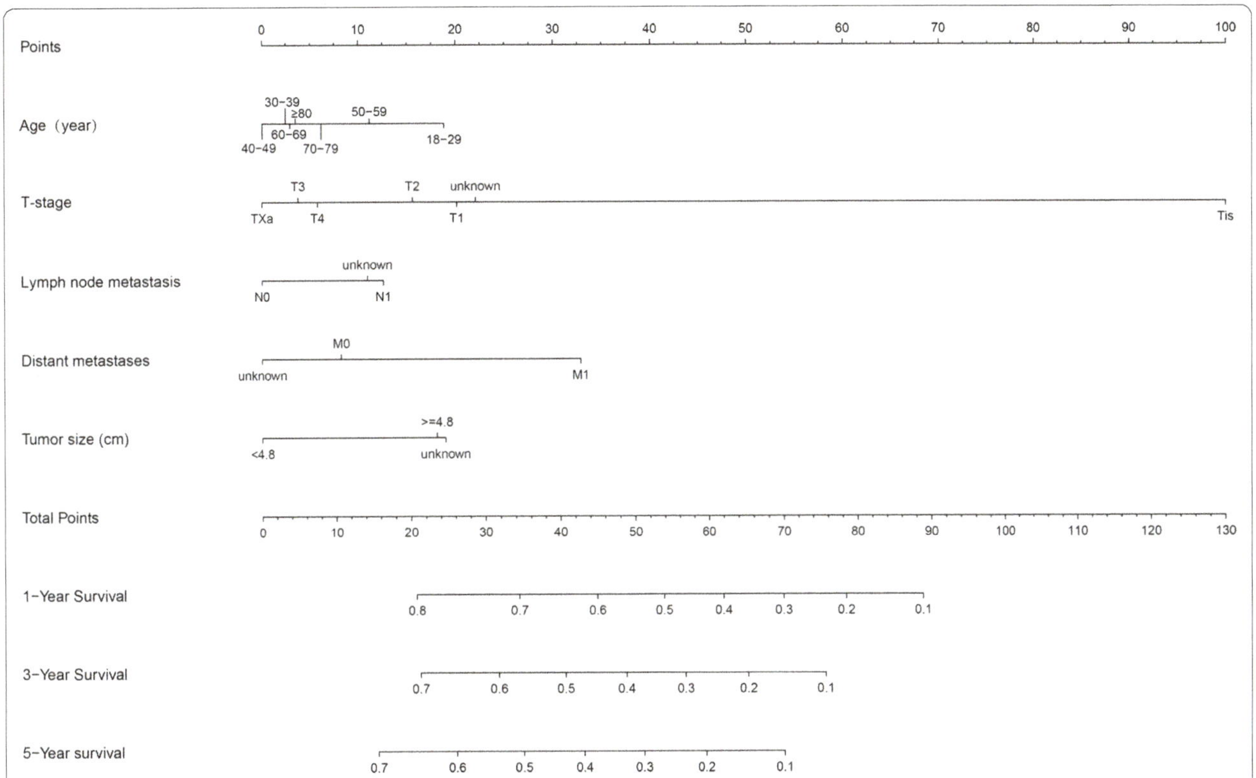

Fig. 4 Nomogram model constructed using the independent prognostic factors predicting the 1-, 3- and 5-year OS for patients with PBS. OS, overall survival; PBS, primary bladder sarcoma

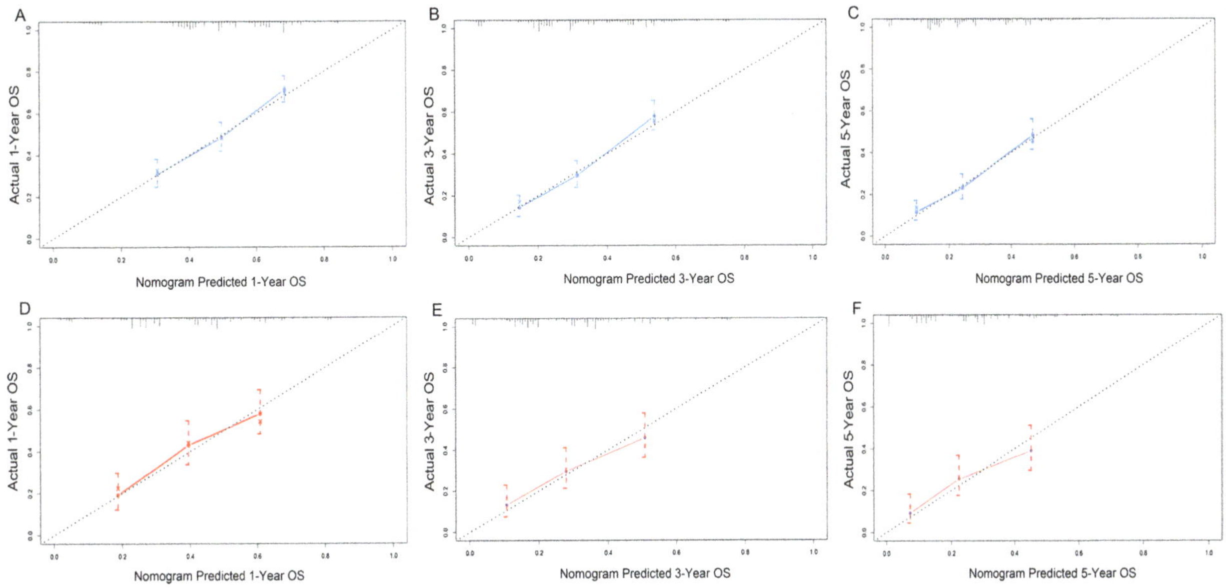

Fig. 5 Calibration plots for the nomogram. Calibration plots of 1-year (**A**), 3-year (**B**), and 5-year (**C**) OS in the training cohort; Calibration plots of 1-year (**D**), 3-year (**E**), and 5-year (**F**) OS in the validation cohort. OS, overall survival

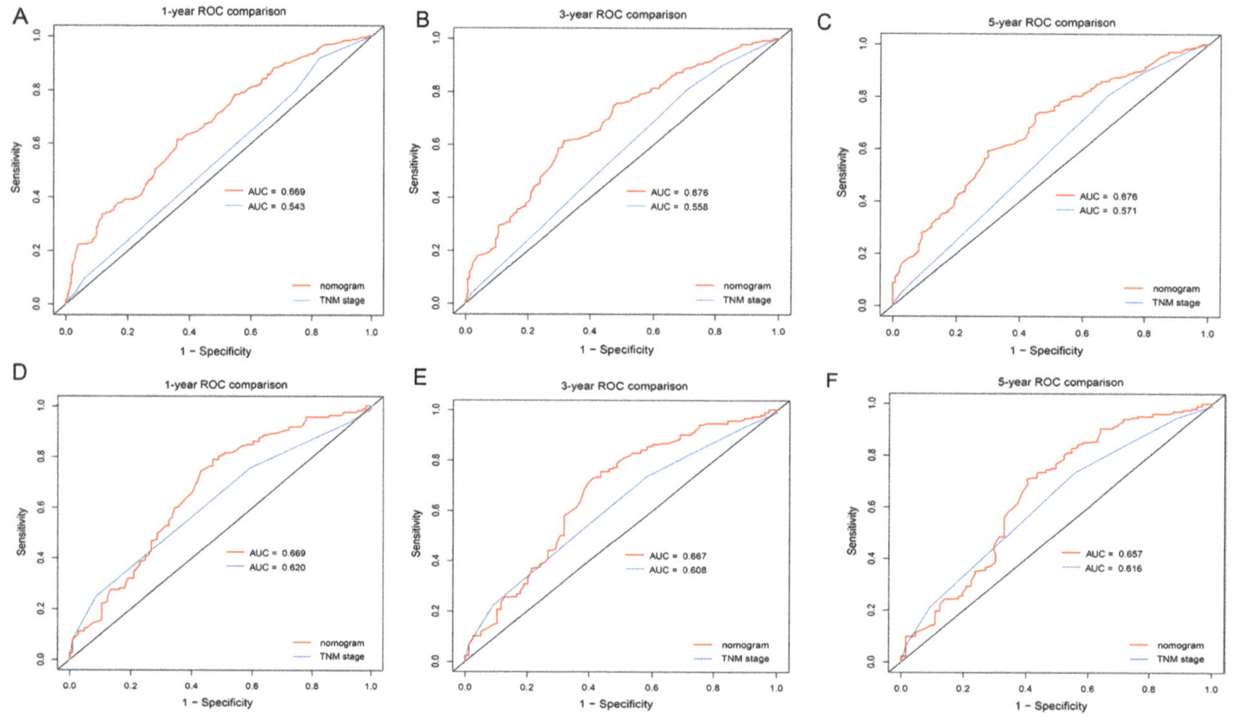

Fig. 6 ROC curves of the nomogram for OS compared with TNM staging. ROC curves comparation of the nomogram and TNM staging for 1-year (**A**), 3-year (**B**) and 5-year (**C**) OS in the training cohort. ROC curves comparation of the nomogram and TNM staging for 1-year (**D**), 3-year (**E**) and 5-year (**F**) OS in the validation cohort. AUC: area under the curve; ROC, receiver operating characteristic; OS, overall survival

have emphasized the poor prognosis of PBS. Rosser et al. [19] reported one of the largest series of 36 adult PBS patients treated between 1986 and 1998. The 5-year disease-specific survival rate was 62.0%. In another systematic review and meta-analysis that included by far the largest number of cases containing 210 patients with PBS between 1970 and 2018, Zieschang et al. [20] determined a 5-year cancer-specific cumulative mortality rate of 38% for patients with PBS. We found that the prognosis of PBS was poor and did not change significantly over decades. In addition, previous studies have shown that the vast majority of PBS patients are elderly men with significant pain. However, hematuria is rare, which is very different from the presentation of urothelial tumors [21, 22]. The treatment of this rare tumor was challenging. The most promising treatment options still seemed to be radical cystectomy over the past few decades, possibly supplemented by chemotherapy or radiotherapy. However, as time migrated and technology developed, partial cystectomy was one of the surgical options available for smaller tumors.

To date, there are no large, prospective, randomized controlled trials on PBS treatment strategies worldwide. Therefore, it is unknown whether the survival rate of the patients depends upon the type of treatment modality. Due to the specificity of PBS, there is no specially designed or widely accepted grading system or prediction model. However, early identification of the disease and effective treatment can significantly improve the prognosis. Hence, efforts to establish predictive models to promote the management of these patients according to their individualized prognosis are justified. In our study, we established and validated a novel predictive tool based on age, tumor stage, lymph node status, distant metastasis, and tumor size that can be used to guide clinical practice.

In recent years, nomograms, developed using the SEER database, have been widely used to predict the prognosis of various malignancies, such as Ewing sarcoma, penile carcinoma, and cardiac sarcoma [23–25]. Our current study was the first to construct a well-validated nomogram including several clinical features and risk scores for patients with PBS, which can predict the clinical prognosis of PBS intuitively and effectively. The variables in the nomogram were independent factors affecting OS, which led to a better prediction of the survival of patients with

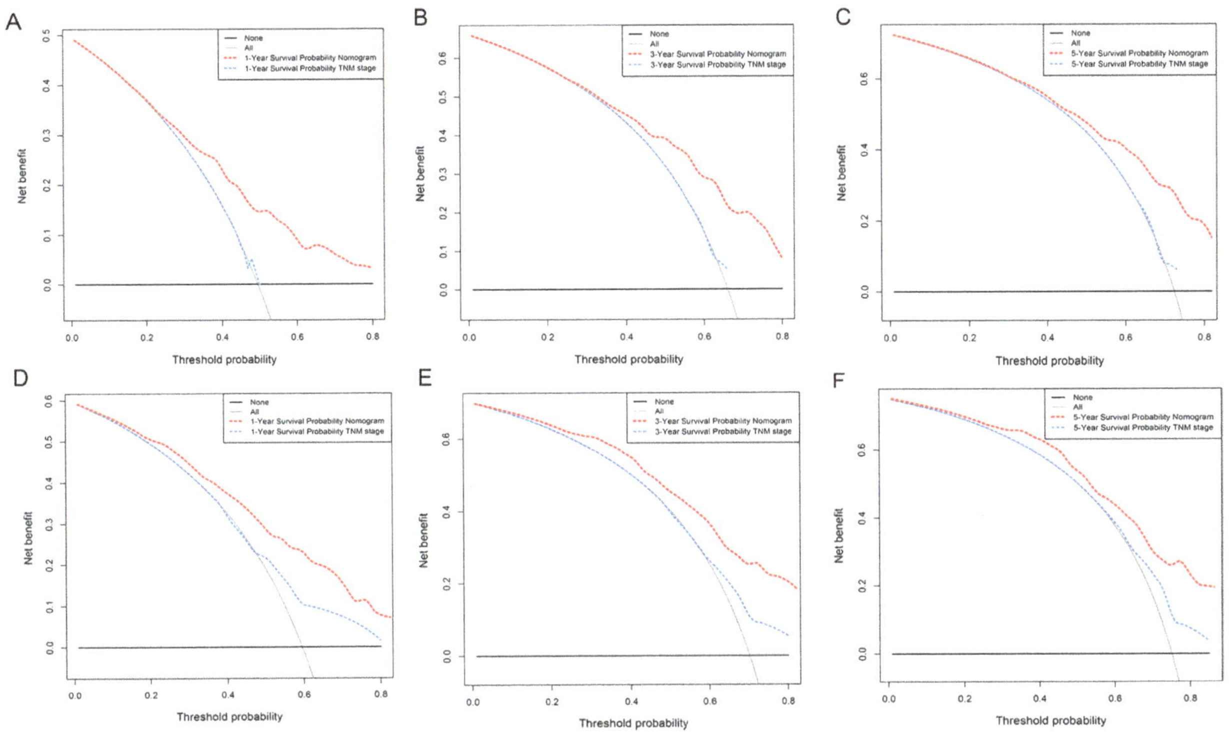

Fig. 7 DCA of the nomogram and AJCC TNM staging for 1-year (**A**), 3-year (**B**) and 5-year (**C**) OS in training cohort, and for 1-year (**D**), 3-year (**E**) and 5-year (**F**) OS in the validation cohort. The red dashed line represents the nomogram. The blue dashed line represents AJCC TNM stage. OS, overall survival; DCA, decision curve analyses; AJCC, American Joint Committee on Cancer

Table 3 NRI and IDI of the nomogram in survival prediction for PBS patients compared with TNM staging

Index	Training cohort			Validation cohort		
	Estimate	95% CI	*P*-value	Estimate	95% CI	*P*-value
NRI (vs. TNM staging)						
For 1-year OS	0.153	0.048–0.238	< 0.01*	0.198	0.072–0.367	< 0.01*
For 3-year OS	0.210	0.084–0.297	< 0.01*	0.165	0.026–0.343	0.02*
For 5-year OS	0.212	0.084–0.304	< 0.01*	0.179	0.029–0.362	0.01*
IDI (vs. TNM staging)						
For 1-year OS	0.033	0.015–0.058	< 0.01*	0.079	0.037–0.149	< 0.01*
For 3-year OS	0.046	0.019–0.081	< 0.01*	0.079	0.033–0.151	< 0.01*
For 5-year OS	0.044	0.017–0.081	< 0.01*	0.086	0.032–0.169	< 0.01*

NRI, net reclassification improvement; IDI, integrated discrimination improvement; PBS, primary bladder sarcoma; OS, overall survival

*$P < 0.05$ indicating statistical significance

PBS. Using this nomogram, we will be able to predict the future survival rate of the patients more accurately. Although the C-indexes and AUCs of the nomogram in the training and validation cohort were not high enough, the predictive ability of the model was more accurate than using the current TNM staging to predict the prognosis. Further DCA, NRI and IDI analyses demonstrated its clear clinical application advantages over the TNM staging system. A risk stratification model based on this nomogram can effectively classify patients in the training or validation cohort into two risk groups (high risk and low risk) and OS can be distinguished. The results of this study could be particularly helpful in predicting postoperative survival of the PBS patients.

Our nomogram is innovative and reasonable in the following aspects: firstly, to the best of our knowledge,

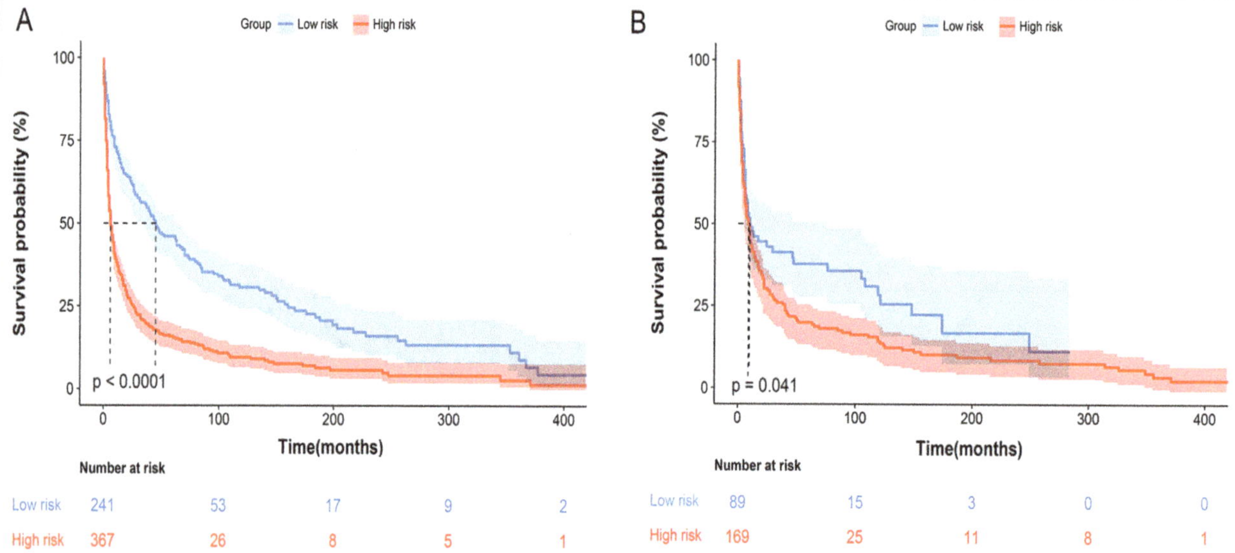

Fig. 8 Kaplan–Meier survival analyses to test the risk stratification system within the training (**A**) and the validation cohort (**B**). The blue line represents low-risk group, and the red line represents high-risk group

this study is the first to attempt to develop a prognostic nomogram for OS of the PBS patients using population-based data, which can provide individualized treatment guidance. Secondly, variables like age, T/N/M stage, and tumor size were used to develop this nomogram. It is worth noting that in order to maintain the integrity of the data, factors containing negative or unknown information were also included in the analysis. Taking tumor size as an example, 414 cases (47.8%) had unknown tumor size. In addition, according to the multivariate Cox regression analysis and nomogram, unknown tumor size seemed to reduce the survival rate, which may be due to the heterogeneity of these tumors. However, we could not exclude this group of patients from the study; otherwise, potential selection bias could have been introduced. On the contrary, using continuous queues and complete information can guarantee more accurate results. Finally, the nomogram based on the SEER database was able to predict the prognosis of PBS. ROC curve, DCA, NRI and IDI analyses of this study showed that the nomogram could predict the death of patients with PBS more accurately, which has clinical applicability. The results of the internal validation of nomogram prediction were found to be consistent.

There are some limitations in our research. Firstly, this is a population-based retrospective analysis using the SEER database, which does not include certain important variables, such as preoperative laboratory results and socio-economic status, which are also reported related to the prognosis of patients with bladder malignant tumor [26]. Secondly, although the selection bias is avoided to some extent, a large amount of information is missing in the SEER database, which may have affected the prediction model. Thirdly, this study only considered OS as the primary endpoint and did not include disease-specific survival, which may partly limit the broad application of the results. Fourthly, there are no data available for external validation and due to the nature of retrospective studies; the nomogram needs to be validated for a prospective cohort.

Conclusion

In this study, we developed and validated a nomogram to predict the OS rate of patients with PBS, and it showed consistent reliability and clinical applicability. The nomogram can assist clinicians in evaluating the risk factors for poor prognosis in patients with PBS and formulating optimal individualized treatment strategies. However, further evaluation in other patient groups is needed to establish the external validity of our findings.

Abbreviations

OS: Overall survival; PBS: Primary bladder sarcoma; CI: Confidence interval; SEER: Surveillance, Epidemiology, and End Results; DCA: Decision curve analysis; ROC: Receiver operating characteristics; AUC: The area under the curve; C-index: Concordance index; AJCC: American Joint Committee on Cancer; NRI: Net reclassification improvement; IDI: Integrated discrimination improvement.

Supplementary Information

Additional file 1: Figure S1. Nomogram is used to evaluate a 70-year-old patient with T2N0M0 and a tumor size of 5 cm. Based on the total score, the survival probability 1-year, 3-year, and 5-year of the patient is 57.5%, 42%, and 34.5%, respectively.

Acknowledgements

We thank Jie Liu, PhD (Department of Vascular and Endovascular Surgery, Chinese PLA General Hospital) for his helpful review and comments regarding the manuscript. We would like to thank Editage for English language editing.

Authors' contributions

XC and SL conceived and designed the study, SL contributed to the data collection and analyses of the data. SL drafted and revised the manuscript. SL and XL prepared figures and tables, XL and XC edited the manuscript. All authors read and approved the final manuscript.

References

1. Robinson SP, Farooq A, Laniado M, Motiwala H. The demographic features, clinical outcomes, prognosis and treatment options for patients with sarcomatoid carcinoma of the urinary bladder: a single centre experience. Int Braz J Urol. 2018;44(1):45–52.
2. Guo CC, Majewski T, Zhang L, Yao H, Bondaruk J, Wang Y, et al. Dysregulation of EMT drives the progression to clinically aggressive sarcomatoid bladder cancer. Cell Rep. 2019;27(6):1781–93.
3. Kadouri Y, Ouskri S, El Sayegh H, Benslimane L, Nouini Y. Sarcomatoid carcinoma of the urinary bladder: analysis of five cases and literature review. Pan Afr Med J. 2020;36:369.
4. Dali KM, Kacem A, Ben Rhouma S, Chaker K, Sellami A, Nouira Y. Carcinosarcoma of the urinary bladder with cartilaginous differentiation: about a case report. Urol Case Rep. 2020;28:101053.
5. Ribeiro JGA. Giant leiomyosarcoma of the urinary bladder. J Clin Diagn Res. 2016;10(5):PD14.
6. Alwan MH, Sayed M, Kamal MM. Schistosomiasis and sarcoma of the urinary bladder. Eur Urol. 1988;15(1–2):139.
7. Hendry WF, Parslow JM, Stedronska J. Exploratory scrototomy in 168 azoospermic males. Br J Urol. 1983;55(6):785–91.
8. Mills SE, Fechner RE, Cantrell RW. Aggressive sinonasal lesion resembling normal intestinal mucosa. Am J Surg Pathol. 1982;6(8):803–9.
9. Navon JD, Rahimzadeh M, Wong AK, Carpenter PM, Ahlering TE. Angiosarcoma of the bladder after therapeutic irradiation for prostate cancer. J Urol. 1997;157(4):1359–60.
10. Helpap B. Nonepithelial neoplasms of the urinary bladder. Virchows Arch. 2001;439(4):497–503.
11. Zieschang H, Koch R, Wirth MP, Froehner M. Leiomyosarcoma of the urinary bladder in adult patients: a systematic review of the literature and meta-analysis. Urol Int. 2019;102(1):96–101.
12. Malla M, Wang JF, Trepeta R, Feng A, Wang J. Sarcomatoid carcinoma of the urinary bladder. Clin Genitourin Cancer. 2016;14(5):366–72.
13. Taylor RE, Busuttil A. Case report: adult rhabdomyosarcoma of bladder, complete response to radiation therapy. J Urol. 1989;142(5):1321.
14. Ahlering TE, Weintraub P, Skinner DG. Management of adult sarcomas of the bladder and prostate. J Urol. 1988;140(6):1397–9.
15. Camp RL, Dolled-Filhart M, Rimm DL. X-tile: a new bio-informatics tool for biomarker assessment and outcome-based cut-point optimization. Clin Cancer Res. 2004;10(21):7252–9.
16. Bray F, Ferlay J, Soerjomataram I, Siegel RL, Torre LA, Jemal A. Global cancer statistics 2018: GLOBOCAN estimates of incidence and mortality worldwide for 36 cancers in 185 countries. CA Cancer J Clin. 2018;68(6):394–424.
17. Alvarez ZR. Bladder sarcoma. Arch Esp Urol. 1947;3(3):217–26.
18. Parekh DJ, Jung C, O'Conner J, Dutta S, Smith ER. Leiomyosarcoma in urinary bladder after cyclophosphamide therapy for retinoblastoma and review of bladder sarcomas. Urology (Ridgewood, NJ). 2002;60(1):164.
19. Rosser CJ, Slaton JW, Izawa JI, Levy LB, Dinney C. Clinical presentation and outcome of high-grade urinary bladder leiomyosarcoma in adults. Urology. 2003;61(6):1151–5.
20. Zieschang H, Koch R, Wirth MP, Froehner M. Leiomyosarcoma of the urinary bladder in adult patients: a systematic review of the literature and meta-analysis. Urol Int. 2018;102(1):96–101.
21. Ro JY, El-Naggar AK, Amin MB, Sahin AA, Ordonez NG, Ayala AG. Pseudosarcomatous fibromyxoid tumor of the urinary bladder and prostate: immunohistochemical, ultrastructural, and DNA flow cytometric analyses of nine cases. Hum Pathol. 1993;24(11):1203–10.
22. Lee TK, Miyamoto H, Osunkoya AO, Guo CC, Weiss SW, Epstein JI. Smooth muscle neoplasms of the urinary bladder: a clinicopathologic study of 51 cases. Am J Surg Pathol. 2010;34(4):502–9.
23. Zhou Z, Wang J, Fang L, Ma J, Guo M. A nomogram for predicting overall survival in patients with E. BMC Musculoskel Dis. 2020;21(1):1–8.
24. Zheng W, Li K, Zhu W, Ding Y, Wu Q, Tang Q, et al. Nomogram prediction of overall survival based on log odds of positive lymph nodes for patients with penile squamous cell carcinoma. Cancer Med-US. 2020;9(15):5425–35.
25. Yin K, Luo R, Wei Y, Wang F, Zhang Y, Karlson KJ, et al. Survival outcomes in patients with primary card. J Thorac Cardiovasc Surg. 2020;162(1):107–15.
26. Weiner AB, Keeter M, Manjunath A, Meeks JJ. Discrepancies in staging, treatment, and delays to treatment may explain disparities in bladder cancer outcomes: an update from the National Cancer Data Base (2004–2013). Urol Oncol: Semin Orig Investig. 2018;36(5):237–9.

22

Integrated mRNA-miRNA transcriptome analysis of bladder biopsies from patients with bladder pain syndrome identifies signaling alterations contributing to the disease pathogenesis

Ali Hashemi Gheinani[1,2,3,4], Akshay Akshay[1], Mustafa Besic[1], Annette Kuhn[5], Irene Keller[6], Rémy Bruggmann[6], Hubert Rehrauer[7], Rosalyn M. Adam[2,3,4], Fiona C. Burkhard[8] and Katia Monastyrskaya[1*]

Abstract

Background: Interstitial cystitis, or bladder pain syndrome (IC/BPS), is a chronic bladder disorder characterized by lower abdominal pain associated with the urinary bladder and accompanied by urinary frequency and urgency in the absence of identifiable causes. IC/PBS can be separated into the classic Hunner's ulcerative type and the more prevalent non-ulcerative disease. Our aim was to unravel the biological processes and dysregulated cell signaling pathways leading to the bladder remodeling in non-ulcerative bladder pain syndrome (BPS) by studying the gene expression changes in the patients' biopsies.

Methods: We performed paired microRNA (miRNA) and mRNA expression profiling in the bladder biopsies of BPS patients with non-Hunner interstitial cystitis phenotype, using comprehensive Next-generation sequencing (NGS) and studied the activated pathways and altered biological processes based on the global gene expression changes. Paired mRNA-miRNA transcriptome analysis delineated the regulatory role of the dysregulated miRNAs by identifying their targets in the disease-induced pathways.

Results: EIF2 Signaling and Regulation of eIF4 and p70S6K Signaling, activated in response to cellular stress, were among the most significantly regulated processes during BPS. Leukotriene Biosynthesis nociceptive pathway, important in inflammatory diseases and neuropathic pain, was also significantly activated. The biological processes identified using Gene Ontology over-representation analysis were clustered into six main functional groups: cell cycle regulation, chemotaxis of immune cells, muscle development, muscle contraction, remodeling of extracellular matrix and peripheral nervous system organization and development. Compared to the Hunner's ulcerative type IC, activation of the immune pathways was modest in non-ulcerative BPS, limited to neutrophil chemotaxis and IFN-γ-mediated signaling. We identified 62 miRNAs, regulated and abundant in BPS and show that they target the mRNAs implicated in eIF2 signalling pathway.

*Correspondence: katia.monastyrskaia@dbmr.unibe.ch
[1] Functional Urology Research Group, Department for BioMedical Research DBMR, University of Bern, Bern, Switzerland
Full list of author information is available at the end of the article

Conclusions: The bladders of non-ulcerative BPS patients recruited in this study had alterations consistent with a strong cell proliferative response and an up-regulation of smooth muscle contractility, while the contribution of inflammatory processes was modest. Pathway analysis of the integrated mRNA-miRNA NGS dataset pinpointed important regulatory miRNAs whose dysregulation might contribute to the pathogenesis. Observed molecular changes in the peripheral nervous system organization and development indicate the potential role of local bladder innervation in the pain perceived in this type of BPS.

Keywords: Bladder, Pain, Cystitis, Gene, miRNA, Signaling pathway, Next-generation sequencing

Background

Interstitial cystitis, or bladder pain syndrome (IC/BPS), is a chronic bladder disorder characterized by lower abdominal pain associated with the urinary bladder and accompanied by day-time and/or night-time urinary frequency and urinary urgency, in the absence of identifiable causes such as bacterial infection [1]. BPS affects people of different age groups with a higher prevalence in women (45 cases per 100,000) compared to men (8 cases per 100,000) [2]. An estimated 2.70% to 6.53% (or 3.3 to 7.9 million) of US women 18 years old or older reported BPS/IC symptoms [3]. IC/PBS can be separated into two subtypes: classic Hunner's ulcerative type, characterized by Hunner's ulcers or haemorrhages in the bladder and the more prevalent non-ulcerative disease [4]. The aetiology of BPS is unknown, and its treatment is largely empiric. The main cause of IC/PBS is thought to be a persistent bladder inflammation, possibly brought about by the deficiency of the glycosaminoglycan covering the urothelium surface that results in leaky urothelium and subsequent activation of afferent nerves and neurogenic inflammation. Growing evidence suggests that there is a morphological and functional distinction between IC/BPS with Hunner lesions and IC/BPS without Hunner lesions: IC/BPS with Hunner lesions is an inflammatory disorder characterized by B cell abnormalities and epithelial denudation, while IC/BPS without Hunner lesions shows minimal histological changes [5].

Studying gene expression changes in disease might shed light on the underlying biological processes and help developing specific therapies. Previously, investigating the expression levels of genes implicated in epithelial permeability, bladder contractility, and inflammation, and the associated regulatory microRNAs in BPS patients' bladder biopsies, we showed a significant down-regulation of tight junction proteins zona occludens-1, junctional adherins molecule-1, and occludin, indicative of increased urothelial permeability, and concomitant up-regulation of bradykinin B(1) receptor, cannabinoid receptor CB1 and muscarinic receptors M3-M5, pointing to the inflammation-driven smooth muscle contractility activation []. BPS induced an up-regulation of acid-sensing ion channel 2a and 3 mRNA in the bladder [6], while causing a decrease in the levels of anti-inflammatory annexin A1 in the urothelium [7].

Recent advances in Next-Generation Sequencing (NGS) allow comprehensive characterization of the gene expression profiles in different disease states, with subsequent pathway analysis revealing the involved pathogenetic mechanisms. To date, several transcriptome studies were carried out in human IC/BPS patients using gene expression microarrays in biopsies [8] and urine sediment [9]; QPCR panels of 96 inflammatory mediators [10], NGS in urine sediment [11] and bladder biopsies [12].

In order to investigate the pathogenetic changes and study the regulatory role of miRNAs in BPS, we performed an integrated analysis of miRNA and mRNA paired expression profiling in the bladder biopsies of BPS human patients with non-Hunner IC phenotype, previously characterized by other methodology [7, 13], using comprehensive Next-generation sequencing (NGS)-derived transcriptome data. We studied the activated pathways and altered biological processes based on the global gene expression changes and explored the presence and regulatory role of the individual miRNA targets in these pathways.

Methods

Patient selection

Patient recruitment and cold cup bladder dome biopsy collection from 14 controls and 22 BPS patients was described in our earlier published study [13]. Permission to conduct this study was obtained from the Ethics Committee of the Canton of Bern (KEK 146/05), and all subjects gave written informed consent. All subjects underwent a complete urological evaluation (including medical history, physical examination, urine culture, flexible urethrocystoscopy). In addition, all subjects with the BPS underwent uroflowmetry, post void residual (PVR) and multichannel urodynamic investigations including filling cystometry and pressure-flow studies. All patients had confirmed BPS without Hunner's lesions. Patient selection and evaluation was described previously [13]. Full information on patients is given in the Additional file 1. Patients were divided in 2 groups:

1. Group 1: Control—asymptomatic patients undergoing cystoscopy for other reasons (e.g. stent placement for stone disease, microhematuria evaluation, fistula closure) (n = 6 for NGS, n = 8 for QPCR validation). All QPCR controls and 2 out of 4 NGS controls were female, average age was 51.8 ± 21 (QPCR) and 46.8 ± 6.7 (NGS).
2. Group 2: BPS—patients with pain (> 3 months) considered to be located in the bladder and/or frequency, urgency and nocturia (n = 6 for NGS, n = 16 for QPCR validation). All patients were female, average age 45.7 ± 15 (QPCR) and 38 ± 11 (NGS).

Biopsy samples from all subjects underwent a routine microscopic examination by a trained pathologist (H&E staining, staining for mast cell tryptase, staining for S100 proteins and PGP 9.5 for nerve fibres). No patient had an increased postvoid residual. Urodynamic studies showed a median cystometric bladder volume of 200 ml (range 60 – 1000), one patient had a high capacity bladder with a volume > 1000 ml and 2 patients had a normal capacity, all of the remaining ones had low capacity bladders. Histopathological evaluation showed chronic inflammation (lymphoplasmocytic infiltration, interstitial edema and/or hyperemia of the blood vessels with dilated lumina) in all but 4 patients, and 17 demonstrated increased mast cells (MC) in the smooth muscle (≥ 20 MC/mm^2) (Additional file 1). Cold cup biopsies from the bladder dome, two biopsies per subject were collected and stored in RNAlater (Qiagen) at − 70 °C until RNA isolation. Total RNA was isolated from bladder dome biopsies using the miRVana miRNA isolation kit (Ambion) and the RNA quality controlled by BioAnalyzer. Six high-quality (RIN ≥ 9) RNA samples were randomly selected for NGS.

miRNA and mRNA sequencing and pathway analysis

Illumina miRNA and mRNA Sequencing

Both miRNA and mRNA sequencing was performed on the Illumina HiSeq 2000 using RNA isolated from the same patient's biopsy. NGS protocol is described in our previous study [14]. Briefly, sequencing was performed on the Illumina HiSeq 2000 single end 100 bp using the TruSeq SBS Kit v3-HS (Illumina, Inc, California, USA). For mRNA-seq, read mapping to human reference genome hg19 was done using Tophat 2.0.9. Counting the number of reads/gene was done using HTSeq v.0.5.4p3. The Bioconductor packages DESeq2 and edgeR (Bioconductor version: Release (3.2)) were used to identify differentially expressed genes. We set the threshold for FDR-adjusted *p* value to 0.15 in order to maximize the number of genes used to build the pathways. The miRNA Target Filter tool in IPA (IPA®, QIAGEN Redwood City, http://www.qiagen.com/ingenuity was used to associate miRNAs from our miRNA sequencing datasets with experimentally observed and predicted mRNA targets. The predicted relationships are from TargetScan (v7.0; targetscan.org) and the experimentally observed relationships are from TarBase.

Hierarchical clustering and heatmaps

Hierarchical clustering and the associated heatmaps for miRNA and mRNA sequencing data were generated with the function heatmap2 in the R package gplots or GENE-E R package. Pairwise correlation matrix between items was computed (based on Pearson correlation method) and then converted as a distance matrix and finally clustering was computed on the resulting distance matrix. Average linkage method used average to calculate the distance matrix. For the heatmap visualization, the log2-expression values were used.

Principal component analysis (PCA)

For a principal component analysis on log2 fold change of mRNA and microRNA expression of patients compared to controls, 'prcomp' function implemented in R (R Core Team, 2016), rgl and scatterplot3d R package was used for the principal component analysis of three-dimensions plots. To achieve a better numerical accuracy, the calculation was done by a singular value decomposition of the (centered and scaled) data matrix.

Gene and miRNA clouds (tag clouds, word clouds)

To condense and visualize gene enrichment data from a pathway analysis dataset a cloud was created using Wordle.net and Word cloud R package. The font size of a gene or miRNA (tag) is determined by its incidence in the pathway analysis dataset.

Functional enrichment analysis

Gene Ontology (GO) over-representation analysis (ORA) [15] methods were used to gain biological insight on the DEGs. We used clusterProfiler (version 3.18.1) package [16] in R to perform GO-ORA and GO-GSEA on biological process (BP) terms associated with DEGs. Results obtained at a threshold of *p* value below 0.1 were considered statistically significant.

QPCR validation of NGS studies

Total RNA was isolated from bladder dome biopsies using the miRVana miRNA isolation kit (Ambion). The reverse transcription reactions were carried out using the High Capacity cDNA Reverse Transcription Kit (Applied Biosystems) with random hexamer primers. TaqMan assays were from Applied Biosystems. QPCR was carried out in triplicates using 7900HT Fast Real-time PCR System (Applied Biosystems). The Ct values obtained after the real time-QPCR were normalized to 18S expression and fold differences compared to the average of controls calculated.

NanoString nCounter analysis

miRNA presence and content were analysed with the nCounter Human miRNA Expression Assay kit (NanoString, Seattle, WA) according to manufacturer's instructions with some modifications, as described in our earlier publication [17]. Briefly, 3 µl of each total RNA sample was used as input into the nCounter Human miRNA sample preparation. Hybridization was conducted for 12 h at 65 °C. Subsequently, the strip tubes were placed into the nCounter Prep Station for automated sample purification and subsequent reporter capture. Each sample was scanned for 600 FOV on the nCounter Digital Analyzer. The R Packages were used for NanoString Data Analysis: "NanoStringNorm" and "NanoStringDiff" (Available in CRAN). Background correction was performed based on the detected values of negative control probes, a within-sample normalization was calculated based on the observed values of positive control probes and normalization across samples using reference (housekeeping) genes. Additionally, we used a new algorithm called Removing Unwanted Variation-III (RUV-III) [18] which employs technical replicates and suitable control genes to normalise the data. "EdgeR" was used for expression profiling.

Statistics

Hierarchical clustering and heatmaps

Hierarchical clustering and the associated heatmaps for miRNA and mRNA sequencing data were generated with the function heatmap2 in the R package gplots or GENE-E R package. Pairwise correlation matrix between items was computed based on Pearson correlation method. Average linkage method used average to calculate the distance matrix. For the heatmap visualization the log2-expression values were used. We used dendextend R package to create and compare visually appealing tree diagrams. *Principal Component analysis (PCA).* 'Prcomp' function implemented in R (R Core Team, 2016), rgl and scatterplot3d R package were used for the principal component analysis of three-dimensions plots. The calculation was done by a singular value decomposition of the (centered and scaled) data matrix. For *QPCR validation* the log2 fold change differences to the average of control samples were calculated. A one-way analysis of variance (ANOVA) was employed and the Tukey correction used to correct p values. The p value < 0.05 was considered statistically significant (GraphPad Prism (version 7.01)). *Contingency analysis.* Graphical matrix was drawn using the function balloonplot() in gplots package in R.

Results

Differentially expressed genes in BPS compared to control

Differentially expressed genes (DEGs, mRNAs and miRNAs) were determined in BPS group using DESeq2 (with p value < 0.05, absolute log2 fold change > 0.5 and mean of read counts > 50 reads). Figure 1A shows the heatmap and hierarchical clustering based on normalized read counts of all significantly regulated mRNAs. Patients with BPS ("pain1-5") cluster away from controls, although patient "pain6" more closely resembles controls in its DEGs profile. Selection of the 84 top regulated mRNAs (p value < 0.05, absolute log2 fold change > 1 and mean of read counts > 50 read) helped to cluster the two groups better (see the dendrogram in Additional file 8: Fig. S1A). PCA based on mRNAseq data shows good separation of BPS patients from controls (Fig. 1B). The scree plot in Additional file 8: Fig. S1B shows that component 1 and 2 can cover more than 75% of variation between samples.

(See figure on next page.)

Fig. 1 Differentially expressed mRNAs and miRNAs in BPS patients. **A** Heatmap and hieratical clustering based on normalized read counts of all mRNA (829) with p value < 0.05, absolute log2 fold change > 0.5 and mean of read counts > 50 reads. Genes are represented in y-axis and patients with BPS and controls are shown in x-axis. Normalized read counts were used for this heatmap. Minimum and maximum renormalized read counts for each mRNA were used to construct a relative color scheme by convert values to colors. One minus Pearson correlation metric was used for clustering accompanied with average linkage method. **B** Principal component analysis of the RNA sequencing data in a 2D graph of PC1 and PC2 based on normalized read counts of all mRNA (829) with p value < 0.05, absolute log2 fold change > 0.5 and mean of read counts > 50 reads. The bi-plot shows samples as labelled dots. Values of cos2 (square cosine, squared coordinates) for each sample indicate the quality of representation of the variables on the factor map. Samples are colour coded according to cos2 scale shown in the bar. **C** Volcano plot of all mRNAs. Up-regulated mRNAs are visualized in red color, and down-regulated in green. mRNAs with p value < 0.05, absolute log2 fold change > 0.5 were selected for further analysis. **D** Heatmap and hieratical clustering of all miRNA (62) with p value < 0.05, absolute log2 fold change > 0.5 and mean of read counts > 50 read. miRNAs are represented in y-axis and patients with BPS and controls are shown in x-axis. Normalized read counts were used for this heatmap. Minimum and maximum renormalized read counts for each miRNA were used to construct a relative color scheme by convert values to colors. One minus Pearson correlation metric was used for clustering accompanied with average linkage method. **E** Principal component analysis of the miRNA data in a 2D graph of PC1 and PC2. PC2 based on normalized read counts of all miRNA (62) with p value < 0.05, absolute log2 fold change > 0.5 and mean of read counts > 50 reads. The bi-plot shows samples as labelled dots. Samples are colour-coded according to the quality of representation of the variables on factor map (cos2, square cosine, squared coordinates) as shown on the side-bar. **F** Volcano plot of all miRNAs. All up-regulated miRNAs are visualized in red color, and all down-regulated in green. miRNAs with p value < 0.05, absolute log2 fold change > 0.5 were selected for further analysis

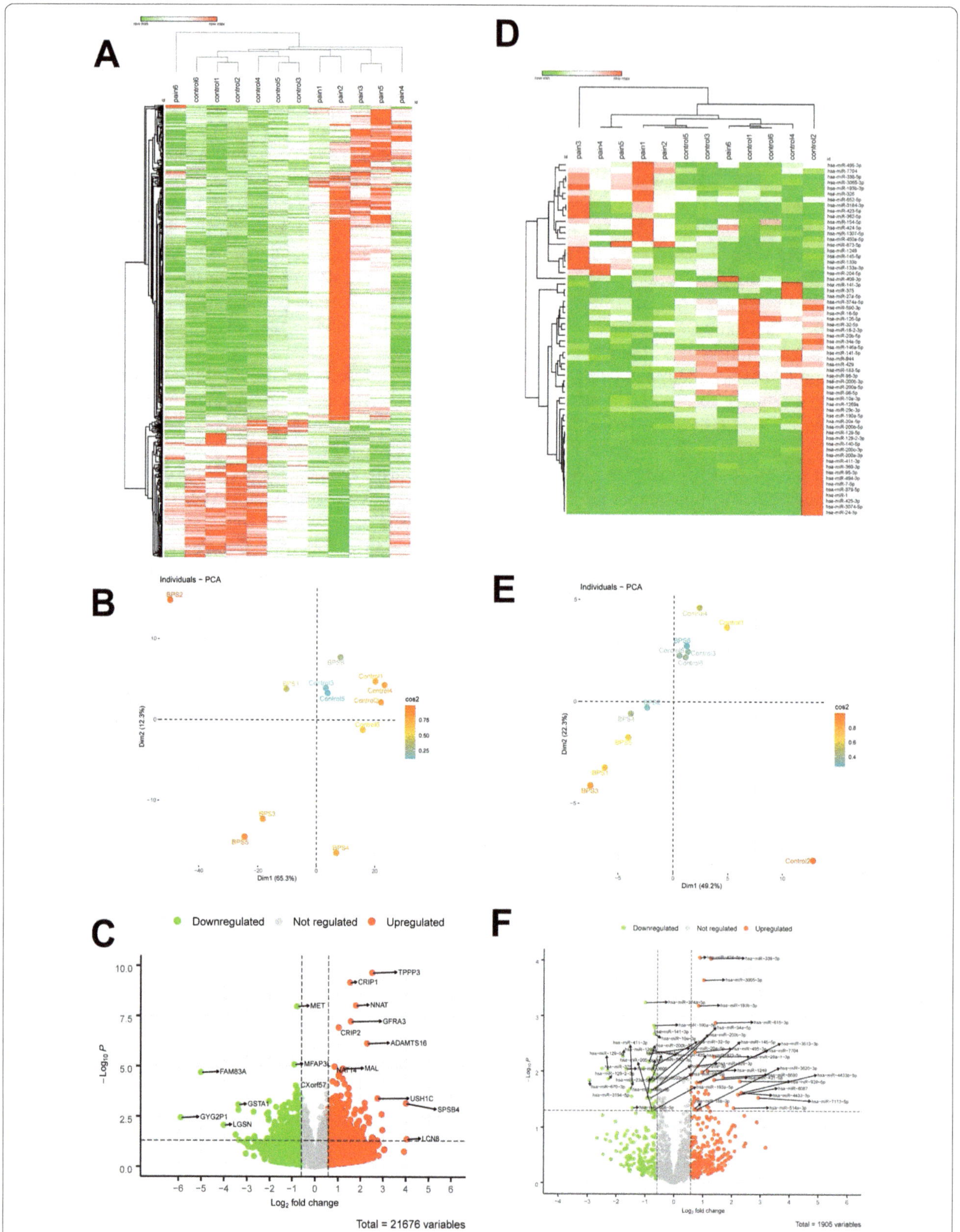

Fig. 1 (See legend on previous page.)

To characterize the relationship between 15 top regulated genes and each single patient in mRNA data set, a contingency analysis was performed. TPPP3, CRIP1, and MFAP5 showed a higher the probability of being indicative for BPS group (Additional file 8: Fig. S1C). DESeq2 analysis resulted in 829 differentially expressed mRNAs (Additional file 2). Overall, we identified 574 up-regulated and 255 down-regulated genes. Volcano plot of significantly regulated mRNAs based on p value (Fig. 1C) or adjusted p value (Additional file 8: Fig. S1) showed that TPPP3 and CRIP1 are the most up-regulated genes while, MET and FAM83A are most down-regulated genes.

The hierarchical clustering of samples based of differentially expressed miRNAs was very similar to the one based on mRNAs (Fig. 1D), likewise sample "pain6" was more similar to the controls than the rest of the samples. In totals, 62 miRNAs were changed during BPS, and PCA based on their normalized read counts clearly differentiated BPS from controls (Fig. 1E). The scree plot shown in Additional file 8: Fig. S2B shows that component 1 and 2 can cover more than 72% of variation between samples. The significant differentially expressed miRNAs are shown as a volcano plot (Fig. 1F). The background data to the miRNA analysis are shown in Additional file 8: Fig. S2.

Functional enrichment analysis and identification of dysregulated biological processes in BPS

Using IPA, 31 significant pathways were built, though most did not have a defined z-score indicative of whether the activity of canonical pathways, including functional end-points, is increased or decreased based on DEGs in the datasets. Top 5 canonical IPA pathways based on mRNA datasets are shown in Table 1 (full list of pathways in Additional file 3). The two pathways involved in translational regulation, EIF2 Signalling and Regulation of eIF4 and p70S6K Signalling, are among the most significantly regulated processes during BPS. Fibrotic pathway important for bladder remodelling is also significant but without a z-score indicative of up- or down-regulation. Leukotriene Biosynthesis nociceptive pathway is significantly activated (positive z-score).

In order to gain insight into the biological processes underlying BPS, we resorted to Gene Ontology (GO) Over Representation Analysis (ORA). The GO terms and associated genes, obtained from the ORA result are listed Additional file 4. To gain a better insight into the GO terms network, we created a semantic similarity matrix for a given list of GO terms depending on the information content of their closest common ancestor term. After removing the redundant GO terms based on semantic similarity score threshold of 0.7, remaining GO terms were grouped by clustering the semantic similarity matrix using binary cut method. A treemap view of GO-term clusters, where each tile and colour represent a term and cluster respectively, is shown in Fig. 2A. In the treemap plot, tile size and group representatives of each cluster corresponds to the GO terms' size. Processes involved in cell division are highly represented in the BPS dataset, based on the abundance of mitosis-connected GO terms (Fig. 2A), followed by ECM reorganisation, neutrophil chemotaxis and muscle contractility. Notably, peripheral nervous system development is a prominent feature of this dataset. Figure 2B represents these

Table 1 Top 5 canonical IPA pathways regulated in BPS based on p value

Ingenuity canonical pathways	−log(p value)	Ratio	z-score	Molecules
EIF2 signalling	9.15	0.125	3.771	DDIT3 EIF2AK3 EIF3G FAU MAP2K2 RPL10A RPL13 RPL18 RPL18A RPL24 RPL27 RPL28 RPL29 RPL35 RPL36 RPL37 RPL38 RPLP1 RPLP2 RPS15 RPS15A RPS16 RPS19 RPS21 RPS4X RPS7 RPS9 RRAS
Hepatic fibrosis/hepatic stellate cell activation	4.54	0.0968	NA	CCL2 CCL21 CCN2 COL18A1 COL19A1 COL22A1 COL4A2 COL6A1 COL6A2 COL9A3 CXCL9 IGFBP4 MET MYL6 MYL9 STAT1 TIMP1 VEGFB
Leukotriene biosynthesis	3.24	0.308	2	DPEP2 GGT1 GGT5 LTC4S
Regulation of eIF4 and p70S6K Signalling	2.81	0.0828	NA	EIF3G FAU ITGA2 MAP2K2 RPS15 RPS15A RPS16 RPS19 RPS21 RPS4X RPS7 RPS9 RRAS
Cholesterol biosynthesis	2.69	0.172	−2.236	HMGCR HMGCS1 MSMO1 SC5D SQLE

(See figure on next page.)

Fig. 2 Gene ontology over-representation analysis of regulated mRNAs in BPS patients. **A** A treemap view of GO-term clusters, where each tile and colour represent a term and cluster, respectively. The list of GO terms was converted into a semantic similarity matrix using binary cut method. Tile size and group representatives of each cluster are corresponding to the GO terms' size. **B** GO terms as clusters. Regulation of cell cycle, neutrophil chemotaxis and muscle and nervous system development are the top 3 clusters for BPS

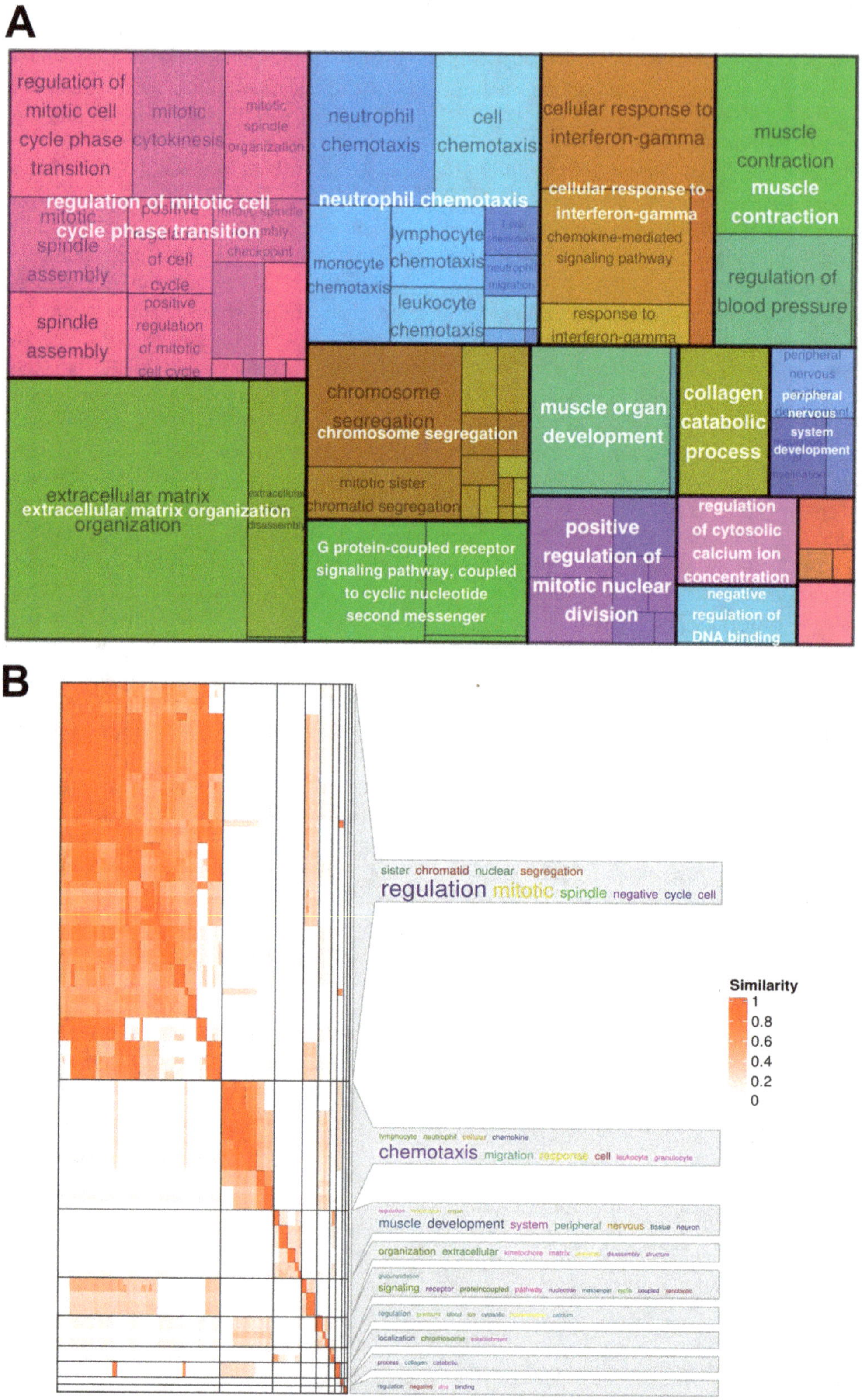

Fig. 2 (See legend on previous page.)

GO terms as clusters, clustered by binary cut method. There, regulation of cell cycle, neutrophil chemotaxis and muscle and nervous system development are the top 3 clusters for BPS. We identified functional modules using Enrichment Map plot (Fig. 3). The network of enriched terms with edges connecting overlapping gene sets clustered mutually overlapping gene sets, visualizing the six main functional modules for BPS: cell cycle regulation, chemotaxis of immune cells, muscle development, muscle contraction, remodelling of extracellular matrix and peripheral nervous system organization and development (Fig. 3). To confirm the NGS results, we investigated the expression levels of 4 selected mRNAs, including the top regulated FAM83A and TPPP3 (Fig. 1C) in the bladder biopsies of a larger independent patient cohort (n = 8 controls and n = 16 BPS). mRNAs for TPPP3, ANGPTL17 and MFAP5 were significantly up-regulated ($p < 0.05$), whereas FAM83A was down-regulated in BPS, in accordance with the NGS data (Fig. 4).

Identification of functionally important miRNAs altered in BPS dataset

We identified 62 microRNAs, regulated and abundant in BPS (Additional file 5) and determined which of their target mRNAs were present and correctly regulated in the mRNA dataset (Additional file 6). The word cloud in Fig. 5A illustrates the miRNAs, with the font size reflecting the number of correctly regulated target mRNAs. Up-regulated miR-424-5p and down-regulated miR-34a-5p have 40 and 45 regulated target genes in mRNA dataset, respectively, and potentially play the highest regulatory role in BPS. Word cloud of the miRNA targets includes TNFSF15, TSPAN4 and WDFY4 mRNAs which are targeted by multiple miRNAs (Fig. 5B). MiRNA-regulated genes fall into multiple categories, the majority being enzymes, transcriptional regulators, transporters and kinases.

Multiple cytokines differentially expressed in the BPS dataset are paired with their regulatory miRNAs

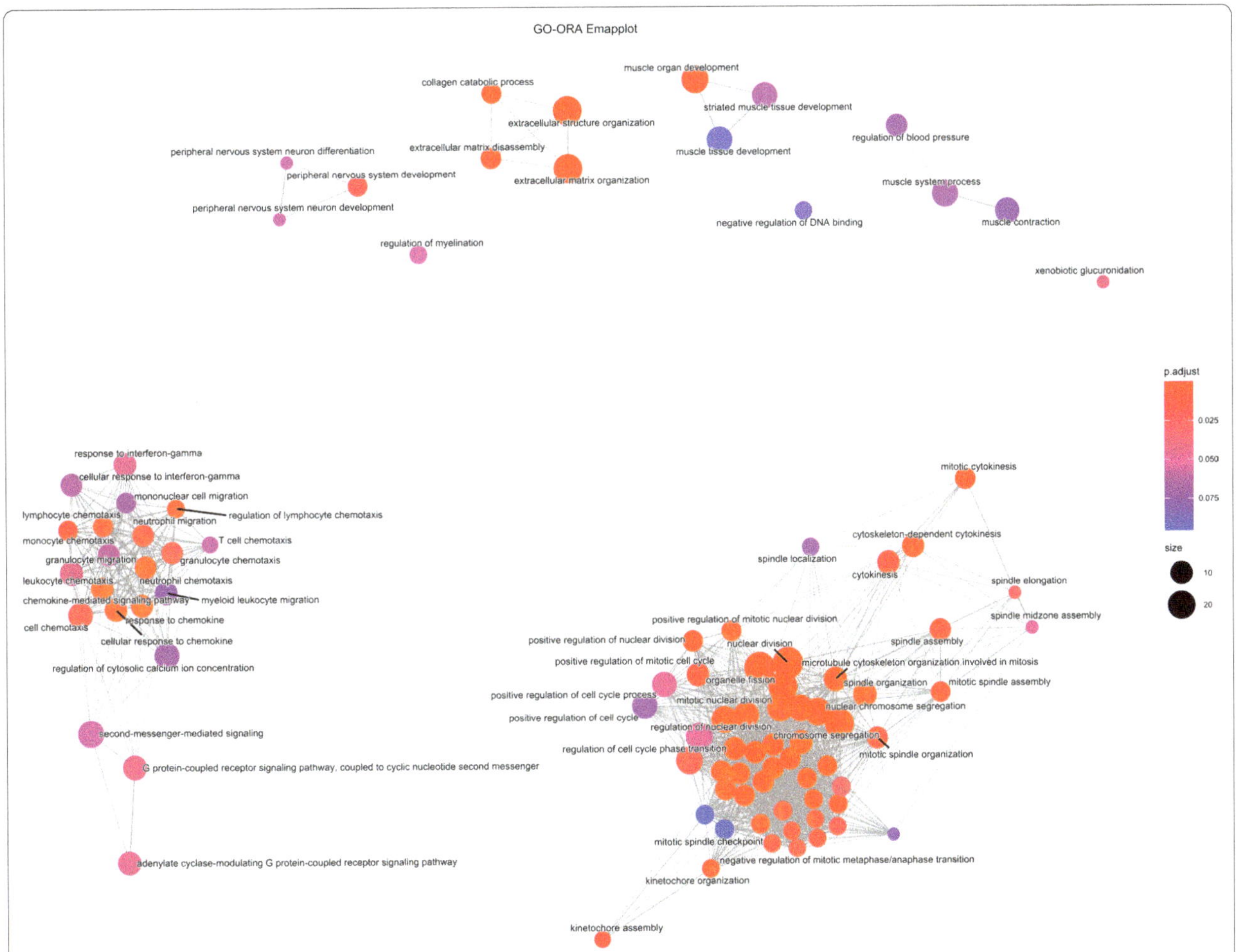

Fig. 3 Enrichment Map plot of GO ORA (mRNA dataset). The network of enriched terms with edges connecting overlapping gene sets clusters mutually overlapping gene sets, visualizing the six main functional modules for BPS

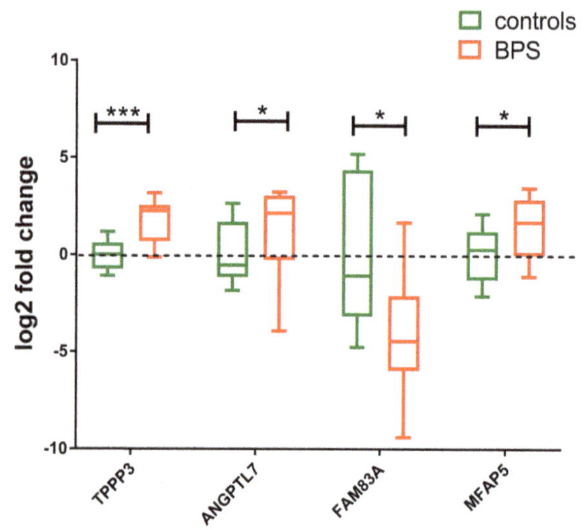

Fig. 4 QPCR validation of selected DEGs based on NGS mRNA dataset. QPCR results for 4 mRNAs, regulated and significant ($p < 0.05$) in NGS mRNA dataset. Gene expression was determined in RNA samples isolated from controls (n = 8) and BPS patients' biopsies (n = 16) using TaqMan gene expression The Ct values obtained after the real time-QPCR were normalized to 18S rRNA expression and fold differences compared to the average of controls calculated. Boxplot of log2 fold changes relative to the average normalized Ct values in the control group is shown. Statistically significant differences (*$p < 0.05$, ***$p < 0.001$, ANOVA)

(Fig. 5C): CCL21 is increased, while miR-205-5p which is predicted to target it, is down-regulated; the same correct behaviour was observed for the down-regulated CCL2, CXCL10, CXCL9, whose regulatory miRNAs were all increased (Fig. 5C). Similarly, the up-regulated components of the activated EIF2 signalling pathway are regulated by miRNAs which are decreased in the biopsies of patients with BPS (Fig. 5D). Top ten significant IPA pathways built using appropriately regulated targets of miRNAs are shown in Fig. 5E. Like in the mRNA dataset shown in Fig. 5F for comparison, eIF2 signalling is the main activated pathway, targeted by miRNAs regulated in BPS.

To validate the miRNA expression results, we carried out a profiling study using NanoString nCounter Human miRNA Expression Assay kit (Additional file 7) using n = 7 controls and n = 16 BPS samples. Comparative regulation of 16 miRNAs, robustly detected by NanoString in all samples, is shown in Additional file 8: Fig. S3. We confirmed the down-regulation of miR-205-5p, and up-regulation of muscle-specific miR-145-5p, miR-143-3p and miR-133a-3p in BPS patients.

Discussion

IC/BPS is a chronic disease of unknown etiology, it is a multifactorial, heterogeneous disorder with several clinical phenotypes. A variety of pathophysiological origins have been proposed for BPS, ranging from autoimmunity, inflammation caused by recurrent bladder injury, neurogenic inflammation with the contributing increase of urothelial permeability and disruption of the GAG layer, and altered central nociception [4, 5]. Emerging gene expression studies, using human tissue (bladder biopsies or urine sediment) or tissue from animal models of IC have shed some light on bladder alterations during BPS, however, no consensus exists regarding the molecular drivers of this dysfunction. Recent findings indicate that IC/BPS with Hunner's lesions is a distinct histological and molecular phenotype of the disease, characterized by pancystitis, frequent clonal B-cell expansion and epithelial denudation [19]. Therefore, current guidelines [20] suggest that Hunner-type interstitial cystitis and bladder pain syndrome should be considered separate entities, because bladder pain syndrome shows minimal pathological changes in the bladder [20]. While the gene expression profile of Hunner-type IC seems quite distinct from the controls, both in the biopsies and urine sediment [11, 12], the patients with non-ulcerative BPS/IC are less clearly definable, and often show no or slight differences in gene expression compared to control either in the biopsies [12], or urine sediment [9].

In this study we analyzed the NGS mRNA and miRNA gene expression profiles in the bladder dome biopsies of female patients with BPS. Unlike many earlier gene expression studies, performed using low throughput

(See figure on next page.)

Fig. 5 Pathway analysis using mRNAs, targeted by miRNAs regulated in BPS. **A** Role of miRNAs depending on the number of their appropriately regulated targets. Word cloud of up-regulated (in red) and down-regulated (in green) miRNAs, font size corresponding to the number of correctly regulated mRNAs, targeted by each specific miRNA. **B** Word cloud of mRNAs, targeted by dysregulated miRNAs; font size corresponds to the number of miRNAs affecting the expression of a particular mRNA. The coloured circle shows the functional groups of the affected mRNAs: most are enzymes and transcription regulators, kinases and cytokines. **C** Cytokines up-regulated (red) and down-regulated (green) and the targeting miRNAs. Note that some cytokines are affected by several miRNAs, and some miRNAs regulate multiple cytokine mRNAs. **D** EIF2 signalling pathway might be activated due to the down-regulation of miRNAs, targeting its elements. Down-regulated miRNAs are shown in green, up-regulated target genes in red. **E** Pathway analysis based on genes, predicted to be targeted by dysregulated miRNAs and differentially expressed in BPS. Top 10 IPA Pathways are shown (based on p value). **F** Pathway analysis based on all regulated mRNAs in BPS, top 10 pathways are shown

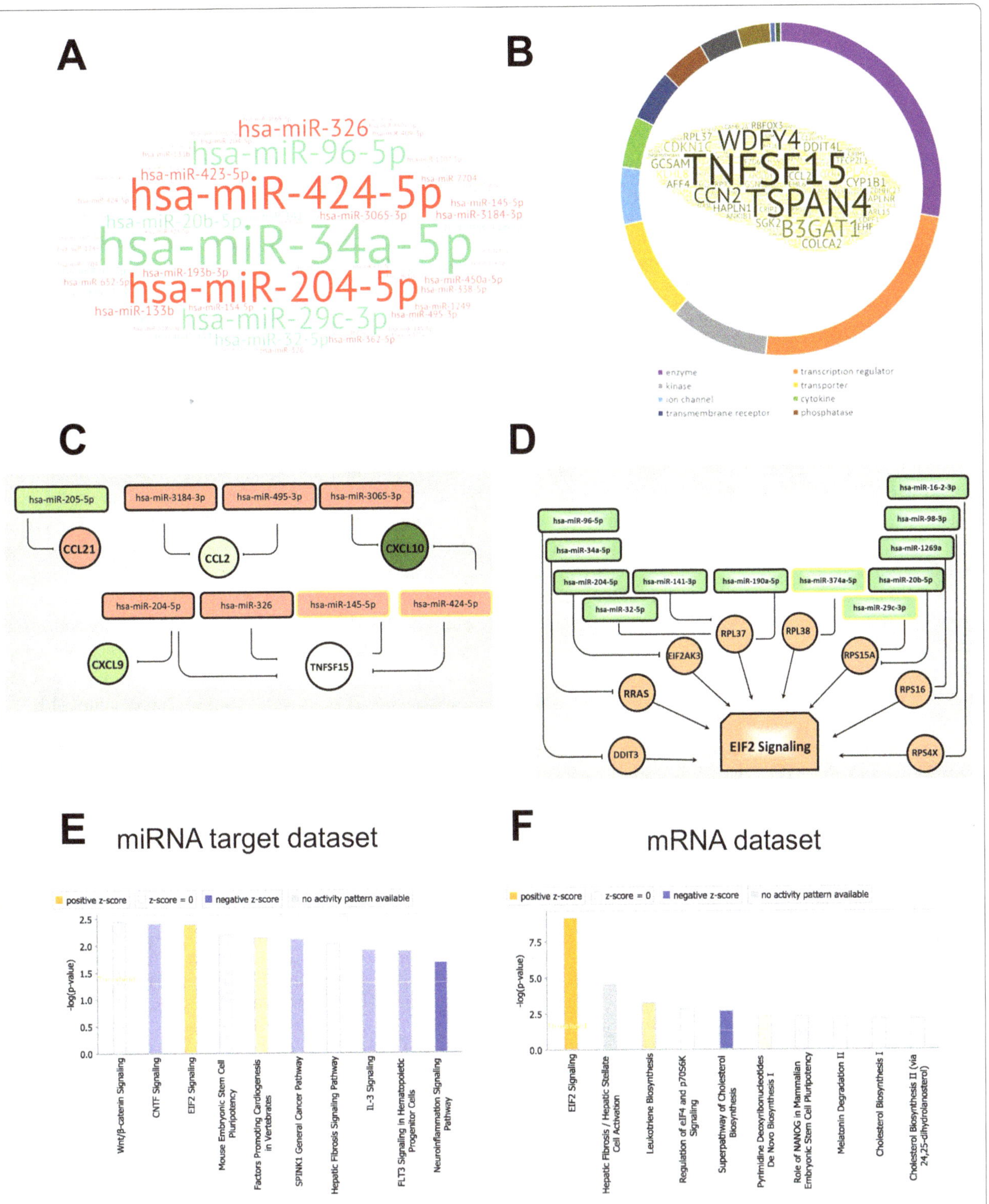

Fig. 5 (See legend on previous page.)

methodology (microarrays, PCR arrays with selected genes), we carried out a comprehensive paired mRNA and miRNA transcriptome analysis from the same patient, allowing us to discern the involvement of particular miRNA targets in the signalling events. The patient group selected in our trial was not specifically recruited based on the presence of Hunner's ulcers, our patients did not have the ulcerative phenotype, and therefore we refer to them as BPS. Most patients in our study had a low bladder capacity with median cystometric bladder volume of 200 ml, and a measurable infiltration of neutrophils and mast cells in the bladder submucosa. The NGS mRNA and miRNA gene expression profiles in our BPS patients (n = 6) were distinct from the controls. This is in agreement with previous findings, pointing to the correlation of gene expression with bladder capacity [8], where the patients with normal bladder capacity were similar to controls, and patients whose bladder volume ranged from 300 to 175 ml were significantly different.

We could use the DEGs mRNA dataset to build IPA pathways, though only a limited number of significant pathways could be assigned a z-score. Nevertheless, two out of top 5 pathways were involved in translational regulation. EIF2 Signalling and Regulation of eIF4 and p70S6K Signalling are among the most significantly regulated processes during BPS. They are activated in response to cellular stress and regulate proinflammatory cytokine expression [21]. Importantly, both pathways were previously described in the urine sediment cells from BPS patients [11], highlighting the importance of cellular stress in the pathogenesis of BPS. Fibrotic pathway appears to be involved, pointing to organ remodelling. Leukotriene Biosynthesis nociceptive pathway, important in a variety of allergic/inflammatory diseases and in neuropathic pain [22], is also significantly activated (positive z-score). Leukotrienes are produced and released by neutrophils and mast cells, which are increased in our population of BPS patients. Mast cell marker tryptase (TPSAB1 gene) was strongly and significantly upregulated in the BPS NGS dataset (Log2 fold change (log2 FC) of 1.16, p value 0.004).

Previously, attempts have been made to distinguish BPS/IC from OAB using immunohistochemistry with antibodies to the nerve cell marker PGP9.5 (neuron-specific protein gene product 9.5), p75NTR (p75 neurotrophin receptor), the B-lymphocyte marker CD20 and mast cell tryptase [23]. Clinically, patients with OAB are similar to patients with BPS/IC regarding frequency and urgency as well as low bladder capacity but usually do not suffer from pain. In addition to the increase of tryptase mRNA, we observed an up-regulation of PGP9.5 gene UCHL1 (log2 FC 0.56), and p75 neurotrophin receptor gene NTRK1 (log2 FC 1.24) in our dataset, indicative of sensory hyperinnervation in BPS. Similarly, several inflammatory mediators, identified earlier by QPCR in trigone biopsies of BPS patients using TaqMan microfluidic cards [10], showed similar regulation of expression: CCL21 (log2 FC 1.15, p value 0.01) and CXCL1 (log2 FC 0.76) mRNAs were both significantly up-regulated in our NGS dataset. We observed that many regulatory miRNAs, altered during BPS, were involved in the regulation of inflammatory mediators, and that the levels of CCL21 and its regulatory miR-205-5p were inversely correlated. Chemokine CCL21 activates microglia in the central nervous system and is expressed in neurons after an insult or mechanical injury, implicated in neuropathic pain [24], rheumatoid arthritis [25] and pulmonary fibrosis [26]. CCR7, the receptor for CCL21, was also up-regulated in the NGS dataset (log2 FC 0.66, n.s.), so it is possible that at least in some BPS patients, the relevant signalling cascade is activated, contributing to the activation of the ERK and JNK pathways. Recent studies have linked bladder inflammation with mood disorders [27]. Although we did not specifically examine this, it is tempting to speculate that the up-regulation of CCL21 reported here might have a bearing on the higher than average incidence of depression, common in BPS [28, 29].

We performed GO ORA using DEGs from the BPS mRNAseq dataset to reveal the biological processes contributing to bladder remodelling. The pathways were clustered into six main functional groups: cell cycle regulation, chemotaxis of immune cells, muscle development, muscle contraction, remodelling of extracellular matrix and peripheral nervous system organization and development. Generally, immune pathways activation, which was a prominent feature of BOO-induced bladder overactivity, and BPH-induced bladder remodelling [14] was modest in our dataset, limiting itself to neutrophil chemotaxis and IFN-γ-mediated signalling. Our data support the notion that, unlike Hunner-type IC, inflammation is less pronounced in non-ulcerative BPS, although it might play an important role in disease pathogenesis. Activation of mitosis, catabolic connective tissue remodelling and muscle tissue development, observed on the molecular level in our dataset, are in line with the bladder morphology of the majority of our subjects, who had thick-walled, low capacity bladders.

Our study has its limitations: only female patients have been recruited; controls for QPCR were also female, but NGS controls included 4 male subjects. To overcome the last limitation, the expression of the Y chromosome-linked genes was not considered in the DEG analysis. The study has a relatively small number of patients, which might have a bearing on our results, given the heterogeneity of BPS.

In conclusion, we studied the gene expression profiles of mRNA and miRNA in bladder biopsies of BPS patients, and identified the key biological functions, contributing to organ remodelling. Non-ulcerative BPS patients, recruited in this study, had strong smooth muscle contractile and cell proliferative phenotype, indicative of smooth muscle hyperplasia. The contribution of inflammatory processes was modest, but we observed molecular changes indicative of neuroinflammation and peripheral nervous system reorganization and development. Pathway analysis of the integrated mRNA-miRNA NGS dataset shed some light on the molecular changes in the bladders of patients with BPS, and pinpointed important regulatory miRNAs whose dysregulation might contribute to the pathogenesis.

Abbreviations

IC/BPS: Interstitial cystitis/bladder pain syndrome; NGS: Next-generation sequencing; DEGs: Differentially expressed genes; mRNA: Messenger RNA; miRNA: MicroRNA; GO ORA: Gene ontology over-representation analysis; QPCR: Quantitative real-time polymerase chain reaction; eIF2(4): Eukaryotic Initiation Factor 2 (4); FC: Fold change; n.s.: Not significant.

Supplementary Information

Additional file 1. Demographical and clinical information about the subjects participating in the study.

Additional file 2. List of differentially expressed genes with p-value<0.05, absolute log2 fold change>0.5 and mean of read counts>50 reads.

Additional file 3. List of significant Ingenuity Canonical Pathways

Additional file 4. Gene Ontology (GO) terms and associated genes, obtained from the Over Representation Analysis (ORA) with adjusted p value < 0.1

Additional file 5. List of abundant microRNAs, significantly regulated in the BPS patients compared to controls

Additional file 6. List of the mRNA targets of 62 miRNAs, abundant and regulated in BPS

Additional file 7. All data on miRNAs, detected in the profiling using NanoString nCounter Human miRNA Expression Assay kit

Additional file 8: Supplementary Figures. Fig. S1. Characterization of regulated mRNAs. (A) Sample clustering based on the expression of the 84 top regulated mRNAs (p value<0.05, absolute log2 fold change>1 and mean of read counts>50 read). (B) Scree plot for visualization of the percentage of variances explained for each principle component (eigenvalues) in RNA sequencing data (C) Contingency table of the 18 top regulated mRNAs displaying the (multivariate) frequency distribution of the variables. The diameter of the orange circle for each gene per patient provides an estimate of the probability for that particular gene to represent that particular patient. (D) Volcano plot of all mRNAs using adjusted P value. **Fig. S2**. Characterization of regulated miRNAs. (A) Sample clustering based on the expression of the 18 top regulated miRNAs (p-value<0.05, absolute log2 fold change>1 and mean of read counts>50 read) (B) Scree plot for visualization of the variances in miRNA sequencing data (C) Contingency table of the 8 top regulated miRNAs displaying the (multivariate) frequency distribution of the variables. The diameter of the orange circle for each miRNA per patient provides an estimate of the probability for that particular miRNA to represent that particular patient. (D) Volcano plot of all miRNAs using adjusted P value. **Fig. S3**. Validation of regulated miRNAs by NanoString. Radar graph visualizing the average log2 fold change of 16 miRNAs significantly regulated in NanoString or sequencing dataset (p-value<0.05, absolute log2 fold change>1 and mean of read counts>300 read). The red line represents the NGS miRNA sequencing data and purple line represents the NanoString data. Red area is showing the upregulation and green area is representing downregulation.

Acknowledgements

Authors thank Dr Veronica Sanchez Freire for expert technical support at the beginning of this work.

Authors' contributions

KM, FCB and AHG planned the study; AK and FCB recruited the patients, MB and KM performed sample preparation and QPCR validation; AHG and AA analysed the data; IK, RB and HR performed NGS and provided bioinformatic support, AHG, RMA and KM wrote the manuscript. All authors read and approved the final manuscript.

Author details

[1]Functional Urology Research Group, Department for BioMedical Research DBMR, University of Bern, Bern, Switzerland. [2]Urological Diseases Research Center, Boston Children's Hospital, Boston, MA, USA. [3]Department of Surgery, Harvard Medical School, Boston, MA, USA. [4]Broad Institute of MIT and Harvard, Cambridge, MA, USA. [5]Department of Gynaecology, Inselspital University Hospital, 3010 Bern, Switzerland. [6]Interfaculty Bioinformatics Unit, University of Bern, Bern, Switzerland. [7]Functional Genomics Center Zurich, ETH Zurich/ University of Zurich, Zurich, Switzerland. [8]Department of Urology, Inselspital University Hospital, 3010 Bern, Switzerland.

References

1. van de Merwe JP, Nordling J, Bouchelouche P, Bouchelouche K, Cervigni M, Daha LK, et al. Diagnostic criteria, classification, and nomenclature for painful bladder syndrome/interstitial cystitis: an ESSIC proposal. EurUrol. 2008;53(1):60–7.
2. Clemens JQ, Meenan RT, Rosetti MC, Gao SY, Calhoun EA. Prevalence and incidence of interstitial cystitis in a managed care population. J Urol. 2005;173(1):98–102; discussion https://doi.org/10.1097/01.ju.0000146114.53828.82.
3. Berry SH, Elliott MN, Suttorp M, Bogart LM, Stoto MA, Eggers P, et al. Prevalence of symptoms of bladder pain syndrome/interstitial cystitis among adult females in the United States. J Urol. 2011;186(2):540–4. https://doi.org/10.1016/j.juro.2011.03.132.
4. Karamali M, Shafabakhsh R, Ghanbari Z, Eftekhar T, Asemi Z. Molecular pathogenesis of interstitial cystitis/bladder pain syndrome based on gene expression. J Cell Physiol. 2019;234(8):12301–8. https://doi.org/10.1002/jcp.28009.
5. Akiyama Y, Luo Y, Hanno PM, Maeda D, Homma Y. Interstitial cystitis/bladder pain syndrome: the evolving landscape, animal models and future perspectives. Int J Urol. 2020;27(6):491–503. https://doi.org/10.1111/iju.14229.
6. Sanchez-Freire V, Blanchard MG, Burkhard FC, Kessler TM, Kellenberger S, Monastyrskaya K. Acid-sensing channels in human bladder: expression, function and alterations during bladder pain syndrome. J Urol. 2011;186(4):1509–16. https://doi.org/10.1016/j.juro.2011.05.047.
7. Monastyrskaya K, Babiychuk EB, Draeger A, Burkhard FC. Down-regulation of annexin A1 in the urothelium decreases cell survival after bacterial toxin exposure. J Urol. 2013. https://doi.org/10.1016/j.juro.2013.01.088.
8. Colaco M, Koslov DS, Keys T, Evans RJ, Badlani GH, Andersson KE, et al. Correlation of gene expression with bladder capacity in interstitial cystitis/bladder pain syndrome. J Urol. 2014;192(4):1123–9. https://doi.org/10.1016/j.juro.2014.05.047.
9. Blalock EM, Korrect GS, Stromberg AJ, Erickson DR. Gene expression analysis of urine sediment: evaluation for potential noninvasive markers of interstitial cystitis/bladder pain syndrome. J Urol. 2012;187(2):725–32. https://doi.org/10.1016/j.juro.2011.09.142.
10. Offiah I, Didangelos A, Dawes J, Cartwright R, Khullar V, Bradbury EJ, et al. The expression of inflammatory mediators in bladder pain syndrome. Eur Urol. 2016;70(2):283–90. https://doi.org/10.1016/j.eururo.2016.02.058.
11. Izquierdo L, Mateu L, Lozano JJ, Montalbo R, Ingelmo-Torres M, Gómez A, et al. Urine gene expression profiles in bladder pain syndrome patients treated with triamcinolone. Eur Urol Focus. 2020;6(2):390–6. https://doi.org/10.1016/j.euf.2018.10.001.

12. Akiyama Y, Maeda D, Katoh H, Morikawa T, Niimi A, Nomiya A, et al. Molecular taxonomy of interstitial cystitis/bladder pain syndrome based on whole transcriptome profiling by next-generation RNA sequencing of bladder mucosal biopsies. J Urol. 2019;202(2):290–300. https://doi.org/10.1097/ju.0000000000000234.
13. Sanchez Freire V, Burkhard FC, Kessler TM, Kuhn A, Draeger A, Monastyrskaya K. MicroRNAs may mediate the down-regulation of neurokinin-1 receptor in chronic bladder pain syndrome. Am J Pathol. 2010;176(1):288–303. https://doi.org/10.2353/ajpath.2010.090552.
14. Gheinani AH, Kiss B, Moltzahn F, Keller I, Bruggmann R, Rehrauer H, et al. Characterization of miRNA-regulated networks, hubs of signaling, and biomarkers in obstruction-induced bladder dysfunction. JCI insight. 2017;2(2):e89560. https://doi.org/10.1172/jci.insight.89560.
15. Boyle EI, Weng S, Gollub J, Jin H, Botstein D, Cherry JM, et al. GO::TermFinder–open source software for accessing Gene Ontology information and finding significantly enriched Gene Ontology terms associated with a list of genes. Bioinformatics. 2004;20(18):3710–5. https://doi.org/10.1093/bioinformatics/bth456.
16. Yu G, Wang LG, Han Y, He QY. clusterProfiler: an R package for comparing biological themes among gene clusters. OMICS. 2012;16(5):284–7. https://doi.org/10.1089/omi.2011.0118.
17. Gheinani AH, Vogeli M, Baumgartner U, Vassella E, Draeger A, Burkhard FC, et al. Improved isolation strategies to increase the yield and purity of human urinary exosomes for biomarker discovery. Sci Rep. 2018;8(1):3945. https://doi.org/10.1038/s41598-018-22142-x.
18. Molania R, Gagnon-Bartsch JA, Dobrovic A, Speed TP. A new normalization for Nanostring nCounter gene expression data. Nucleic Acids Res. 2019;47(12):6073–83. https://doi.org/10.1093/nar/gkz433.
19. Maeda D, Akiyama Y, Morikawa T, Kunita A, Ota Y, Katoh H, et al. Hunner-type (classic) interstitial cystitis: a distinct inflammatory disorder characterized by pancystitis, with frequent expansion of clonal B-cells and epithelial denudation. PLoS ONE. 2015;10(11):e0143316. https://doi.org/10.1371/journal.pone.0143316.
20. Homma Y, Akiyama Y, Tomoe H, Furuta A, Ueda T, Maeda D, et al. Clinical guidelines for interstitial cystitis/bladder pain syndrome. Int J Urol. 2020;27(7):578–89. https://doi.org/10.1111/iju.14234.
21. Shrestha N, Bahnan W, Wiley DJ, Barber G, Fields KA, Schesser K. Eukaryotic initiation factor 2 (eIF2) signaling regulates proinflammatory cytokine expression and bacterial invasion. J Biol Chem. 2012;287(34):28738–44. https://doi.org/10.1074/jbc.M112.375915.
22. Noguchi K, Okubo M. Leukotrienes in nociceptive pathway and neuropathic/inflammatory pain. Biol Pharm Bull. 2011;34(8):1163–9. https://doi.org/10.1248/bpb.34.1163.
23. Regauer S, Gamper M, Fehr MK, Viereck V. Sensory hyperinnervation distinguishes bladder pain syndrome/interstitial cystitis from overactive bladder syndrome. J Urol. 2017;197(1):159–66. https://doi.org/10.1016/j.juro.2016.06.089.
24. Honjoh K, Nakajima H, Hirai T, Watanabe S, Matsumine A. Relationship of inflammatory cytokines from M1-Type microglia/macrophages at the injured site and lumbar enlargement with neuropathic pain after spinal cord injury in the CCL21 knockout (plt) mouse. Front Cell Neurosci. 2019;13:525. https://doi.org/10.3389/fncel.2019.00525.
25. Pickens SR, Chamberlain ND, Volin MV, Pope RM, Talarico NE, Mandelin AM 2nd, et al. Role of the CCL21 and CCR7 pathways in rheumatoid arthritis angiogenesis. Arthritis Rheum. 2012;64(8):2471–81. https://doi.org/10.1002/art.34452.
26. Pierce EM, Carpenter K, Jakubzick C, Kunkel SL, Flaherty KR, Martinez FJ, et al. Therapeutic targeting of CC ligand 21 or CC chemokine receptor 7 abrogates pulmonary fibrosis induced by the adoptive transfer of human pulmonary fibroblasts to immunodeficient mice. Am J Pathol. 2007;170(4):1152–64. https://doi.org/10.2353/ajpath.2007.060649.
27. Hirshman NA, Hughes FM Jr, Jin H, Harrison WT, White SW, Doan I, et al. Cyclophosphamide-induced cystitis results in NLRP3-mediated inflammation in the hippocampus and symptoms of depression in rats. Am J Physiol Renal Physiol. 2020;318(2):F354–62. https://doi.org/10.1152/ajprenal.00408.2019.
28. Crawford A, Tripp DA, Nickel JC, Carr L, Moldwin R, Katz L et al. Depression and helplessness impact interstitial cystitis/bladder pain syndrome pain over time. Canadian Urological Association journal = Journal de l'Association des urologues du Canada. 2019;13(10):328–33. https://doi.org/10.5489/cuaj.5703.
29. McKernan LC, Walsh CG, Reynolds WS, Crofford LJ, Dmochowski RR, Williams DA. Psychosocial co-morbidities in Interstitial Cystitis/Bladder Pain syndrome (IC/BPS): a systematic review. Neurourol Urodyn. 2018;37(3):926–41. https://doi.org/10.1002/nau.23421.

23

Overexpression of miR-340 inhibits cell proliferation and induces apoptosis of human bladder cancer via targeting Glut-1

Gang Xu, Shouhua Pan*, Zhirong Zhu and Junlong Li

Abstract

Background: Bladder cancer (BC) has high mortality due to distant metastasis. Previous works suggested that microRNA (miRNA)-340 is a critical regulator for the development and progression of various cancers. The specific biological function of miR-340 in BC is little known.

Methods: In the present study, RT-qPCR was performed to measure the expression of miR-340 in paired BC tissues and adjacent non-tumor tissues. Next, the target gene of miR-340 was identified using dual-luciferase reporter assay and its level was also tested in tissues. Moreover, cell proliferation and apoptosis were analyzed by CCK-8 and flow cytometry. Finally, the expression of PCNA, Bax was detected by RT-qPCR and western blotting, as well as PI3K/AKT signaling measured by western blotting.

Result: The results demonstrated that miR-340 expression was downregulated and its target Glut-1 level was upregulated in BC tissues. Functionally, overexpression of miR-340 suppressed the proliferation and induced apoptosis in BC cells, while Glut-1 reversed the suppression of proliferation or induction of apoptosis induced by miR-340. Additionally, miR-340 repressed PCNA, p-PI3K and p-AKT levels but enhanced Bax level, while Glut-1 rescued the effects.

Conclusion: In conclusion, miR-340 functions as a tumor suppressor of BC, which inhibited proliferation and induced apoptosis by targeting Glut-1 partly through regulating PCNA, Bax expression and PI3K/AKT pathway. This study suggested that miR-340 is a potential target for the treatment of BC.

Keywords: Bladder cancer, miR-340, Glut-1, Proliferation, Apoptosis

Introduction

Bladder cancer (BC) is the ninth most general malignancy in the worldwide with the thirteenth deadliest [1]. BC can be divided into most common type: transitional cell carcinoma (more than 90%) and less common type: squamous cell carcinoma (5%) and adenocarcinoma (less than 2%) [2]. The incidence of this disease is higher in males than females because of the high prevalence of smoking [3]. The other risk factors for BC include age, body weight, lifestyle, and heredity [4]. Most patients with advanced disease develop metastasis including lymph nodes, bone, lung, liver, and peritoneum, and the 5-year survival rate is 96% for preinvasive carcinoma, but only 5% in distant metastasis unfortunately [5]. Although diagnosis and treatment for BC has little progress in recent 30 years [6], the emergence of immunotherapy, biomarkers and advanced imaging is hopeful for improving treatment effects for patients with BC [7]. To data, only a few of BC biomarkers are approved for clinical use [8], so it is urgent to find more meaningful targets for early screening and treatment of BC.

*Correspondence: 13606550587@163.com
Department of Urology, Shaoxing People's Hospital (Shaoxing Hospital, Zhejiang University School of Medicine), No. 568, Zhongxing North Road, Shaoxing 312000, Zhejiang, China

MicroRNAs (miRNAs) are a class of 20–30 nucleotides (nt), noncoding RNAs that regulate endogenous genomes expression and function [9]. They regulate gene expression through targeting mRNA cleavage or translational repression, and mediate cell proliferation, apoptosis, differentiation and metabolism [10]. Aberrantly expressed miRNAs are usually observed in clinical tissues, urine and blood of patients with BC, which is associated with tumor stage, recurrence and chemosensitivity [11]. These abnormal miRNAs play important role in BC development, progression and metastasis, as well as diagnostic and prognostic biomarkers [12]. MiR-340 is a multifunctional miRNA, which is involved in several diseases' programs, such as activity-based anorexia [13], Parkinson's disease [14], endometrial fibrosis [15] and human cancers [16–18]. For example, in pediatric patients with osteosarcoma, Cai et al. reported that miR-340-low/ROCK1-high mRNA is associated with poorer OS and PFS, which is an independent prognostic factor according to multi-variants analysis [19]. Danilo Fiore et al. reported that miR-340 could predict glioblastoma survival and modulates key cancer hallmarks through down-regulation of NRAS in glioblastoma [20]. Huang et al. reported that MiR-340 could inhibit prostate cancer cell proliferation and metastasis by targeting the MDM2-p53 pathway [21]. MicroRNA-340 could induce apoptosis and inhibit metastasis of ovarian cancer cells by inactivation of NF-κB1 [22]. MicroRNA-340 could inhibit the growth and invasion of angiosarcoma cells by targeting SIRT7 [23]. Loss of miR-340 function could enhanced lactate secretion and glucose uptake rate [16]. Jian et al. suggested that knockdown of Glut-1 in osteosarcoma cell could inhibited cell growth in vitro [7]. Xu and coworkers reported that miR-340 could accelerate tumor cell glycolysis and promote cell growth and proliferation via increasing the expression of Glut-1 in oral squamous cell carcinoma [24]. Though promising, most miR-340 related studies are still in early stage currently and it is little known about the role of miR-340 in BC. In the present study, we studied the relationship between miR-340 expression and Glut-1 in BC tissues cells.

Materials and methods

Tissue samples collection

BC tissues and adjacent normal tissues were obtained after resection from 30 cases of patients who underwent surgery at Shaoxing People's Hospital. These samples were immediately frozen in liquid nitrogen and stored at -80°C refrigerator. Written informed consent was provided by all patients participated in our study. This study was approved by the Ethic Committee of Shaoxing People's Hospital.

Cell culture

Human BC cell line T24 was purchased from American Type Culture Collection (ATCC; Manassas, VA, USA). T24 cells were cultured in RPMI 1640 medium supplemented with 10% fetal bovine serum (FBS) and 1% penicillin–streptomycin (All reagents were acquired from Hyclone, South Logan, UT, USA). The cultured condition of cells was maintained at 37°C in a humidified atmosphere containing 5% CO_2.

Dual-luciferase reporter assay

The target of miR-340 was predicted by bioinformatics online tool TargetScan Human 7.2 (http://www.targetscan.org/vert_72/) and verified by dual-luciferase reporter assay. MiR-340 mimics and its matched negative control (miR-NC mimics) were purchased from GeneCopoeia (Rockville, MD, USA). pGL3 vector (Promega, Madison, WI, USA) containing wild-type (WT) binding site of Glut-1 or mutant type of Glut-1 was co-transfected with miR-340 mimics or miR-NC mimics into T24 cells using Lipofectamine 2000 (Invitrogen, Carlsbad, CA, USA). 48 h later, Luc-Pair Duo-Luciferase Assay Kit was used to detect Firefly luciferase and Renilla luciferase activities (GeneCopoeia). Renilla luciferase activity was performed as the endogenous control.

Transient transfection

The coding sequence of Glut-1 was cloned into pcDNA3.1 plasmid, termed as pcDNA3.1-Glut-1. T24 cells were seeded into 6-well plates at the density of 2×10^5 cells/well. After cells growth to 80% confluence, miR-340 mimics, miR-NC mimics, pcDNA3.1 and pcDNA3.1-Glut-1 were transfected into T24 cells using Lipofectamine 2000 (Invitrogen) following manufacturer's protocol. After transfection of 48 h, the cells were collected for further study.

RT-qPCR

Total RNA was isolated from tissues and T24 cells using RNAsimple Total RNA Kit (Tiangen, Beijing, China). The purity of RNA was detected at OD260/OD280, and the integrality was visualized by agarose gel electrophoresis. The reverse transcription was determined by FastQuant RT Super Mix (Tiangen). Then SuperReal PreMix Plus (SYBR Green) (Tiangen) was used to examine the miR-340, Glut-1, PCNA and Bax expression through ABI PRISM 7700 Real-time PCR system (Applied Biosystems, Foster City, CA, USA) with the reaction condition as follows: 95°C for 15 min, 40 cycles of 95°C for 10 s and 60°C for 32 s. The expression of U6 and GAPDH was detected as the normalization for miR-340 and other mRNAs, respectively. The fold change of relative expression was calculated by using $2^{-\Delta\Delta Ct}$ method.

Western blotting

Total protein was extracted from tissues and cells using RIPA lysis buffer (Solarbio, Beijing, China) and the concentration was estimated by BCA Protein Assay Kit (Solarbio). Equal amount of extracted protein samples was loaded on 10% SDS-PAGE and subsequently transferred to PVDF membrane (Millipore, Billerica, MA, USA). Afterwards, the membranes were blocked with TBST mixed with 5% non-fat milk, incubated with primary antibodies overnight at 4°C, and then incubated with secondary antibodies for 1 h at room temperature. All primary antibodies including anti-Glut-1, anti-PCNA, anti-Bax, anti-PI3K, anti-p-PI3K, anti-AKT, anti-p-AKT, anti-GAPDH and secondary antibody were purchased from Abcam (Cambridge, MA, USA). GAPDH was used as the loading control. Finally, each protein signals were visualized using ECL chemiluminescence detection kit (Jining Shiye, Shanghai, China).

Cell proliferation and apoptosis analysis

After cells were trandfected with miR-340 mimics, miR-NC mimics and pcDNA3.1-Glut-1, cell proliferation and apoptosis were assessed by Cell Counting Kit-8 (CCK-8; Dojindo, Kumamoto, Japan) and Annexin V-APC/7-AAD Apoptosis Detection Kit (MultiSciences, Hangzhou, China). Briefly, cell proliferation was detected at cells incubated at 37°C with 5% CO_2 for 0 h, 12 h, 24 h and 48 h. Each well was added with 10 μl CCK-8 solution and continued to incubate for 2 h. A microplate reader was used to measure the OD value at the wavelength of 450 nm. For cell apoptosis, transfected cells were washed twice with PBS and resuspended with 100 μl binding buffer. After that, 5 μl Annexin V-APC and 10 μl 7-AAD staining solution were added to incubated with cells for 15 min at room temperature. After adding 380 μl binding buffer, the samples were analyzed using flow cytometry.

Data analysis

All data was analyzed by Graphpad Prism 6.0 La Jolla, CA, USA) from at least three independent experiments, and showed as mean ± SEM. The differences were assessed by Student's t-test and one-way ANOVA between two groups or multiple groups. The statistical significance was defined by $P < 0.05$.

Results

Downregulation of miR-340 is found in BC tissues

To investigate the role of miR-340 in BC, 30 pairs of tumor tissues and matched non-tumor tissues were collected from patients with BC. The corresponding baseline characteristics was shown in Additional file 14: Table S1. The results of RT-qPCR showed that the expression of miR-340 was decreased in BC tissues, compared with adjacent tissues ($P < 0.01$; Fig. 1A).

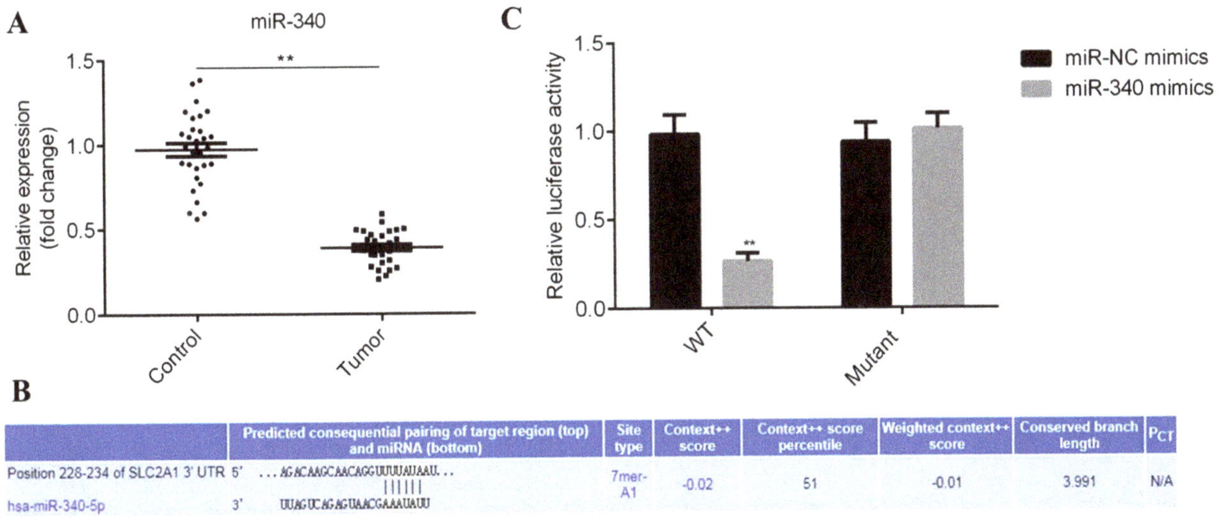

Fig. 1 Glut-1 is a potential target of miR-340. **A** MiR-340 expression is downregulated in BC tissues, which was detected by RT-qPCR in both tumor tissues and corresponding adjacent normal tissues collected a total of 30 cases of patients with BC. **$P < 0.01$. **B** The binding site between miR-340 and 3'UTR of Glut-1 was predicted by TargetScan. **C** The relative luciferase reporter assay was measured after T24 cells co-transfection of miR-340 mimics or miR-NC mimics together with WT-Glut-1 or mutant-Glut-1with dual-luciferase reporter assay. **$P < 0.01$

MiR-340 targets Glut-1 in BC cells

Through the bioinformatics online tool TargetScan Human 7.2, Glut-1 was screened as a potential target of miR-340. Glut-1 is an integral membrane protein providing glucose pass through plasma membrane down its concentration gradient. As shown in Fig. 1B, miR-340 could bind to the 3'-UTR of Glut-1 at the position of 228–234 nt, but not the mutant position of 3'UTR. Moreover, the results of dual-luciferase reporter assay demonstrated that the relative luciferase activity was weakened by overexpression of miR-340 when cells cotransfected with WT type of Glut-1 3'UTR, compared with miR-NC mimics ($P<0.01$), which was not affected when Glut-1 3'UTR was mutant (Fig. 1C).

The expression of Glut-1 is increased in BC tissues and negatively regulated by miR-340 in BC cells

Then we detected the expression of Glut-1 in BC tissues by RT-qPCR and western blotting. The mRNA level of Glut-1 is upregulated in tumor tissues, compared with corresponding para-carcinoma tissues ($P<0.01$; Fig. 2A). Similarly, Glut-1 protein level was also elevated in BC tissues (Fig. 2B). In addition, after T24 teansfected with miR-340 mimics and miR-NC mimics, the level of miR-340 is significantly increased in miR-340 mimics group, compared with miR-NC mimics ($P<0.01$; Fig. 2C), meanwhile the expression of Glut-1 was downregulated in miR-340 mimics group ($P<0.01$; Fig. 2D, E).

Overexpression of miR-340 inhibits BC cell proliferation and enhances apoptosis through targeting Glut-1 in vitro

To explore the function role of miR-340 and Glut-1, pcDNA3.1-Glut-1 and pcDNA3.1 were also transfected into T24 cells, and transfection efficiency was examined. Glut-1 level was increased in pcDNA3.1-Glut-1 group, compared with pcDNA3.1 group ($P<0.01$; Fig. 3A, B). Importantly, the results of CCK-8 demonstrated that cell proliferation was suppressed after 48 h by overexpression of miR-340, compared with miR-NC mimics ($P<0.01$), which was reversed by restoration of Glut-1 (Fig. 3C). Inversely, the data of flow cytometry indicated that cell apoptosis was induced by miR-340 mimics ($P<0.01$), which was abolished by pcDNA3.1-Glut-1 (Fig. 3D).

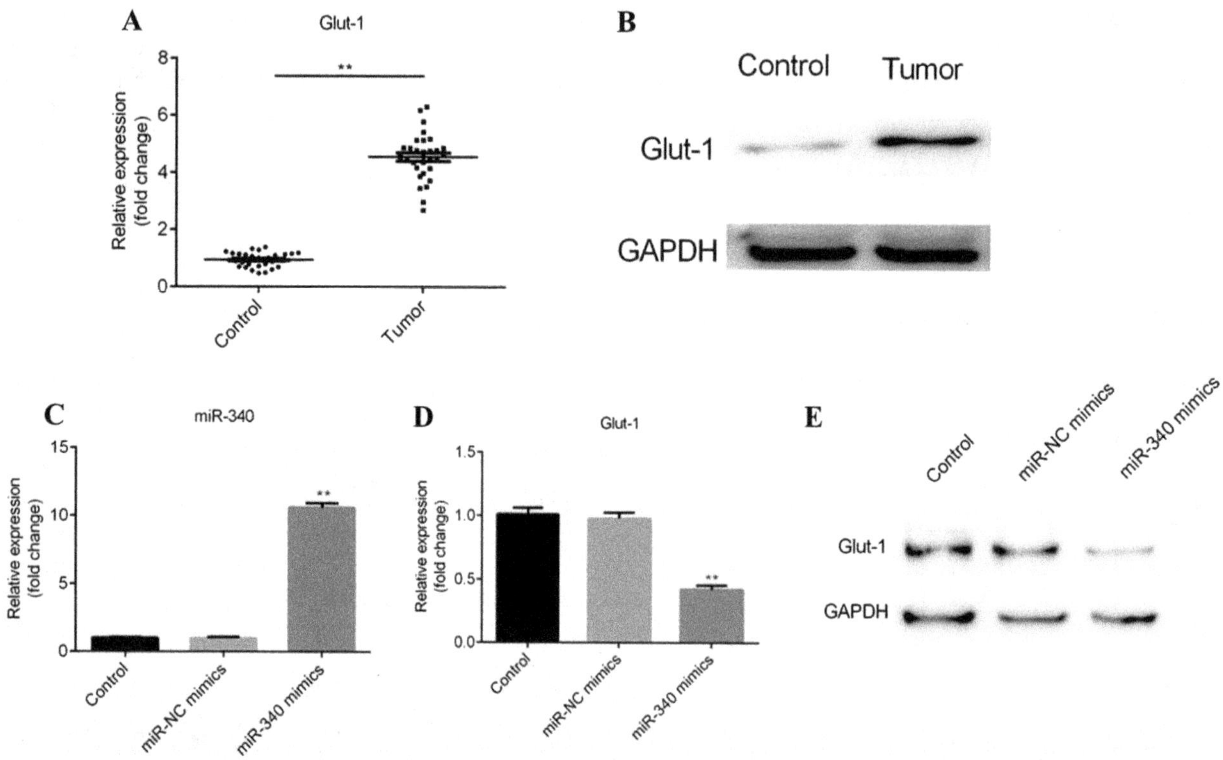

Fig. 2 The level of Glut-1 was found to be upregulated in BC tissues and negatively regulated by miR-340 overexpression. **A** and **B** The mRNA and protein expression of Glut-1 was tested in 30 pairs of BC tissues and adjacent normal tissues by RT-qPCR and western blotting, respectively. Full length blots/gels are presented in Additional file 1: Fig. S1–Additional file 2: Fig. S2. **C** The transfection efficiency was examined by RT-qPCR after T24 cells transfection of miR-340 mimics and miR-NC mimics for 48 h. **D** and **E** The mRNA and protein levels of Glut-1 were detected using RT-qPCR and western blotting after T24 cells transfection of miR-340 mimics and miR-NC mimics. $^{**}P<0.01$. Full length blots/gels are presented in Additional file 3: Fig. S3–Additional file 4: Fig. S4

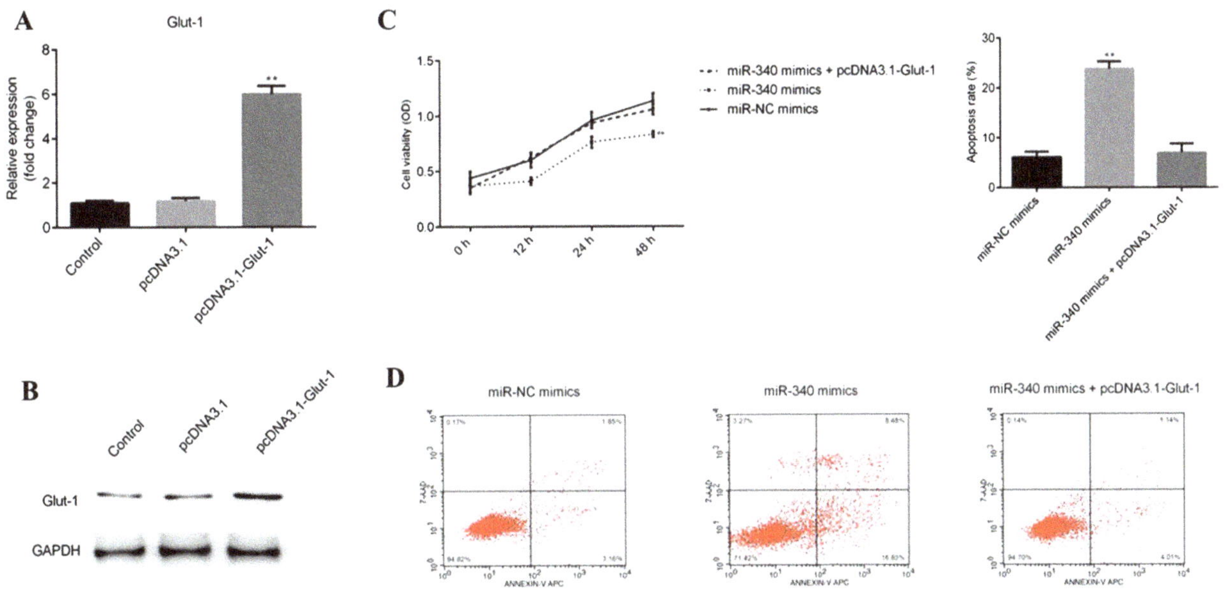

Fig. 3 MiR-340 targets Glut-1 to suppress the proliferation and promote apoptosis in BC cell line. **A** and **B** The transfection efficiency was tested after T24 cells transfected with pcDNA3.1 and pcDNA3.1-Glut-1 using RT-qPCR and western blotting. Full length blots/gels are presented in Additional file 5: Fig. S5–Additional file 6: Fig. S6. **C** Cell proliferation was measured at transfected cells incubated for 0, 12, 24 and 48 h using CCK-8 assay. **D** Cell apoptosis was tested by flow cytometry after transfected cells incubated for 24 h, and cell apoptosis rate was quantified. **P < 0.01

MiR-340 regulates PCNA, Bax expression and PI3K/AKT signaling pathway through targeting Glut-1

Finally, the expression of PCNA and Bax was tested by RT-qPCR and western blotting. As shown in Fig. 4A, B, overexpression of miR-340 repressed PCNA level but enhanced Bax level ($P<0.01$), while Glut-1 reversed the inhibitory effects on PCNA and the enhancement on Bax induced by miR-340. Similarly, the changes of protein expression of PCNA and Bax were consistent with those of mRNA (Fig. 4C). In addition, overexpression of mir-340 resulted in a decreased phosphorylation of PI3K and AKT, which was rescued by Glut-1 restoration, while total PI3K and AKT expression was not affected by miR-340 and Glut-1 (Fig. 4C).

Discussion

MiR-340 is commonly functions as a tumor suppressor in human cancers, which regulates cellular processes such as proliferation, apoptosis, migration and invasion. For example, miR-340 reduced cell viability and proliferation, and induced cell apoptosis of gastric cancer [25]. Additionally, overexpression of miR-340 suppressed cell proliferation, migration and invasion through targeting NT5E of gallbladder cancer [26]. Moreover, miR-340 could block hepatocellular carcinoma cell proliferation and promote apoptosis via regulating DcR3 expression [27]. Similarly, in the present study, miR-340 expression was lower in BC tissues than that in matched normal tissues, and overexpression of miR-340 inhibited T24 cell proliferation and enhanced apoptosis, which suggested that miR-340 also functions as a tumor suppressor in BC.

This study also revealed the underlying molecular mechanism. Glut-1 is a potential target of miR-340, which was predicted by TargetScan and verified by dual-luciferase reporter assay. Glucose transporter (Glut) proteins are the first rate-limiting step for glucose metabolism in mammalian cells, and overexpression of Glut-1 is associated with increased glucose transport, thus accelerating metabolism and accelerating glucose uptake and promoting malignant cell growth [28]. Recent years, Glut-1 is reported to be highly expressed in several human cancer types including but not limited to nasopharyngeal cancer [29], gastric cancer [30] and breast cancer [31]. Also, overexpressed of Glut-1 in malignant predicts poor prognosis [32–34]. In BC, the upregulation of Glut-1 is an independent prognostic factor and related to a low survival rate [35, 36]. However, the biological function of Glut-1 in BC is still unknown. In the present study, we confirmed that Glut-1 level was increased in BC tissues. Moreover, overexpression of miR-340 induced the downregulation of Glut-1, and restoration of Glut-1 reversed the inhibition of proliferation and the promotion of apoptosis induced by miR-340 in BC cells. These results suggested that miR-340 has suppressive effects on BC through targeting Glut-1.

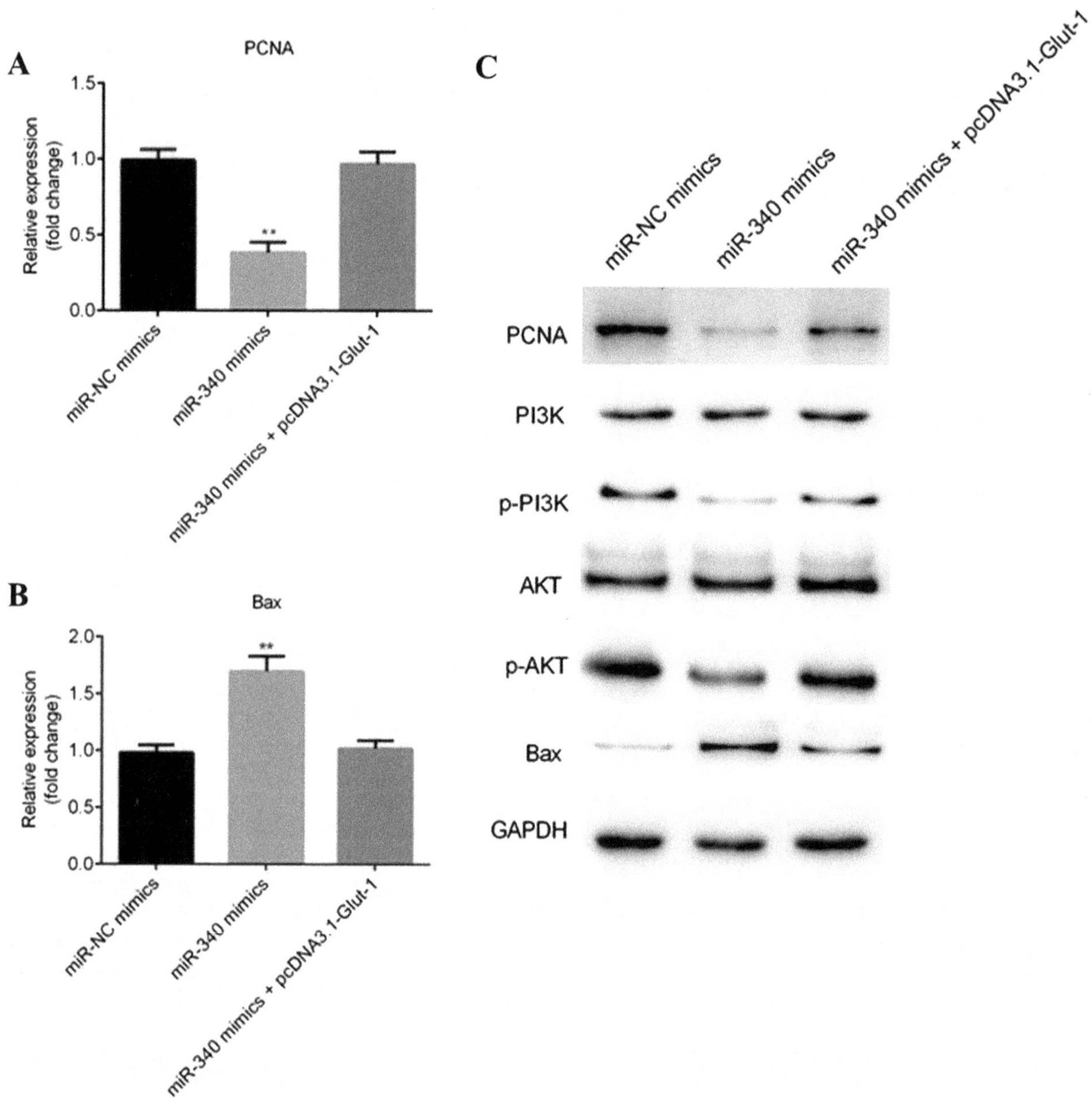

Fig. 4 Upregulation of miR-340 targets Glut-1 to regulate PCNA and Bax levels, as well as PI3K/AKT pathway. **A** and **B** The expression of PCNA and Bcl-2 at mRNA level was detected by RT-qPCR. **C** The protein levels of PCNA, Bcl-2 and PI3K/AKT pathway related factors such as PI3K, p-PI3K, AKT and p-AKT were detected by western blotting. GAPDH was used as the internal control. $^{**}P < 0.01$. Full length blots/gels are presented in Additional file 7: Fig S7–Additional file 13: Fig. S13

Accumulating evidence shows that numerous miRNAs are related to molecular and cellular mechanism of BC, besides miR-340. Previous works suggested that down-regulation of miR-145 and upregulation of miR-21 in bladder cancer. Prognostic relationships were seen with miRs-133b/129/518c. High-grade tumors were characterized by upregulation of miR-21, which probably reflected a p53-targeting role. Prognostic relationships were seen with miRs-133b/129/518c. MiRNAs appear to be important modulators of urologic cancer.

In this study, PCNA, p-PI3K and p-AKT levels were repressed, and Bax level was elevated by miR-340 but reversed by Glut-1, which suggested that miR-340 has suppressive effect on proliferation and promoting effect on apoptosis through decreasing PCNA expression, increasing Bax expression and inactivating PI3K/AKT signaling pathway. PCNA, a eukaryotic replication accessory factor, plays a critical role in cell cycle, apoptosis and proliferation in many types of human cancers [37]. Bax is a pro-apoptotic member of the Bcl-2 family, which is important for tumor therapy by regulating its expression [38]. The PI3K/AKT pathway is a commonly altered signaling network in cancers, and inhibition of AKT activity contributes to anticancer therapy [39]. These results suggested that PCNA, Bax and PI3K/AKT pathway associated with the cell growth and cell apoptosis, even though the potential mechanism between miR-340 and PCNA, Bax or PI3K/AKT pathway is still unclear. In view of the intrinsic property of pre-clinical study, several limitations existed, such as the small number of BC tissue samples and lack of analysis per grade, tumor stage and cancer type (invasiveness vs non-invasiveness) in the present work. Lack of animal experiment is another limitation, which should be investigated in next step.

In conclusion, our study revealed that miR-340 in BC functions as a tumor suppressor. Overexpression of miR-340 resulted in the decreased expression of target gene Glut-1, subsequently inhibited the proliferation and induced apoptosis partly through repressing PCNA, promoted Bcl-2 expression and inactivating PI3K/AKT signaling pathway of BC. This study revealed that miR-340 is a potential therapeutic target for the treatment of BC.

Supplementary Information

Additional file 1. Fig. S1: GAPDH.
Additional file 2. Fig. S2: Glut-1.
Additional file 3. Fig. S3: GAPDH.
Additional file 4. Fig. S4: Glut-1.
Additional file 5. Fig. S5: GAPDH.
Additional file 6. Fig. S6: Glut-1.
Additional file 7. Fig. S7: GAPDH.
Additional file 8. Fig. S8: Bax.
Additional file 9. Fig. S9: p-AKT.
Additional file 10. Fig. S10: AKT.
Additional file 11. Fig. S11: p-PI3K.
Additional file 12. Fig. S12: PI3K.
Additional file 13. Fig. S13: PCNA.
Additional file 14. Table S1: Baseline characteristics.

Acknowledgements

We especially appreciated Dr. ZQ Yan (3D Medicines Inc., Shanghai) and Dr. J Xia (3D Medicines Inc., Shanghai), who performed manuscript editing and review.

Authors' contributions

SH Pan conceived and designed this study. G Xu made contributions to data analysis and manuscript writing. ZR Zhu and JL Li helped with data collection and summary. All authors read and approved the final manuscript.

References

1. Berdik C. Unlocking bladder cancer. Nature. 2017;551(7679):S34-s35. https://doi.org/10.1038/551S34a.
2. Kaufman DS, Shipley WU, Feldman AS. Bladder cancer. The Lancet. 2009;374(9685):239–49. https://doi.org/10.1016/s0140-6736(09)60491-8.
3. Burger M, Catto JW, Dalbagni G, Grossman HB, Herr H, Karakiewicz P, et al. Epidemiology and risk factors of urothelial bladder cancer. Eur Urol. 2013;63(2):234–41. https://doi.org/10.1016/j.eururo.2012.07.033.
4. Smolensky D, Rathore K, Cekanova M. Molecular targets in urothelial cancer: detection, treatment, and animal models of bladder cancer. Drug Des Dev Ther. 2016;10:3305–22. https://doi.org/10.2147/dddt.S112113.
5. DeGeorge KC, Holt HR, Hodges SC. Bladder cancer: diagnosis and treatment. Am Fam Physician. 2017;96(8):507–14.
6. Grayson M. Bladder cancer. Nature. 2017;551(7679):S33. https://doi.org/10.1038/551S33a.
7. Smith AB. Recent developments in the management of bladder cancer: introduction. Urol Oncol. 2018;36(3):95–6. https://doi.org/10.1016/j.urolonc.2017.10.026.
8. Ghafouri-Fard S, Nekoohesh L, Motevaseli E. Bladder cancer biomarkers: review and update. Asian Pac J Cancer Prev. 2014;15(6):2395–403. https://doi.org/10.7314/apjcp.2014.15.6.2395.
9. Carthew RW, Sontheimer EJ. Origins and mechanisms of miRNAs and siRNAs. Cell. 2009;136(4):642–55. https://doi.org/10.1016/j.cell.2009.01.035.
10. Bartel DP. MicroRNAs: genomics, biogenesis, mechanism, and function. Cell. 2004;116(2):281–97. https://doi.org/10.1016/s0092-8674(04)00045-5.
11. Dong F, Xu T, Shen Y, Zhong S, Chen S, Ding Q, et al. Dysregulation of miRNAs in bladder cancer: altered expression with aberrant biogenesis procedure. Oncotarget. 2017;8(16):27547–68. https://doi.org/10.18632/oncotarget.15173.
12. Enokida H, Yoshino H, Matsushita R, Nakagawa M. The role of microRNAs in bladder cancer. Investig Clin Urol. 2016;57(Suppl 1):S60-76. https://doi.org/10.4111/icu.2016.57.S1.S60.
13. Schroeder M, Jakovcevski M, Polacheck T, Drori Y, Luoni A, Röh S, et al. Placental miR-340 mediates vulnerability to activity based anorexia in mice. Nat Commun. 2018;9(1):1596. https://doi.org/10.1038/s41467-018-03836-2.
14. Li Y, Wu J, Yu X, Na S, Li K, Yang Z, et al. The protective role of brain CYP2J in Parkinson's disease models. Oxid Med Cell Longev. 2018;2018:2917981. https://doi.org/10.1155/2018/2917981.
15. Xiao B, Zhu Y, Huang J, Wang T, Wang F, Sun S. Exosomal transfer of bone marrow mesenchymal stem cell-derived miR-340 attenuates endometrial fibrosis. Biol Open. 2019. https://doi.org/10.1242/bio.039958.
16. Huang D, Qiu S, Ge R, He L, Li M, Li Y, et al. miR-340 suppresses glioblastoma multiforme. Oncotarget. 2015;6(11):9257–70. https://doi.org/10.18632/oncotarget.3288.
17. Huang T, Zhou Y, Zhang J, Wong CC, Li W, Kwan JSH, et al. SRGAP1, a crucial target of miR-340 and miR-124, functions as a potential oncogene in gastric tumorigenesis. Oncogene. 2018;37(9):1159–74. https://doi.org/10.1038/s41388-017-0029-7.
18. Yang L, Men WL, Yan KM, Tie J, Nie YZ, Xiao HJ. MiR-340-5p is a potential prognostic indicator of colorectal cancer and modulates ANXA3. Eur Rev Med Pharmacol Sci. 2018;22(15):4837–45. https://doi.org/10.26355/eurrev_201808_15619.
19. Cai H, Lin L, Cai H, Tang M, Wang Z. Combined microRNA-340 and ROCK1 mRNA profiling predicts tumor progression and prognosis in pediatric osteosarcoma. Int J Mol Sci. 2014;15(1):560–73. https://doi.org/10.3390/ijms15010560.
20. Fiore D, Russo VAA, Donnarumma E, Roscigno G, Adamo A, Quintavalle C, Romano G, Greco A, Brunetti YS, Croce CM, Condorelli G, Iaboni M, De Martino F, Arturo A. miR-340 predicts glioblastoma survival and modulates key cancer hallmarks through down-regulation of NRAS; 2016.
21. Huang K, Tang Y, He L, Dai Y. MicroRNA-340 inhibits prostate cancer cell proliferation and metastasis by targeting the MDM2-p53 pathway. Oncol Rep. 2016;35(2):887–95. https://doi.org/10.3892/or.2015.4458.

22. Li P, Sun Y, Liu Q. MicroRNA-340 induces apoptosis and inhibits metastasis of ovarian cancer cells by inactivation of NF-x03BA;B1. Cell Physiol Biochem. 2016;38(5):1915–27. https://doi.org/10.1159/000445553.
23. Wang X, Song Y. MicroRNA-340 inhibits the growth and invasion of angiosarcoma cells by targeting SIRT7. Biomed Pharmacother. 2018;103:1061–8. https://doi.org/10.1016/j.biopha.2018.04.148.
24. Xu P, Li Y, Zhang H, Li M, Zhu H. MicroRNA-340 mediates metabolic shift in oral squamous cell carcinoma by targeting glucose transporter-1. J Oral Maxillofac Surg. 2016;74(4):844–50. https://doi.org/10.1016/j.joms.2015.09.038.
25. Yu J, Wang R, Chen J, Wu J, Dang Z, Zhang Q, et al. miR-340 inhibits proliferation and induces apoptosis in gastric cancer cell line SGC-7901, possibly via the AKT pathway. Med Sci Monit. 2017;23:71–7. https://doi.org/10.12659/msm.898449.
26. Wang N, Xiang X, Chen K, Liu P, Zhu A. Targeting of NT5E by miR-30b and miR-340 attenuates proliferation, invasion and migration of gallbladder carcinoma. Biochimie. 2018;146:56–67. https://doi.org/10.1016/j.biochi.2017.10.027.
27. Xie L, Chen Z, Liu H, Guan L, Wang Z, Li W. Effects of miR-340 on hepatocellular carcinoma by targeting the DcR3 gene. Dig Liver Dis. 2018;50(3):291–6. https://doi.org/10.1016/j.dld.2017.10.024.
28. Macheda ML, Rogers S, Best JD. Molecular and cellular regulation of glucose transporter (GLUT) proteins in cancer. J Cell Physiol. 2005;202(3):654–62. https://doi.org/10.1002/jcp.20166.
29. Zhou JC, Zhang JJ, Zhang W, Ke ZY, Ma LG, Liu M. Expression of GLUT-1 in nasopharyngeal carcinoma and its clinical significance. Eur Rev Med Pharmacol Sci. 2017;21(21):4891–5.
30. Schlößer HA, Drebber U, Urbanski A, Haase S, Baltin C, Berlth F, et al. Glucose transporters 1, 3, 6, and 10 are expressed in gastric cancer and glucose transporter 3 is associated with UICC stage and survival. Gastr Cancer. 2017;20(1):83–91. https://doi.org/10.1007/s10120-015-0577-x.
31. Jiwa LS, van Diest PJ, Hoefnagel LD, Wesseling J, Wesseling P, Moelans CB. Upregulation of Claudin-4, CAIX and GLUT-1 in distant breast cancer metastases. BMC Cancer. 2014;14:864. https://doi.org/10.1186/1471-2407-14-864.
32. Sharen G, Peng Y, Cheng H, Liu Y, Shi Y, Zhao J. Prognostic value of GLUT-1 expression in pancreatic cancer: results from 538 patients. Oncotarget. 2017;8(12):19760–7. https://doi.org/10.18632/oncotarget.15035.
33. Li CX, Sun JL, Gong ZC, Lin ZQ, Liu H. Prognostic value of GLUT-1 expression in oral squamous cell carcinoma: a prisma-compliant meta-analysis. Medicine. 2016;95(45): e5324. https://doi.org/10.1097/md.0000000000005324.
34. Cho H, Lee YS, Kim J, Chung JY, Kim JH. Overexpression of glucose transporter-1 (GLUT-1) predicts poor prognosis in epithelial ovarian cancer. Cancer Invest. 2013;31(9):607–15. https://doi.org/10.3109/07357907.2013.849722.
35. Palit V, Phillips RM, Puri R, Shah T, Bibby MC. Expression of HIF-1alpha and Glut-1 in human bladder cancer. Oncol Rep. 2005;14(4):909–13. https://doi.org/10.3892/or.14.4.909.
36. Boström PJ, Thoms J, Sykes J, Ahmed O, Evans A, van Rhijn BW, et al. Hypoxia marker GLUT-1 (glucose transporter 1) is an independent prognostic factor for survival in bladder cancer patients treated with radical cystectomy. Bladder Cancer. 2016;2(1):101–9. https://doi.org/10.3233/blc-150033.
37. Park SY, Jeong MS, Han CW, Yu HS, Jang SB. Structural and functional insight into proliferating cell nuclear antigen. J Microbiol Biotechnol. 2016;26(4):637–47. https://doi.org/10.4014/jmb.1509.09051.
38. Czabotar PE, Lessene G, Strasser A, Adams JM. Control of apoptosis by the BCL-2 protein family: implications for physiology and therapy. Nat Rev Mol Cell Biol. 2014;15(1):49–63. https://doi.org/10.1038/nrm3722.
39. Wang Q, Chen X, Hay N. Akt as a target for cancer therapy: more is not always better (lessons from studies in mice). Br J Cancer. 2017;117(2):159–63. https://doi.org/10.1038/bjc.2017.153.

24

Identification of prognostic and therapeutic value of CC chemokines in Urothelial bladder cancer: Evidence from comprehensive bioinformatics analysis

Yuxin Li[1,2], Xiong Chen[1,2], Dongjie Li[1,2], Zhiming Yang[1,2], Yao Bai[1,2], Sheng Hu[1,2], Zhenyu Liu[1,2], Jie Gu[1,2,4*] and XiaoBo Zhang[1,2,3*]

Abstract

Background: Urothelial bladder cancer (BC) is one of the most prevalent malignancies with high mortality and high recurrence rate. Angiogenesis, tumor growth and metastasis of multiple cancers are partly modulated by CC chemokines. However, we know little about the function of distinct CC chemokines in BC.

Methods: ONCOMINE, Gene Expression Profiling Interactive Analysis (GEPIA), Kaplan–Meier plotter, cBioPortal, GeneMANIA, and TIMER were used for analyzing differential expression, prognostic value, protein–protein interaction, genetic alteration and immune cell infiltration of CC chemokines in BC patients based on bioinformatics.

Results: The results showed that transcriptional levels of CCL2/3/4/5/14/19/21/23 in BC patients were significantly reduced. A significant relation was observed between the expression of CCL2/11/14/18/19/21/23/24/26 and the pathological stage of BC patients. BC patients with high expression levels of CCL1, CCL2, CCL3, CCL4, CCL5, CCL8, CCL13, CCL15, CCL17, CCL18, CCL19, CCL22, CCL25, CCL27 were associated with a significantly better prognosis. Moreover, we found that differentially expressed CC chemokines are primarily correlated with cytokine activity, chemokines receptor binding, chemotaxis, immune cell migration. Further, there were significant correlations among the expression of CC chemokines and the infiltration of several types of immune cells (B cells, CD8+ T cells, CD4+ T cells, macrophages, neutrophils, and dendritic cells).

Conclusions: This study is an analysis to the potential role of CC chemokines in the therapeutic targets and prognostic biomarkers of BC, which gives a novel insight into the relationship between CC chemokines and BC.

Keywords: Bioinformatics analysis, CC chemokines, Urothelial bladder cancer, Biomarker, Prognosis

Background

Bladder cancer is one of the most prevalent cancers, with an estimated 549,000 new cases and 200,000 deaths reported in 2018 [1]. Urothelial bladder cancer accounts for more than 90% of bladder cancer [2]. Typically, the main therapy strategies of bladder cancer comprise Transurethral resection of bladder tumor (TURBT), radiotherapy, chemotherapy, and immunotherapy [3–6] and with limited survival [7]. Besides, the high recurrence rate (up to 60–70%) [6] of Bladder cancer patients pose a heavy load on public health system [8]. Moreover, cystectomy, as the most important method of tumor treatment, is an invasive procedure.

*Correspondence: jiegu9292@163.com; zhangxb@csu.edu.cn
[1] Department of Geriatric Urology, Xiangya International Medical Center, Xiangya Hospital, Central South University, Changsha, Hunan 410008, People's Republic of China
Full list of author information is available at the end of the article

Cystectomy was not promising to increase the recurrence-free survival (RFS) and overall survival (OS) in the expected range even with extended removal of lymph nodes [9].

Chemokines, constituting the largest family of cytokines, are chemotactic cytokines that mediate immune cell migration and lymphoid tissue growth [10]. Sequencing and gene expression studies have found the CC chemokines may play an important role in the tumorigenesis and progression of distinct tumors [11–13]. Previous studies have identified several CC chemokines were associated with disease-specific survival [14], tumor growth and progression [12]. Studies interpreted that CC chemokines may affect the abundance, infiltration and accumulation of immune cells [15, 16]. Thus, CC chemokines have multiple functions in tumor progression and invasion, and they serve as prognostic biomarkers for many types of tumors, including BC. However, the expression and prognostic values of CC chemokines in BC still remain unclear.

In this study, we performed a comprehensive analysis of CC chemokines to evaluate their potential value as therapeutic targets and prognostic biomarkers based on several large public databases, thus supplying informative assistance to help clinicians select appropriate therapeutic drugs and more accurately prognosis in BC patients.

Methods

ONCOMINE

The mRNA levels of distinct CC chemokines in diverse cancer types were analysed in ONCOMINE (www.oncomine.org), an online database providing powerful, genome-wide expression analysis with cancer microarray information [17]. In this study, a p-value < 0.05, a fold change of 2, and a gene rank in the top 10% were set as the significance thresholds. The mRNA expression of CC chemokines in clinical cancer specimens were compared with those in normal controls. Student's t-test was used to analyze the difference in the expression of CC chemokines in BC.

GEPIA

GEPIA (http://gepia.cancer-pku.cn/index.html) is a new analytical tool using a standard processing pipeline and consist of thousands of tumors and normal tissue samples data [18]. In this research, a differential gene expression analysis of mRNA expression of tumor and normal tissues, pathological stage analysis, and correlative prognostic analysis through GEPIA. Student's t-test was used to generate a p-value for the expression or pathological stage analysis.

Kaplan–Meier plotter

The prognostic analysis of CC chemokines patients was also performed by using Kaplan–Meier plotter (http://kmplot.com/analysis/) [19], which is an online tool about the association of gene expression with the survival of patients. Data as the number-at-risk cases, median values of mRNA expression levels, HRs, 95% CIs and p-values can be obtained from the K–M plotter webpage. A statistically significant difference was considered when the p-value was < 0.05. Patient samples were split into two groups by median expression (high versus low expression) and assessed by a Kaplan–Meier survival plot.

cBioPortal

cBioPortal (www.cbioportal.org) is a comprehensive web resource, can visualize and analyze multidimensional cancer genomics data [20]. Based on The Cancer Genome Atlas (TCGA) database, genetic alterations, and co-expression of CC chemokines were obtained from cBioPortal.

String

STRING (https://string-db.org/) is a website that provides a comprehensive and objective global network of protein–protein interaction (PPI) [21]. A PPI network analysis was performed to collect and integrate the different expressions of CC chemokines and potential interactions through STRING.

GeneMANIA

GeneMANIA (http://www.genemania.org) is a website about gene information, analyzing gene lists and prioritizing genes for functional assays [22]. The potential interactions between different CC chemokines were analysed on it.

Timer

TIMER (https://cistrome.shinyapps.io/timer/) is web interface that provides systematic evaluations of the infiltration of different immune cells and their clinical impact [23]. In this study, "Gene module" was selected to evaluate the correlation between CC chemokines level and the infiltration of immune cells. "Survival module" was used to evaluate the correlation among clinical outcome and the infiltration of immune cells and CC chemokine expression.

Results

Expression of different CC chemokines BC

A total of 24 CC chemokines were retrieved using the ONCOMINE database. The distinct expression of 24

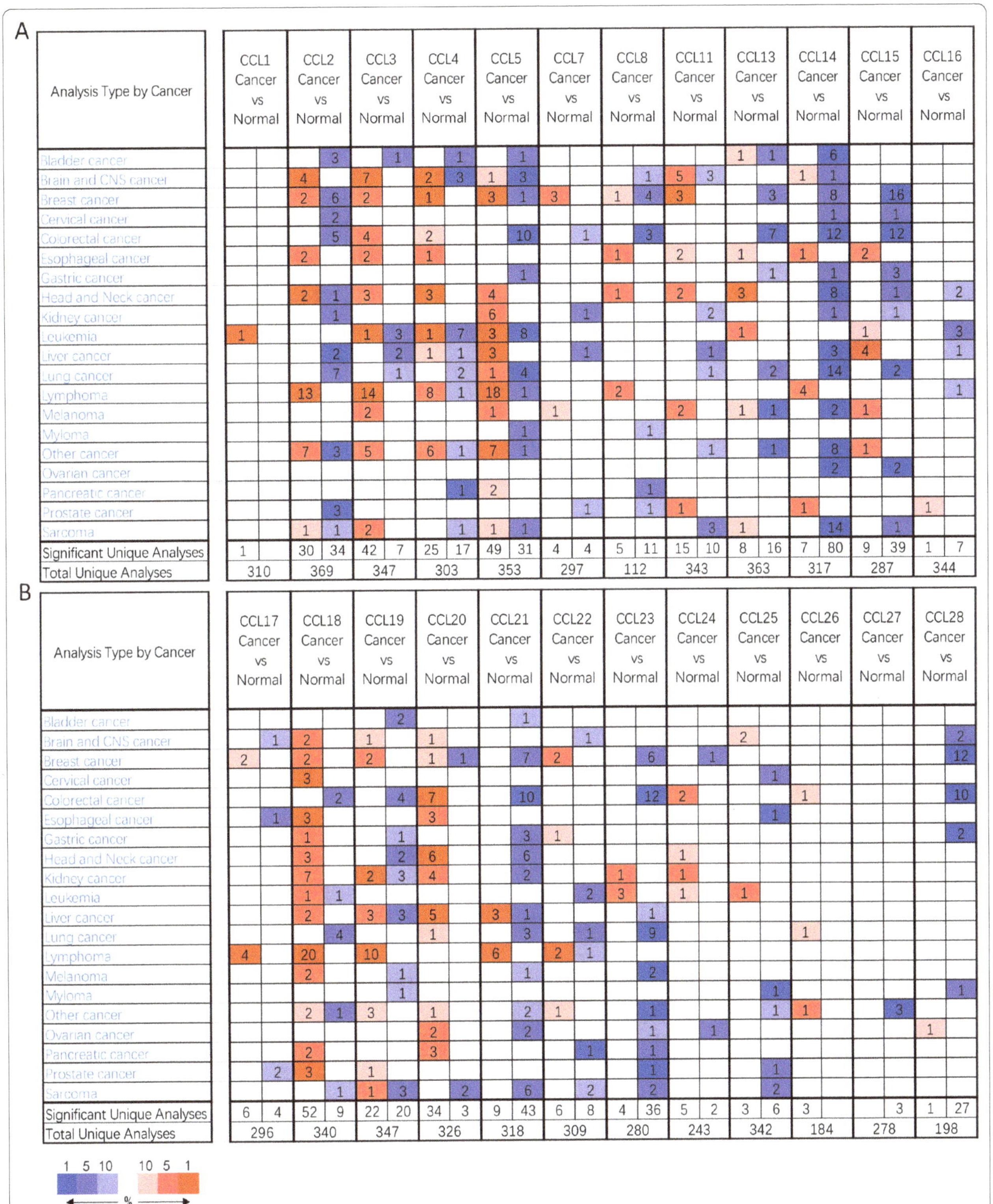

Fig. 1 **A** CCL1-CCL16, **B** CCL17-CCL28 mRNA levels of CC chemokines in BC (ONCOMINE). The figure shows the numbers of datasets with statistically significant mRNA over-expression (red) or downregulated expression (blue) of CC chemokines

CC chemokines in BC were explored. As presented in Fig. 1, the mRNA expression levels of CCL2, CCL3, CCL4, CCL5, CCL13, CCL14, CCL19 and CCL21 were significantly reduced in BC patients. But significantly increased CCL13 (P=0.011, Fold change=2.654) were also observed in BC compared with normal tissue. Similar results were found when we assessed the transcriptional levels of CC chemokines using the GEPIA database, CCL2, CCL14, CCL21 and CCL23 were lower in BC patients than normal patients (Fig. 2). We then evaluated the correlation between the expression of differentially expressed CC chemokines and the pathological stage of BC patients. The results revealed that CCL2 (Pr=2.53e−05), CCL11 (Pr=2.61e−08), CCL14 (Pr=6.35e−06), CCL18 (Pr=0.00218), CCL19 (Pr=0.00868), CCL21 (Pr=0.000135), CCL23 (Pr=0.0134), CCL24 (Pr=0.00147) and CCL26 (Pr=3.78e-06) may play a significant role in the tumorigenesis in BC patients (Fig. 3).

Prognostic value of the mRNA expression of CC chemokines in BC patients

We explored the value of differentially expressed CC chemokines in the progression of BC patients. According to the data from GEPIA (not including CCL1), patients with higher levels of CCL14 (P=0.0036) (Fig. 4) showed shorter overall survival (OS), but OS tended to be longer in patients with higher levels of CCL15 (P=0.00069) (Fig. 4). And current results did not show a significant relation between overall survival (OS) or Disease-free survival (DFS) and other CC chemokines.

Besides, we also analysed the prognostic values of CC chemokines using Kaplan–Meier plotter in BC patients (Fig. 5). Significantly increased OS and DFS were observed in patients with higher levels of CCL3, CCL4, CCL5, CCL13 or CCL27. Patients with higher levels of CCL1, CCL2, CCL8, CCL18, CCL19, CCL22, CCL24, or CCL25 were associated with increased DFS and higher levels of CCL15, CCL17 were correlated with longer OS. However, there is a significant negative correlation between CCL11, CCL24, CCL26 with OS and between CCL28 with DFS.

Genetic alteration, expression, and interaction analyses of CC chemokines in BC patients

We assessed the genetic alterations of CC chemokines in BC patients by using the eBioPortal online tool. CCL1, CCL2, CCL3, CCL4, CCL5, CCL7, CCL8, CCL11, CCL13, CCL14, CCL15, CCL16, CCL17, CCL18, CCL19, CCL20, CCL21, CCL22, CCL23, CCL24, CCL25, CCL26, CCL27 and CCL28 were altered in 2.6, 2.4, 1.8, 1.5, 1.4, 2.8, 2.2, 2.4, 2.7, 1.9, 2.1, 1.7, 0.6, 1.5, 1.6, 2.2, 2, 0.9, 1.6, 1.2, 0.7, 1.3, 1.9 and 5% of the queried BC samples, respectively (Fig. 6A). Furthermore, we conducted a PPI network analysis of the differentially expressed CC chemokines with STRING to evaluate the potential interactions among them. As illustrated in Fig. 6B, 157 edges and 24 nodes were obtained. The CC chemokines were mainly associated with chemokine signaling pathway and immune cell regulation. The GeneMANIA results revealed that these CC chemokines were related to cytokine activity, chemokines receptor binding, chemotaxis immune cell migration (Fig. 6C).

Immune cell infiltration of CC chemokines in BC patients

To explore the relation between immune cell level and cancer cell, the TIMER database are used to perform an analysis. The results (Fig. 7) indicated a high correlation between immune cell infiltration and CC chemokines as follows: CCL1 with $CD8^+$ T cells (ρ=0.10, P=4.71e−02), neutrophils (ρ=0.23, P=8.53e−06), and dendritic cells (ρ=0.168, P=1.19e−03); CCL2 with $CD4^+$ T cells (ρ=0.162, P=1.77e−03), $CD8^+$ T cells (ρ=0.1, P=2.08e−03), macrophages (ρ=0.197, P=1.47e−04), neutrophils (ρ=0.371, P=1.87e−13), and dendritic cells (ρ=0.311, P=1.12e−09); CCL3 with neutrophils (ρ=0.583, P=6.38e−35), and dendritic cells (ρ=0.601, P=1.61e−37); CCL4 with $CD8^+$ T cells (ρ=0.4, P=1.50e−15), neutrophils (ρ=0.671, P=2.12e−49), and dendritic cells (ρ=0.601, P=1.45e−37); CCL5 with $CD8^+$ T cells (ρ=0.359, P=1.26e−12), neutrophils (ρ=0.549, P=2.53e−30), and dendritic cells (ρ=0.471, P=1.12e−21); CCL7 with B cell (ρ=− 0.119, P=2.25e−02), $CD8^+$ T cells (ρ=0.362, P=7.78e−13), neutrophils (ρ=0.485, P=4.26e−23), macrophages (ρ=0.517, P=1.62e−26); CCL8 with $CD8^+$ T cells (ρ=0.388, P=1.06e−14), neutrophils (ρ=0.54, P=2.71e−29), and dendritic cells (ρ=0.541, P=2.45e−29); CC11 with $CD4^+$ T cells (ρ=0.112, P=3.24e−02), $CD8^+$ T cells (ρ=0.11, P=3.05e−02), macrophages (ρ=0.263, P=3.20e−07), neutrophils (ρ=0.158, P=2.40e−03), and dendritic cells (ρ=0.146, P=4.91e−03); CCL13 with $CD8^+$ T cells (ρ=0.302, P=3.46e−09), neutrophils (ρ=0.412, P=1.70e−16), and dendritic cells (ρ=0.468, P=2.00e−21); CCL14 with $CD4^+$ T cells (ρ=0.153, P=3.21e−03), $CD8^+$ T cells (ρ=− 0.204, P=7.81e−05), macrophages (ρ=0.188, P=2.78e−04), neutrophils (ρ=− 0.19, P=2.38e−04), and dendritic cells (ρ=− 0.225, P=1.36e−05); CCL15 with $CD8^+$ T cells (ρ=− 0.264, P=2.91e−07), neutrophils (ρ=− 0.271, P=1.25e−07), and dendritic cells (ρ=-0.304, P=2.68e-09); CCL16 with $CD8^+$ T cells (ρ=− 0.118, P=2.39e−02) and dendritic cells (ρ=− 0.209, P=5.56e−05); CCL17 with B cell (ρ=0.123, P=1.84e−02), $CD4^+$ T cells (ρ=0.247, P=1.67e−06),

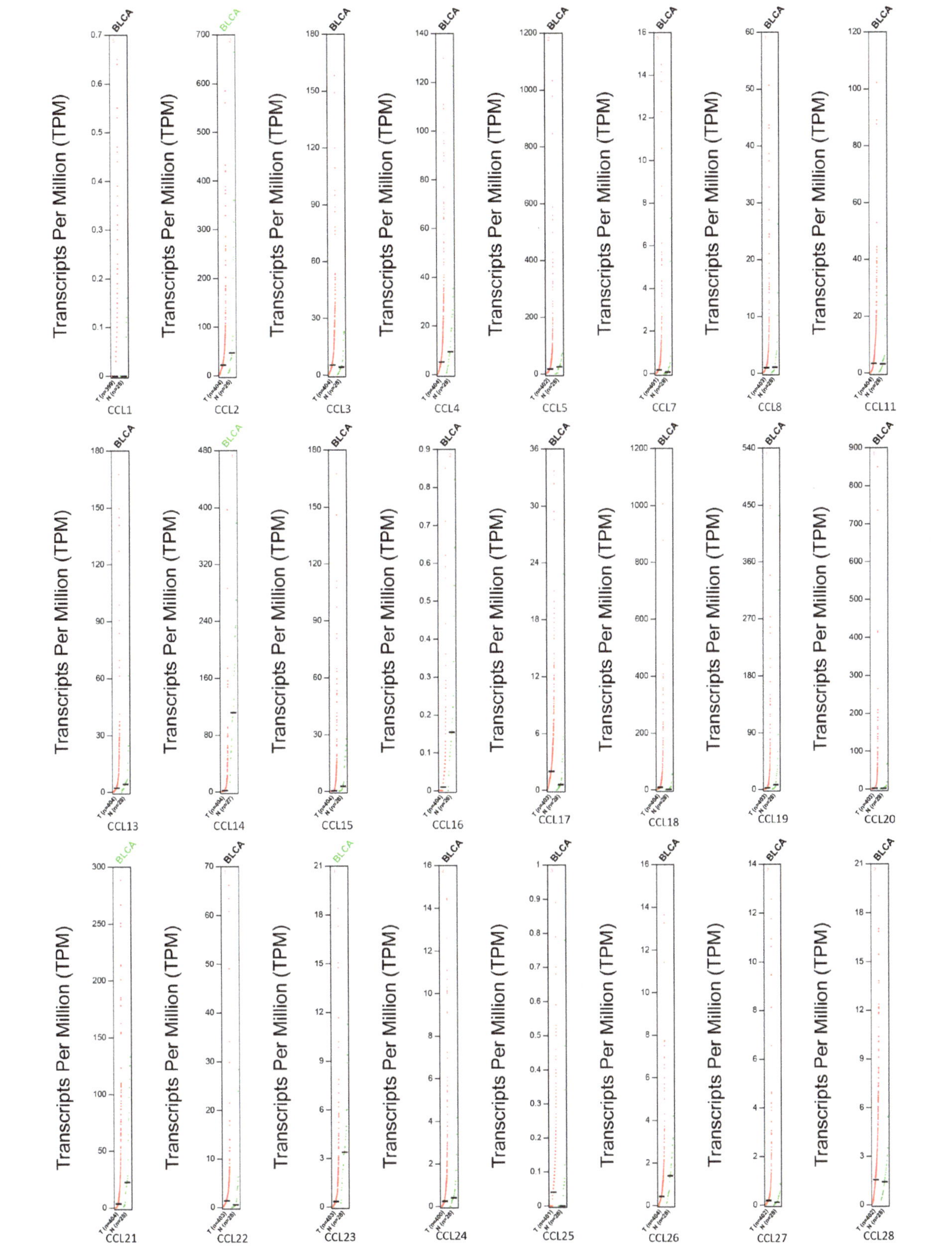

Fig. 2 The expression of CC chemokines in BC (GEPIA)

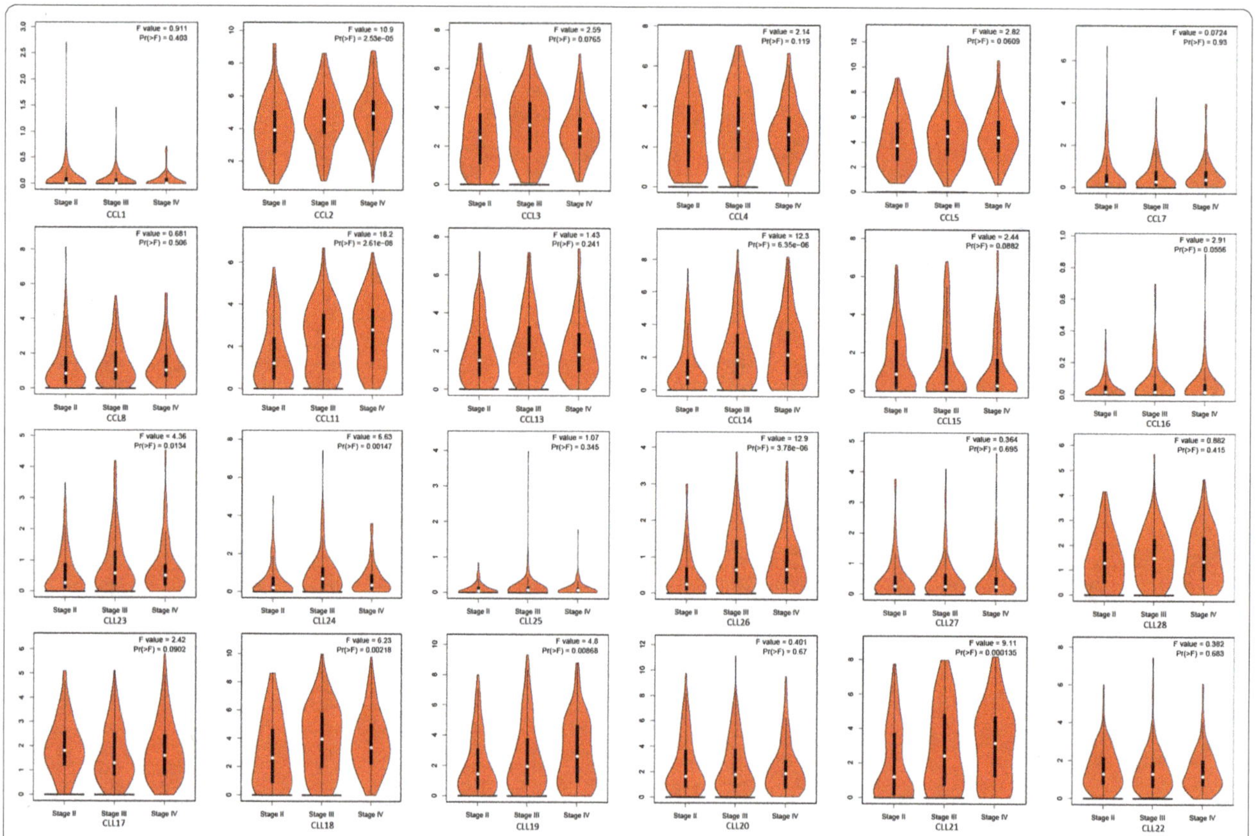

Fig. 3 Correlation between CC chemokines and tumor stage in BC patients (GEPIA)

$CD8^+$ T cells (ρ = − 0.221, P = 1.96e−05), and macrophages (ρ = − 0.197, P = 1.46e−04); CCL18 with $CD8^+$ T cells (ρ = 0.341, P = 1.71e−11), neutrophils (ρ = 0.432, P = 3.42e−18), and dendritic cells (ρ = 0.434, P = 2.42e−18); CCL19 with $CD4^+$ T cells (ρ = 0.281, P = 4.35e−08) and neutrophils (ρ = 0.126, P = 1.37e−02); CCL20 with $CD8^+$ T cells (ρ = 0.231, P = 7.9e−06), macrophages (ρ = − 0.141, P = 6.8e−03), neutrophils (ρ = 0.461, P = 1.02e−20), and dendritic cells (ρ = 0.343, P = 1.25e−11); CCL21 with $CD4^+$ T cells (ρ = 0.173, P = 8.64e−04), $CD8^+$ T cells (ρ = 0.149, P = 4.20e−03), neutrophils (ρ = 0.138, P = 7.96e−03), and dendritic cells (ρ = 0.186, P = 3.35e−04); CCL22 with $CD4^+$ T cells (ρ = 0.189, P = 2.72e−04), macrophages (ρ = −0.179, P = 5.54e−04), neutrophils (ρ = 0.316, P = 5.67e−10), and dendritic cells (ρ = 0.239, P = 3.39e−06); CCL23 with $CD4^+$ T cells (ρ = 0.123, P = 1.86e−02), $CD8^+$ T cells (ρ = 0.159, P = 2.22e−03), neutrophils (ρ = 0.338, P = 2.85e−11), and dendritic cells (ρ = 0.381, P = 4.56e−10); CCL24 with $CD8^+$ T cells (ρ = 0.234, P = 5.56e−06), macrophages (ρ = 0.116, P = 2.60e−02), neutrophils (ρ = 0.344, P = 1.17e−11), and dendritic cells (ρ = 0.275, P = 7.82e−08); CCL25 with B cell (ρ = 0.152, P = 3.51e−03), $CD4^+$ T cells (ρ = 0.104, P = 4.54e−02), neutrophils (ρ = 0.244, P = 2.19e−06), and dendritic cells (ρ = 0.151, P = 3.79e−03); CCL26 with B cell (ρ = − 0.207, P = 6.30e−05), $CD8^+$ T cells (ρ = 0.218, P = 2.49e−05), macrophages (ρ = 0.267, P = 1.99e−07), neutrophils (ρ = 0.189, P = 2.67e−04), and dendritic cells (ρ = 0.247, P = 1.66e−06); CCL27 with macrophages (ρ = − 0.136, P = 9.10e−03) and neutrophils (ρ = − 0.133, P = 1.07e−02); CCL28 with B cell (ρ = 0.103, P = 4.83e−02), $CD8^+$ T cells (ρ = 0.186, P = 3.35e−04), macrophages (ρ = 0.137, P = 8.34e−03), neutrophils (ρ = 0.194, P = 1.76e−04), and dendritic cells (ρ = 0.124, P = 1.74e-02).

Discussion

Bladder cancer is one of the most common causes of cancer-related deaths worldwide [24]. CC chemokines, which can be expressed by tumor cells and other cells, play an important role in the immune cell tumor trafficking [25–27], tumor metastasis [28] and apoptosis [29]. Accumulating evidence has revealed the potential value of CC chemokines in cancer immunotherapy. However, the prognostic and possible therapeutic value of CC chemokines in BC is not yet defined.

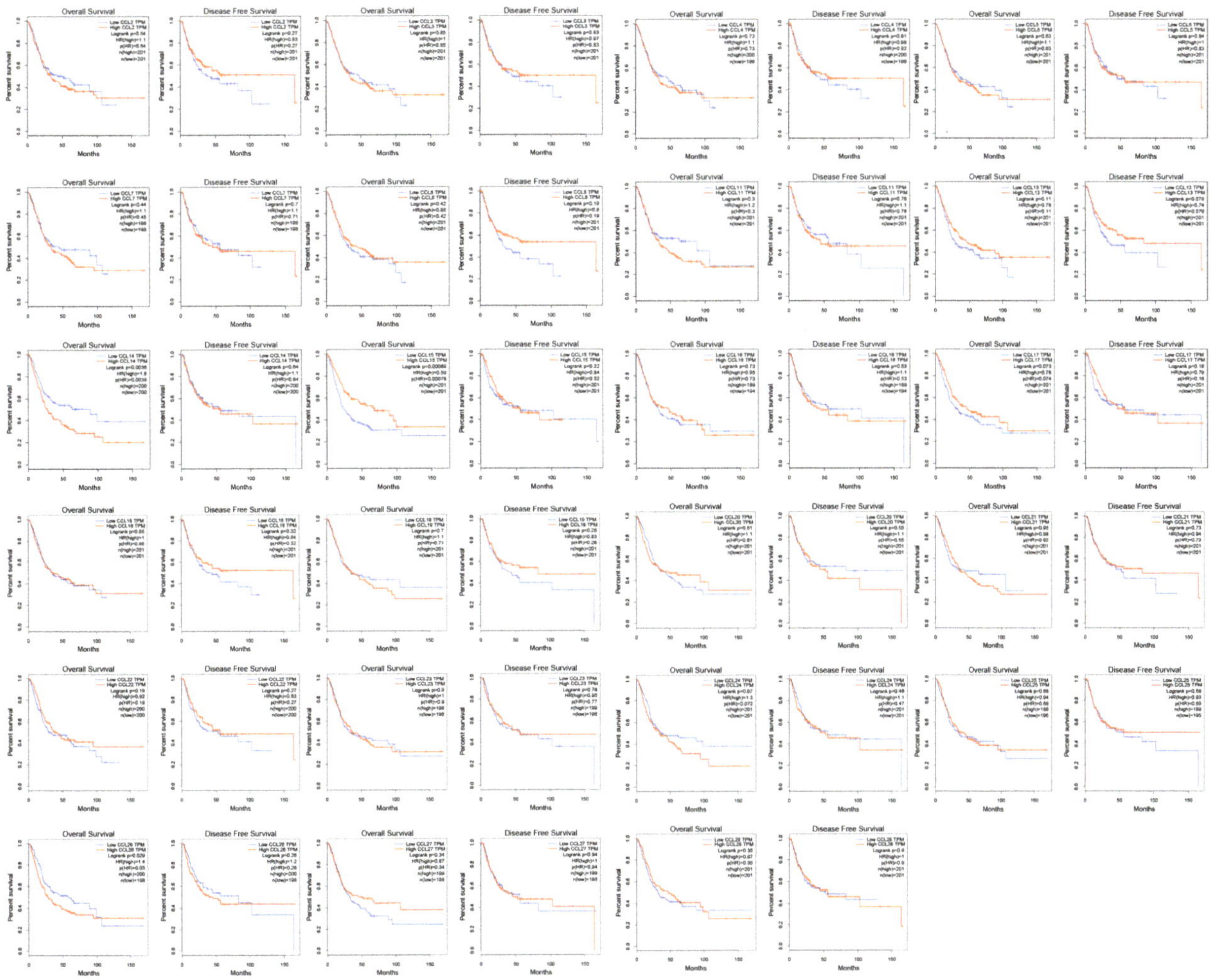

Fig. 4 The prognostic value of mRNA level of CC chemokines in BC patients (GEPIA)

Among the CC chemokines, CCL2 is the most studied in BC. Expression of CCL2 was higher in BC tissues and in human BC cell lines [30]. And this trend was obvious with the stage of BC [30]. The reduced expression of CCL2 downregulated by miR-1-3p could inhibit the metastasis and proliferation of BC cells [30]. Besides, animal experiment also proved the increased CCL2 expression in murine bladder cancer cell line [31]. Recent studies have revealed a negative relationship between prognosis, survival and CCL2 in BC patients received chemotherapy [16, 32]. While gemcitabine-treated BC cells also induced more CCL2 which may recruit more monocyte-myeloid-derived suppressed cells (M-MDSCs) and incurred poor prognosis [33]. Several studies demonstrated overexpression of CCL2 in bladder cancer was correlated with tumor invasion, tumor progression [34] and lymphatic metastasis [35]. HSP47 [36], LNMAT1 [35], ERβ [37] seem to be related to CCL2 directly or indirectly. While in this study, the results indicated that the expression level of CCL2 was reduced in BC than normal sample. Moreover, a low CCL2 expression was significantly correlated with poor DFS.

For the other CC chemokines, a previous study demonstrated that CCL1 can be up-regulated by estrogen receptors alpha and then enhance bladder cancer cell invasion [38]. CCL1/CCR axis was found to be correlated with cancer-related inflammation and immune evasion [39]. Besides, GAS5 may inhibit bladder cancer cell proliferation by suppressing the expression of CCL1 [40]. However, our results did not reveal a significant difference in CCL1 expression between BC and normal patients. In vitro experiments found that upregulated CCL3 inhibits the immune response which would favor tumor growth [31]. Interestingly, a higher CCL3 expression seems to be correlated with a better OS and DFS in our study. Steve et al. [41] found CCL18 was significantly increased in voided urine of BC, but it seems not related with bladder cancer grade nor stage [42]. There

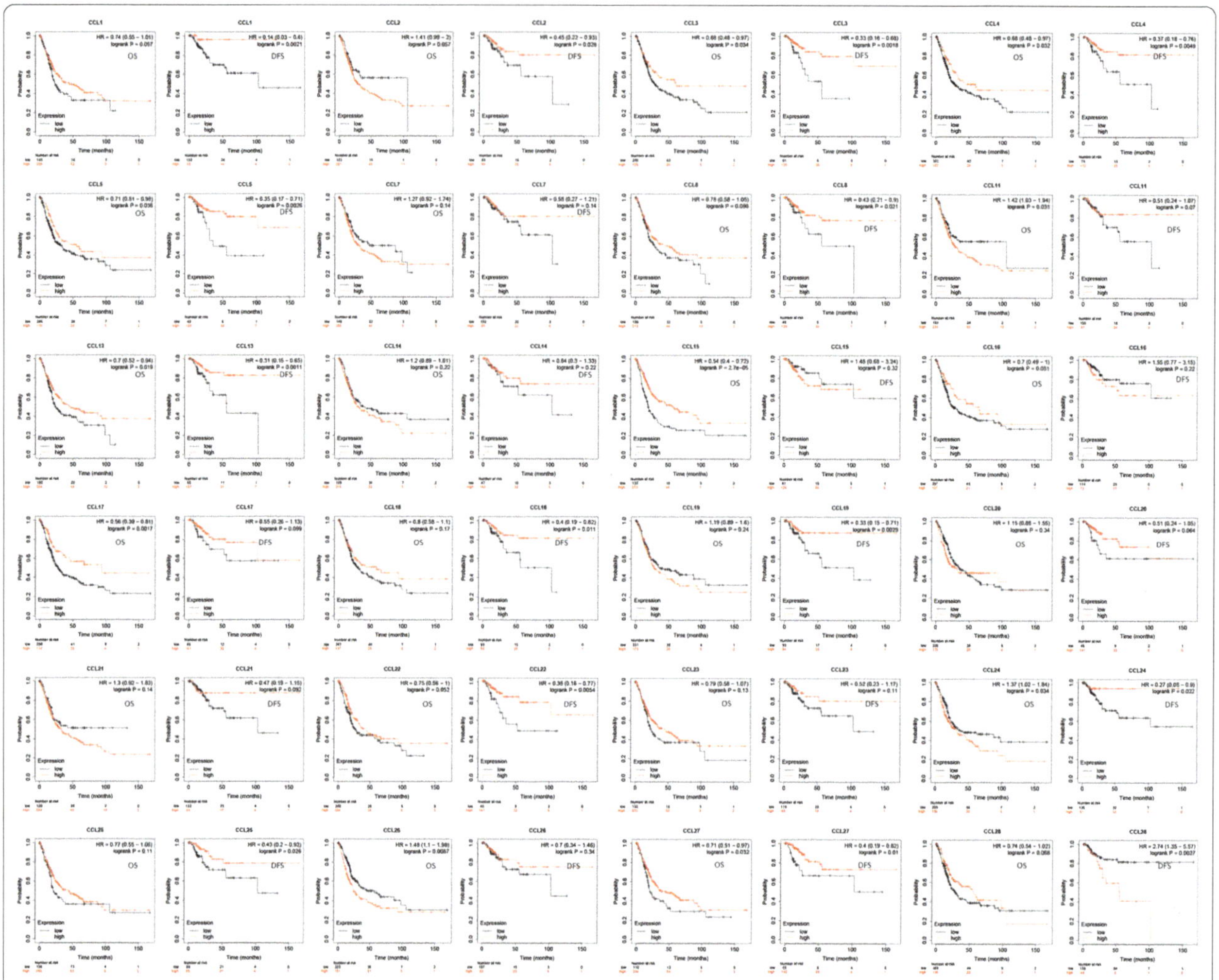

Fig. 5 Prognostic value of CC chemokines in BC Patients (Kaplan–Meier plotter)

are studies showed CCL18 may enhance migration and invasion by binding CCR8 in bladder cancer cells [43]. According to our study, there is no difference in CCL18 expression between normal patients and BC. Different from previous studies, patients with a higher level of CCL18 are associated with a better DFS in this study. Feng et al. [44] found the CCL21/CCR7 axis promotes migration and invasion capacity of urinary bladder cancer cells and induces lymphatic metastatic spread. In the present study, CCL21 did not show a significant influence on OS or DFS. We also found the expression level of CCL4/5/14/19/21/23 were lower in BC patients than normal patients. Whereas in certain data sets CCL13 was increased significantly in BC patients compared with normal patients. Various means of data collection in different studies may be the reason for differentially expressed CCL13. In addition, CCL2, CCL11, CCL14, CCL18, CCL19, CCL21, CCL23, CCL24, CCL26 were markedly related with clinical stage in BC patients and CC chemokines were related to cytokine activity, chemokines receptor binding, chemotaxis immune cell migration. In this study, we found a significant correlation between the expression of CC chemokines and the infiltration of the immune cell types, indicating that CC chemokines may also play a significant role in the immune activity.

One of the limitations of our study was that a detailed description or stratified analysis was missed about characteristics of the patients and clinical subtypes of BC. The data in our study are extracted from several online databases and different studies. Particularly, part of the clinical course of bladder tumors, characteristics of the patients baseline data is not complete in these studies. Among these patients, stage Ois bladder urothelial carcinoma, superficial bladder cancer, infiltrating bladder urothelial carcinoma are included. Therefore, a detailed description or stratified analysis was missed about these items related to diagnosis or therapeutic. Moreover, in the Figs. 4 and 5,

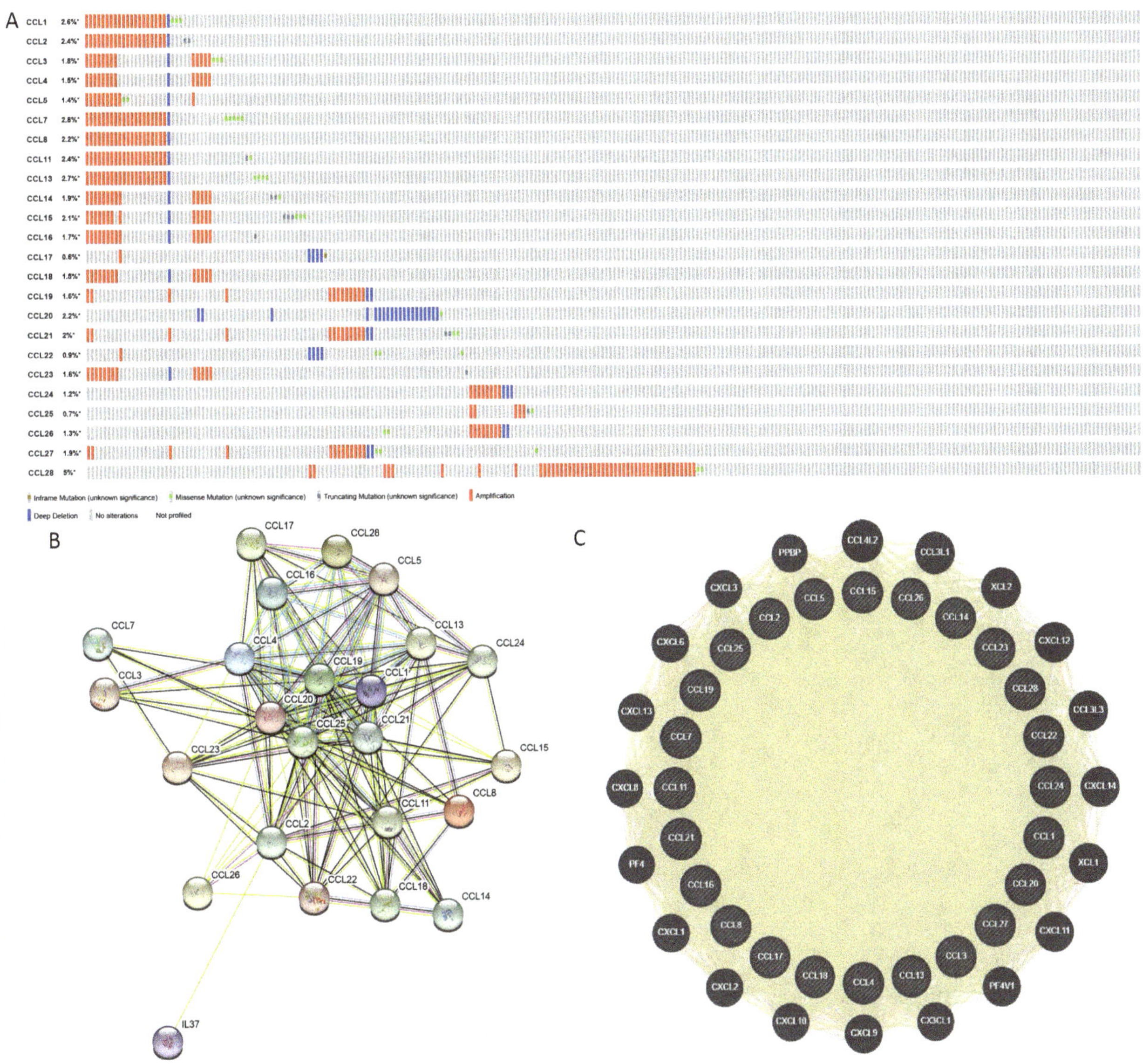

Fig. 6 CC chemokines gene mutation and expression analyses in BC (cBioPortal, GeneMANIA and STRING). **A** Summary of alterations in different expressed CC chemokines in BC. **B, C** Protein–protein interaction network of different expressed CC chemokines

several of the survival curves cross each other, which limit the usefulness of the log-rank test for comparing the survival outcome in our study. Further analysis, like Parametric Regressive Model, should be perform to compare it. Regrettably, we failed to establish a univariate- and multivariable Cox proportional-hazards model due to the fact that some valid information may be missed. What`s more, it`s a limitation of our study that adjusted p-value was not employed to prevent family-wise error rates.

Conclusions

In this research, we analyzed the prognostic and therapeutic value of CC chemokines in BC. Our results provided the information that CC chemokines might play an important role in BC oncogenesis which indicates a potential target of BC. We hope our results provide novel insights on the therapeutic targets of BC and help clinicians make a better personal treatment plan. However, further studies are needed to elucidate the

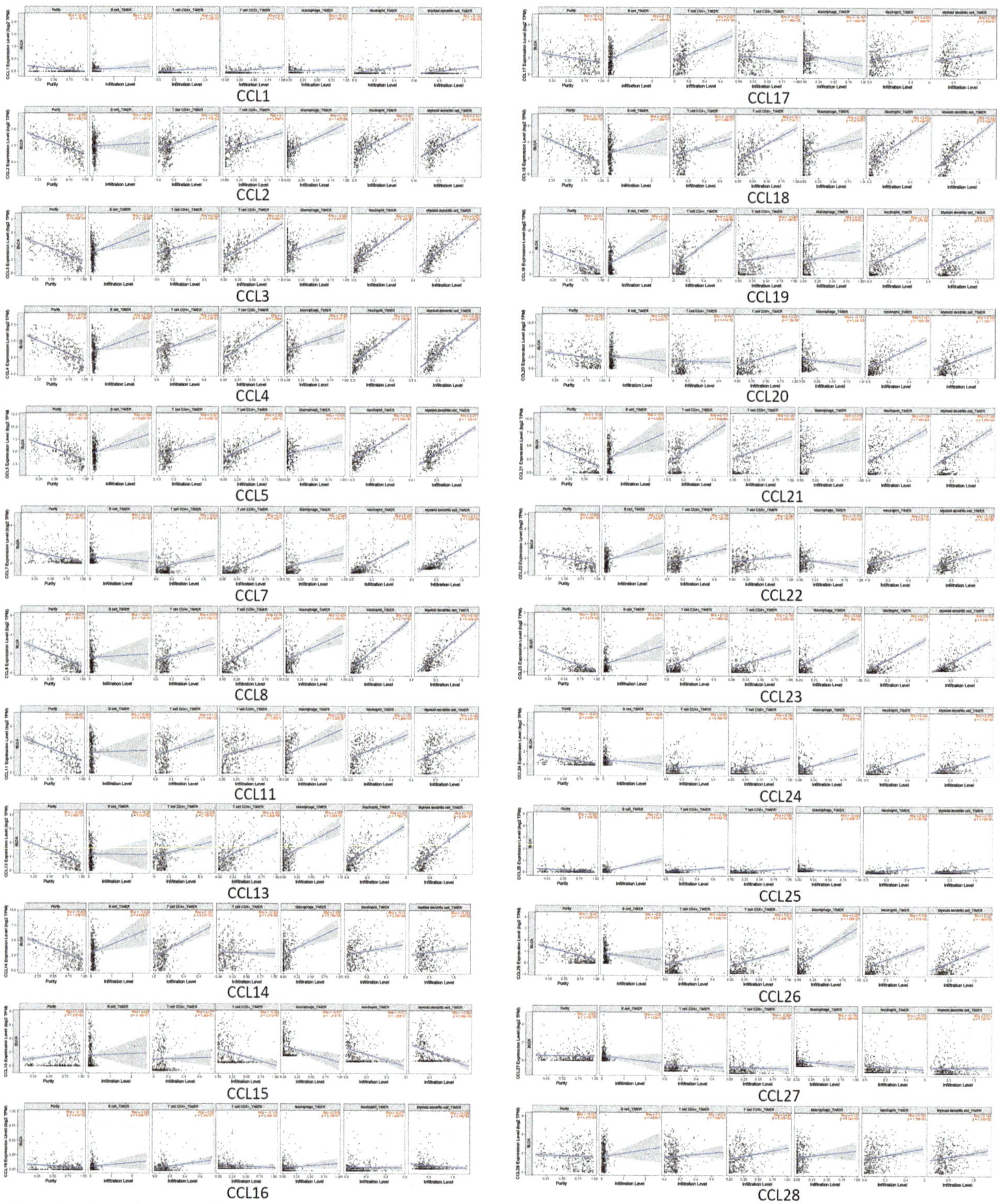

Fig. 7 Correlations between differentially expressed CC chemokines and immune cell infiltration (TIMER). Correlations between the abundance of immune cells and the expression of CCL1-28

difference between subgroup of BC classified by Infiltration degree or grade of these genes in BC.

Abbreviations

BC: Urothelial bladder cancer; GEPIA: Gene Expression Profiling Interactive Analysis; TURBT: Transurethral resection of bladder tumour; RFS: Recurrence-free survival; OS: Overall survival; TCGA: The Cancer Genome Atlas; PPI: Protein–protein interaction; DFS: Disease-free survival; M-MDSCs: Monocyte-myeloid-derived suppressed cells; HSP47: Heat shock protein 47; LNMAT1: Lymph Node Metastasis Associated Transcript 1; ERβ: Estrogen receptor beta; GAS5: Growth arrest-specific 5.

Acknowledgements

Jie Gu is supported by a scholarship from the China Scholarship Council Program (No. 201906370030).

Authors' contributions

YXL performed database analysis and drafted the manuscript. XBZ and JG contributed to all the designs of the study. All authors read and approved the final manuscript.

Author details

[1]Department of Geriatric Urology, Xiangya International Medical Center, Xiangya Hospital, Central South University, Changsha, Hunan 410008, People's Republic of China. [2]National Clinical Research Center for Geriatric Disorders, Xiangya Hospital, Central South University, Changsha, Hunan 410008, People's Republic of China. [3]Urolithiasis Institute of Central South University, Changsha, Hunan 410008, People's Republic of China. [4]Martini-Klinik Prostate Cancer Center, University Hospital Hamburg-Eppendorf, Hamburg, Germany.

References

1. Bray F, Ferlay J, Soerjomataram I, Siegel RL, Torre LA, Jemal A. Global cancer statistics 2018: GLOBOCAN estimates of incidence and mortality worldwide for 36 cancers in 185 countries. CA Cancer J Clin. 2018;68:394–424.
2. Helpap B. New WHO classification of urothelial carcinoma of the urinary bladder. Verh Dtsch Ges Pathol. 2002;86:57–66.
3. Messing EM, Tangen CM, Lerner SP, Sahasrabudhe DM, Koppie TM, Wood DP, et al. Effect of intravesical instillation of gemcitabine vs saline immediately following resection of suspected low-grade non-muscle-invasive bladder cancer on tumor recurrence: SWOG S0337 randomized clinical trial. JAMA. 2018;319:1880–8.
4. Witjes JA, Bruins M, Cathomas R, Compérat E, Cowan NC, Gakis G, et al. EAU guidelines on muscle-invasive and metastatic bladder cancer 2020. In: European Association of Urology Guidelines. 2020 Edition. Arnhem, The Netherlands: European Association of Urology Guidelines Office; 2020. http://uroweb.org/guideline/bladder-cancer-muscle-invasive-and-metastatic/.
5. Babjuk M, Burger M, Compérat E, Gontero P, Mostafid AH, Palou J, et al. EAU guidelines on non-muscle-invasive bladder cancer (TaT1 and CIS) 2020. In: European Association of Urology Guidelines. 2020 Edition. Arnhem, The Netherlands: European Association of Urology Guidelines Office; 2020. http://uroweb.org/guideline/non-muscle-invasive-bladder-cancer/.
6. Berdik C. Unlocking bladder cancer. Nature. 2017;551:S34–5.
7. Abdollah F, Gandaglia G, Thuret R, Schmitges J, Tian Z, Jeldres C, et al. Incidence, survival and mortality rates of stage-specific bladder cancer in United States: a trend analysis. Cancer Epidemiol. 2013;37:219–25.
8. James AC, Gore JL. The costs of non-muscle invasive bladder cancer. Urol Clin North Am. 2013;40:261–9.
9. Gschwend JE, Heck MM, Lehmann J, Rübben H, Albers P, Wolff JM, et al. Extended versus limited lymph node dissection in bladder cancer patients undergoing radical cystectomy: survival results from a prospective. Randomized Trial Eur Urol. 2019;75:604–11.
10. Nagarsheth N, Wicha MS, Zou W. Chemokines in the cancer microenvironment and their relevance in cancer immunotherapy. Nat Rev Immunol. 2017;17:559–72.
11. Qian B-Z, Li J, Zhang H, Kitamura T, Zhang J, Campion LR, et al. CCL2 recruits inflammatory monocytes to facilitate breast-tumour metastasis. Nature. 2011;475:222–5.
12. Chen J, Yao Y, Gong C, Yu F, Su S, Chen J, et al. CCL18 from tumor-associated macrophages promotes breast cancer metastasis via PITPNM3. Cancer Cell. 2011;19:541–55.
13. Zheng J, Zhu X, Zhang J. CXCL5 knockdown expression inhibits human bladder cancer T24 cells proliferation and migration. Biochem Biophys Res Commun. 2014;446:18–24.
14. Park J, Zhang X, Lee SK, Song N-Y, Son SH, Kim KR, et al. CCL28-induced RARβ expression inhibits oral squamous cell carcinoma bone invasion. J Clin Invest. 2019;129:5381–99.
15. Adachi K, Kano Y, Nagai T, Okuyama N, Sakoda Y, Tamada K. IL-7 and CCL19 expression in CAR-T cells improves immune cell infiltration and CAR-T cell survival in the tumor. Nat Biotechnol. 2018;36:346–51.
16. Taubert H, Eckstein M, Epple E, Jung R, Weigelt K, Lieb V, et al. Immune cell-associated protein expression helps to predict survival in muscle-invasive urothelial bladder cancer patients after radical cystectomy and optional adjuvant chemotherapy. Cells. 2021;10:159.
17. Rhodes DR, Yu J, Shanker K, Deshpande N, Varambally R, Ghosh D, et al. ONCOMINE: a cancer microarray database and integrated data-mining platform. Neoplasia. 2004;6:1–6.
18. Tang Z, Li C, Kang B, Gao G, Li C, Zhang Z. GEPIA: a web server for cancer and normal gene expression profiling and interactive analyses. Nucleic Acids Res. 2017;45:W98-102.
19. Nagy Á, Munkácsy G, Győrffy B. Pancancer survival analysis of cancer hallmark genes. Sci Rep. 2021;11:6047.
20. Gao J, Aksoy BA, Dogrusoz U, Dresdner G, Gross B, Sumer SO, et al. Integrative analysis of complex cancer genomics and clinical profiles using the cBioPortal. Sci Signal. 2013;6:pl1.
21. Szklarczyk D, Gable AL, Lyon D, Junge A, Wyder S, Huerta-Cepas J, et al. STRING v11: protein-protein association networks with increased coverage, supporting functional discovery in genome-wide experimental datasets. Nucleic Acids Res. 2019;47:D607–13.
22. Warde-Farley D, Donaldson SL, Comes O, Zuberi K, Badrawi R, Chao P, et al. The GeneMANIA prediction server: biological network integration for gene prioritization and predicting gene function. Nucleic Acids Res. 2010;38:W214–20.
23. Li T, Fan J, Wang B, Traugh N, Chen Q, Liu JS, et al. TIMER: a web server for comprehensive analysis of tumor-infiltrating immune cells. Cancer Res. 2017;77:e108–10.
24. Sung H, Ferlay J, Siegel RL, Laversanne M, Soerjomataram I, Jemal A, et al. Global cancer statistics 2020: GLOBOCAN estimates of incidence and mortality worldwide for 36 cancers in 185 countries. CA Cancer J Clin. 2021;71:209–49.
25. Kryczek I, Zhao E, Liu Y, Wang Y, Vatan L, Szeliga W, et al. Human TH17 cells are long-lived effector memory cells. Sci Transl Med. 2011;3:104ra100.
26. Metelitsa LS, Wu H-W, Wang H, Yang Y, Warsi Z, Asgharzadeh S, et al. Natural killer T cells infiltrate neuroblastomas expressing the chemokine CCL2. J Exp Med. 2004;199:1213–21.
27. Curiel TJ, Coukos G, Zou L, Alvarez X, Cheng P, Mottram P, et al. Specific recruitment of regulatory T cells in ovarian carcinoma fosters immune privilege and predicts reduced survival. Nat Med. 2004;10:942–9.
28. Wolf MJ, Hoos A, Bauer J, Boettcher S, Knust M, Weber A, et al. Endothelial CCR2 signaling induced by colon carcinoma cells enables extravasation via the JAK2-Stat5 and p38MAPK pathway. Cancer Cell. 2012;22:91–105.
29. Sukkurwala AQ, Martins I, Wang Y, Schlemmer F, Ruckenstuhl C, Durchschlag M, et al. Immunogenic calreticulin exposure occurs through a phylogenetically conserved stress pathway involving the chemokine CXCL8. Cell Death Differ. 2014;21:59–68.
30. Wang W, Shen F, Wang C, Lu W, Wei J, Shang A, et al. MiR-1-3p inhibits the proliferation and invasion of bladder cancer cells by suppressing CCL2 expression. Tumour Biol. 2017;39:1010428317698383.
31. Tham SM, Ng KH, Pook SH, Esuvaranathan K, Mahendran R. Tumor and microenvironment modification during progression of murine orthotopic bladder cancer. Clin Dev Immunol. 2011;2011:865684.
32. Eckstein M, Epple E, Jung R, Weigelt K, Lieb V, Sikic D, et al. CCL2 expression in tumor cells and tumor-infiltrating immune cells shows divergent prognostic potential for bladder cancer patients depending on lymph node stage. Cancers Basel. 2020;12:1253.

33. Mu X-Y, Wang R-J, Yao Z-X, Zheng Z, Jiang J-T, Tan M-Y, et al. RS 504393 inhibits M-MDSCs recruiting in immune microenvironment of bladder cancer after gemcitabine treatment. Mol Immunol. 2019;109:140–8.
34. Chiu H-Y, Sun K-H, Chen S-Y, Wang H-H, Lee M-Y, Tsou Y-C, et al. Autocrine CCL2 promotes cell migration and invasion via PKC activation and tyrosine phosphorylation of paxillin in bladder cancer cells. Cytokine. 2012;59:423–32.
35. Chen C, He W, Huang J, Wang B, Li H, Cai Q, et al. LNMAT1 promotes lymphatic metastasis of bladder cancer via CCL2 dependent macrophage recruitment. Nat Commun. 2018;9:3826.
36. Ma W, Ou T, Cui X, Wu K, Li H, Li Y, et al. HSP47 contributes to angiogenesis by induction of CCL2 in bladder cancer. Cell Signal. 2021;85:110044.
37. Rao Q, Chen Y, Yeh C-R, Ding J, Li L, Chang C, et al. Recruited mast cells in the tumor microenvironment enhance bladder cancer metastasis via modulation of ERβ/CCL2/CCR2 EMT/MMP9 signals. Oncotarget. 2016;7:7842–55.
38. Yeh C-R, Hsu I, Song W, Chang H, Miyamoto H, Xiao G-Q, et al. Fibroblast ERα promotes bladder cancer invasion via increasing the CCL1 and IL-6 signals in the tumor microenvironment. Am J Cancer Res. 2015;5:1146–57.
39. Eruslanov E, Stoffs T, Kim W-J, Daurkin I, Gilbert SM, Su L-M, et al. Expansion of CCR8(+) inflammatory myeloid cells in cancer patients with urothelial and renal carcinomas. Clin Cancer Res. 2013;19:1670–80.
40. Cao Q, Wang N, Qi J, Gu Z, Shen H. Long non-coding RNA-GAS5 acts as a tumor suppressor in bladder transitional cell carcinoma via regulation of chemokine (C-C motif) ligand 1 expression. Mol Med Rep. 2016;13:27–34.
41. Urquidi V, Kim J, Chang M, Dai Y, Rosser CJ, Goodison S. CCL18 in a multiplex urine-based assay for the detection of bladder cancer. PLOS ONE. 2012;7:e37797.
42. Miyake M, Ross S, Lawton A, Chang M, Dai Y, Mengual L, et al. Investigation of CCL18 and A1AT as potential urinary biomarkers for bladder cancer detection. BMC Urol. 2013;13:42.
43. Liu X, Xu X, Deng W, Huang M, Wu Y, Zhou Z, et al. CCL18 enhances migration, invasion and EMT by binding CCR8 in bladder cancer cells. Mol Med Rep. 2019;19:1678–86.
44. Xiong Y, Huang F, Li X, Chen Z, Feng D, Jiang H, et al. CCL21/CCR7 interaction promotes cellular migration and invasion via modulation of the MEK/ERK1/2 signaling pathway and correlates with lymphatic metastatic spread and poor prognosis in urinary bladder cancer. Int J Oncol. 2017;51:75–90.

25

Comparison between 5-aminolevulinic acid photodynamic diagnosis and narrow-band imaging for bladder cancer detection

Hiroki Hagimoto*, Noriyuki Makita, Yuta Mine, Hidetoshi Kokubun, Shiori Murata, Yohei Abe, Masashi Kubota, Naofumi Tsutsumi, Toshinari Yamasaki and Mutsushi Kawakita

Abstract

Background: To compare 5-aminolevulinic acid (5-ALA)-mediated photodynamic diagnosis (PDD) with narrow-band imaging (NBI) for cancer detection during transurethral resection of bladder tumour (TURBT).

Methods: Between June 2018 and October 2020, 114 patients and 282 lesions were included in the analysis. Patients were orally administered 5-ALA (20 mg/kg) 2 h before TURBT. The bladder was inspected with white light (WL), PDD, and NBI for each patient, and all areas positive by at least one method were resected or biopsied. The imaging data were then compared to the pathology results.

Results: The sensitivities of WL, PDD, and NBI for detecting urothelial carcinoma were 88.1%, 89.6%, and 76.2%, respectively. The specificity, positive predictive value, and negative predictive value for detecting urothelial carcinoma were 47.5%, 80.9%, and 61.3%, respectively, for WL; 22.5%, 74.5%, and 46.2%, respectively, for PDD; and 46.3%, 78.2%, and 43.5%, respectively, for NBI. PDD was significantly more sensitive than NBI for all lesions ($p < 0.001$) and carcinoma in situ (CIS) lesions (94.6% vs. 54.1%, $p < 0.001$).

Conclusions: PDD can increase the detection rate of bladder cancer, compared to NBI, by greater than 10%. Therefore, 100% of CIS lesions can be detected by adding PDD to WL.

Keywords: Bladder cancer, 5-aminolevulinic acid, Narrow-band imaging, Photodynamic diagnosis, Transurethral resection of bladder tumour

Introduction

Bladder cancer is the ninth most frequently diagnosed malignancy in the world [1] and is the fourth leading cause of death among men [2]. The 5-year recurrence rate of non-muscle-invasive bladder cancer ranges from 50 to 70%, and the reported 5-year progression rate ranges from 10 to 30% [3]. Transurethral resection of bladder tumour (TURBT) with intraoperative detection of the cancer by white light (WL) is the standard treatment for non-muscle invasive bladder cancer [4]. However, it is difficult to detect flat lesions, including carcinoma in situ (CIS), with WL alone, and the high rate of intravesical recurrence of CIS is problematic. Therefore, it is important to accurately detect CIS in order to be able to eliminate any residual tumour, and more importantly to identify the patients who require further treatment such as intravesical BCG. It is known that the addition of photodynamic diagnosis (PDD) and narrow-band imaging (NBI) to WL increases the detection rate of cancer in flat lesions that do not appear as distinct lesions with conventional WL [5–8]. They also are associated

*Correspondence: hiroki1104hagimoto@gmail.com
Department of Urology, Kobe City Medical Center General Hospital, 2-1-1 Minatojima-Minamimachi, Chuo-ku, Kobe, Hyogo 650-0047, Japan

with lower recurrence rates compared to WL only [2, 9–11]. PDD is a technique that exploits the property of tumours or rapidly proliferating cells to emit red fluorescence during cystoscopy using blue light, after oral or intravesical administration of a photosensitizing precursor such as 5-aminolevulinic acid (5-ALA). NBI is a technique that utilises the fact that tissue penetration by light depends on its wavelength. By exposing the bladder wall to light with two narrow-banded wavelengths, that are easily absorbed by haemoglobin, capillaries on the surface of the mucosa are displayed as brown and blood vessels inside the submucosa as blue-green, highlighting the tumour. PDD using 5-ALA (5-ALA-PDD) for non-muscle invasive bladder cancer reduces the risk of recurrence [12], and has a real-world sensitivity and specificity of 90.1% and 61.2%, respectively [13]. For NBI, a meta-analysis showed that the pooled sensitivity and specificity for non-muscle invasive bladder cancer were 94.8% and 65.6%, respectively [14].

The 2021 European Association of Urology (EAU) guidelines strongly recommend taking biopsies from both abnormal-looking urothelium and normal-looking mucosa (mapping biopsies from the trigone, bladder dome, right, left, anterior, and posterior bladder wall) when cytology is positive, in case of a history of high grade (G3) tumours, and for tumours with non-papillary appearance. Moreover, PDD-guided biopsies should be used if equipment is available. However, bladder biopsy using NBI during TURB is weakly recommended [15].

Some studies have examined the usefulness of combining PDD and NBI for the detection of flat lesions [16, 17]. However, no comparative studies exist between 5-ALA-PDD and NBI for the detection of urothelial carcinoma, including both protruded and flat lesions. The purpose of this study was to compare 5-ALA-PDD and NBI in terms of bladder cancer detection capability in the same patients.

Material and methods

Study cohort and design

This single-centre retrospective cohort study was approved by the institutional review board (IRB No. zn210416) and conformed to the provisions of the Declaration of Helsinki (as revised in Fortaleza, Brazil, October 2013). All patients were informed of the efficacy and adverse events associated with 5-ALA-PDD and NBI, and we obtained informed consent from all patients before the operation. A total of 141 patients with primary bladder cancer, who underwent 5-ALA-PDD and NBI-assisted TURBT between June 2018 and October 2020, were included in the study. Eighteen patients with random bladder biopsies, five patients with histology consistent with prostate cancer, squamous cell carcinoma, or renal cell carcinoma, and four patients with no observation records for either NBI or 5-ALA-PDD were excluded. Included in the analysis were 114 patients with 282 lesions. Figure 1 shows the flow diagram of the study. We recorded the data on the surgeons' interpretation of the images prospectively, and analysed them retrospectively.

Surgical procedure

All patients were administered 20 mg/kg of 5-ALA 2 h before the start of surgery. In all cases, the positive and negative lesions were determined by two urologists. At the time of TURBT, the bladder was inspected with WL, 5-ALA-PDD, and NBI, and all lesions deemed positive by at least one modality were resected. WL was used first and was followed by either 5-ALA-PDD or NBI depending on the surgeon's preference. We used AUTOCON® III 400 (KARL STORZ, Tuttlingen) for PDD and OES ELITE 30° optic tube Φ4 mm (Olympus, Tokyo) for NBI. Bladder inspection with each modality occurred consecutively. Figure 2 shows a typical view by each modality. After TURBT, 50 mg of epirubicin hydrochloride in 50 mL of saline solution was instilled into the bladder through a Foley catheter, which was clamped for 30 min. The patients were kept out of direct sunlight for 48 h after surgery. We reviewed the pathology results and the intraoperative detection frequencies of each modality, and, accordingly, determined the cancer detection rate and sensitivity for each modality. Grading was performed according to the 2016 World Health Organization classification.

Safety assessment

We noted the incidence of side effects common with 5-ALA, such as vomiting, liver damage, and hypotension. Grades were determined based on the Common Terminology Criteria for Adverse Events, version 6.

Statistical analysis

The extracted data from the prospective database included age, sex, body mass index, preoperative urine cytology, operation time, surgeon, anaesthetic method, pathological examination, length of hospital stay, readmission, in-hospital complications, and Clavien-Dindo grade [18]. We calculated and compared the sensitivity, specificity, positive predictive value, and negative predictive value for each lesion. Significant differences between the two groups were assessed based on McNemar's odds ratio using standard analysis software (BellCurve for Excel; Social Survey Research Information Co., Ltd.). All

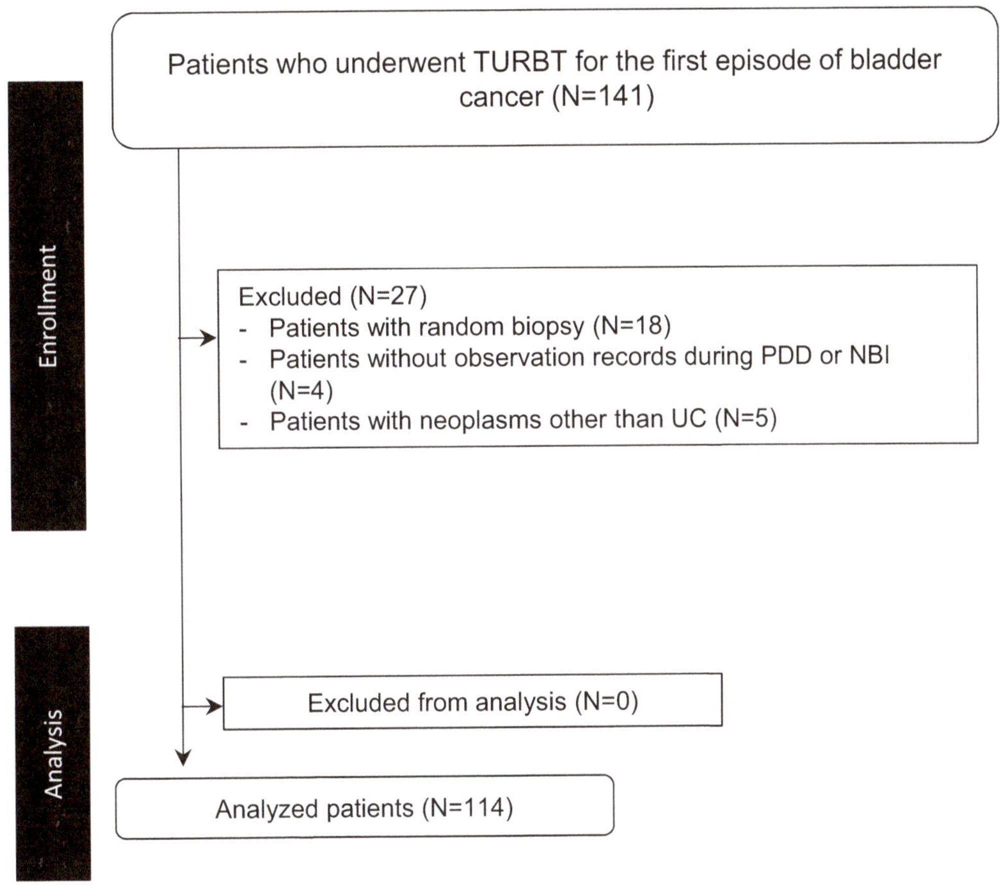

Fig. 1 Flow diagram of patient enrolment

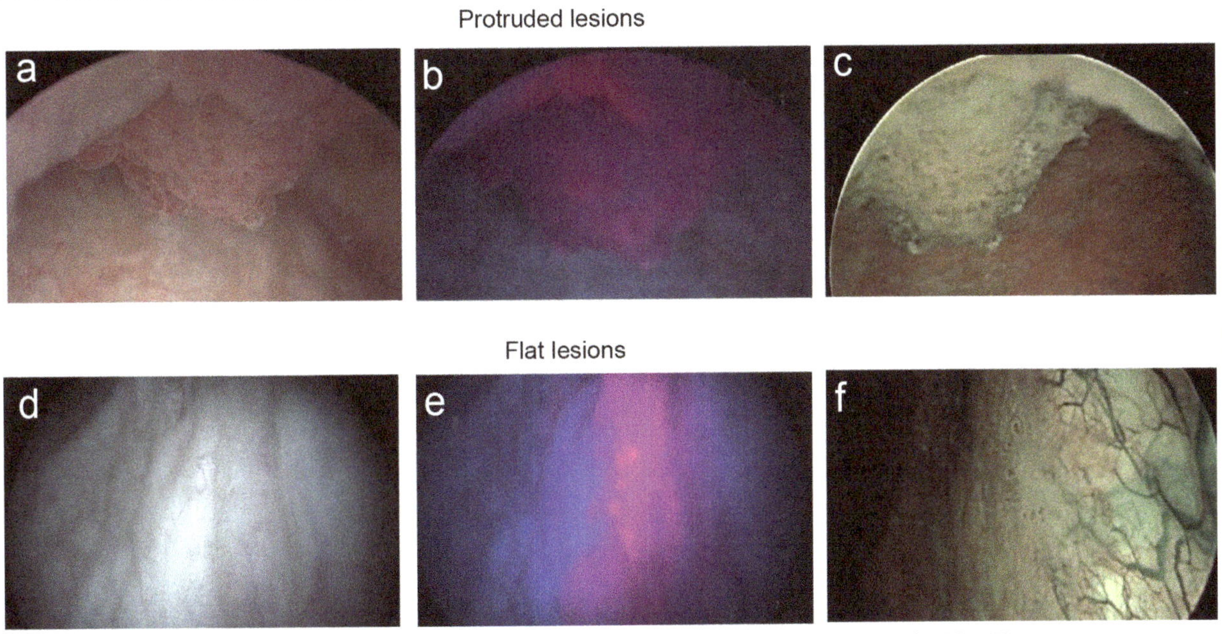

Fig. 2 Representative endoscopy images of positive tumour findings in protruded and flat lesions using **a** WL, **b** PDD, **c** NBI

Table 1 Patients' background and tumour characteristics

Enrolled patients	Total (n = 114)
Age, years (median)	76 (IQR: 60–81)
Gender	
Female, n(%)	35 (30.7%)
Male, n(%)	79 (69.3%)
Body weight, kg, median(IQR)	53 (45.3–62.8)
Operation time, min, median (IQR)	60 (38–79)
Preoperative cytology	
Positive, n(%)	25 (21.9%)
Negative, n(%)	85 (74.6%)
N/A, n(%)	4 (3.5%)
Anesthetic method	
General, n(%)	47(41.2%)
Lumbar, n(%)	67 (58.8%)
5-ALA exposure time, min, median(IQR)	177(157.5–207)
Number of lesions	282
Protruded papillary, n(%)	189 (67.0%)
Protruded non-papillary, n(%)	17 (6.0%)
Flat lesions, n(%)	76 (27.0%)
Number of tumors per person, median(IQR)	2 (2–3)

5-ALA: 5-aminolevulinic acid, IQR: interquartile range

Table 2 Specimen histology

Tumors	N (%)
Total	282
UC	202 (71.6)
Stage	
Ta	125 (44.3)
T1	26 (9.2)
T2	14 (5.0)
CIS	37 (13.1)
Grade	
Low	16 (5.7)
High	186 (66.0)
Benign	80 (28.4)
Dysplasia	3 (1.1)
Papilloma	13 (4.6)
Normal	64 (22.7)

CIS: carcinoma in situ; UC: urothelial carcinoma

statistical tests were two-tailed, with $p < 0.05$ indicating statistical significance.

Results

In total, 282 lesions from 114 patients were included in the study, and all of them were available for data analysis. A total of 24 patients were observed with PDD first followed by NBI, and 90 patients were observed with NBI first followed by PDD. Table 1 shows the patients' characteristics. The specimens' histology is presented in Table 2. Urothelial carcinoma (UC) was diagnosed in 202 specimens, whereas the remaining 80 were benign. Of the benign specimens, 3 were consistent with dysplasia, 13 with papilloma, and the rest were normal tissues. Table 3 shows the sensitivity of each modality for the detection of UC and the specificity for benign lesions. As shown, 5-ALA-PDD had a higher overall sensitivity than NBI (89.6% vs. 76.2%, $p < 0.001$). It also was more sensitive than NBI for CIS lesions (94.6% vs. 54.1%, $p < 0.001$). We were able to detect 100% of the CIS lesions with combined WL + PDD (WP), thus increasing the rate of detection by 35.1% compared with that of WL alone.

Adverse events, including hypotension (N = 61), elevated liver enzyme levels (N = 4), and vomiting (N = 20) were less than grade 3. All incidents (N = 61) of hypotension were of grade 2 or lower according to Common Terminology Criteria for Adverse Events version 5.0. Of the 67 patients who received lumbar anaesthesia, 22 patients (32.8%) received intraoperative vasopressors, and of the 47 patients who received general anaesthesia, 39 patients (83.0%) received vasopressors during induction. None of the patients required vasopressors after the surgery. Elevated levels of aspartate aminotransferase were found in four patients, one of whom was classified as grade 2, and three were classified as grade 1. All the patients who had vomiting were classified as grade 1. They had vomiting postoperatively within a median of 5.9 (interquartile range: 1.3–7.4) hours following 5-ALA administration. In all cases, nausea had disappeared by the next day. Regarding postoperative complications, there were 12 cases of grade 1 or higher as per the Clavien-Dindo classification. There was only one case of grade 3a, which required ERCP for fever due to postoperative recurrence of hepatocellular carcinoma. The remaining 11 cases were grade 2 or lower, including temporary postoperative urinary retention and clot retention requiring manual bladder washing to eliminate the blood clot.

Discussion

In this study, 5-ALA-PDD was superior and considered more useful than NBI in reducing the number of missed tumours. The detection rate of pTis lesions in the WL + PDD group was 100%, and the rate of additionally detected CIS with WL + PDD was increased by 35.1% compared with WL alone. Although this 100% sensitivity is partially due to the fact that we did not sample negative lesions for PDD, NBI, or WL; thus, it is possible that some patients may have had an undetected CIS that we were not aware of; 5-ALA-PDD proved to be particularly useful in detecting flat lesions such as CIS.

Table 3 Sensitivity of each modality for detection of UC and specificity for benign lesions

	WL (%)	NBI (%)	PDD (%)	WN (%)	WP (%)	WNP (%)
Sensitivity						
All UC	178/202 (88.1)	154/202(76.2)	181/202 (89.6)	183/202 (90.6)	201/202 (99.5)	202/202 (100)
CIS	24/37 (64.9)	20/37 (54.1)	35/37 (94.6)	26/37 (70.3)	37/37 (100)	37/37 (100)
Non-CIS	153/165 (92.7)	134/165 (81.2)	145/165 (87.9)	156/165 (94.5)	162/165 (98.2)	163/165 (98.8)

	WL (%)	NBI (%)	*PDD* (%)
Specificity			
All benign	38/80 (47.5)	37/80 (46.3)	18/80 (22.5)

CIS, carcinoma in situ; NBI, narrow-band imaging; PDD, photodynamic diagnosis; UC, urothelial carcinoma; WL, white light; WN, white light with NBI; WNP, white light with NBI and PDD; WP, WL + PDD

The present study determined a lower specificity for PDD than other reports [12, 13]. This may be due to the lack of a systematic biopsy of the negative areas and the exclusion of cases for whom random biopsies were performed, such as cold-cup biopsies of normal appearing lesions, or biopsies on lesions that were even slightly positive for PDD to avoid missing cancer. This is one of the limiting factors that prevented us from examining the specificity in the present study as it was a retrospective study.

According to the literature, transient elevation of liver enzymes of grade 3 or lower, as well as hypotension, can occur due to 5-ALA, and caution is recommended with its use [19, 20]. In this study, there was only one case of grade 3a adverse effects, which was not associated with 5-ALA. Moreover, the rest of the adverse events were grade 2 or lower, and could be easily managed.

The present study has several limitations which are as follows: (1) the small number of patients included; (2) single-centre retrospective design; (3) inter-observer and intra-observer bias, which was due to the subjective nature of visual estimation and could be potentially be addressed by the development of methods to quantify visual information; and (4) procedure bias introduced by the order of use of each modality and the time between 5-ALA administration and bladder inspection in PDD. This study includes the possibility that the sensitivity of PDD was increased because of the bias in which many of the patients were observed first with NBI followed by PDD. There is a phenomenon called photobleaching, in which 5-ALA degrades upon repeated illumination and the detection rate is reduced [21]. Although observation at 2–4 h after 5-ALA oral administration is recommended, the time of 5-ALA exposure to light may be less important, as it has been shown that no significant difference exists between exposure times of 2–3 h and 4 h or more [13]. Recent studies have shown a fluorescence enhancement effect using polyethylene glycol-modified titanium dioxide nanoparticles [21], which may be useful for reducing the bias caused by photobleaching.

Conclusions

5-ALA-PDD at the time of TURBT increased the detection rate of bladder cancer and especially of flat lesions such as CIS, compared to NBI. Furthermore, the combination of PDD with WL, which is the current standard of care, achieves 100% sensitivity in the detection of CIS. Prospective studies will be needed to verify these results.

Abbreviations

5-ALA: 5-Aminolevulinic acid; CIS: Carcinoma in situ; NBI: Narrow-band imaging; PDD: Photodynamic diagnosis; TURBT: Transurethral resection of bladder tumour; WL: White light.

Acknowledgements

Not applicable.

Authors' contributions

All authors participated in creating the study design. HH performed recruitment, clinical follow up, interpretation of data, statistical analyses and writing of the manuscript. NM contributed to the original concept and design of this study. YM, HK, SM, YA, MK, NT, TY and MK provided a critical revision of the manuscript. All the authors have read and approved the final manuscript.

References

1. Antoni S, Ferlay J, Soerjomataram I, Znaor A, Jemal A, Bray F. Bladder cancer incidence and mortality: a global overview and recent trends. Eur Urol. 2017;71:96–108. https://doi.org/10.1016/j.eururo.2016.06.010.
2. Lenis AT, Lec PM, Chamie K. Bladder cancer: a review. JAMA. 2020;324:1980–91. https://doi.org/10.1001/jama.2020.17598.
3. Kamat AM, Hahn NM, Efstathiou JA, Lerner SP, Malmström P, Choi W, et al. Bladder cancer. Lancet. 2016;388:2796–810. https://doi.org/10.1016/S0140-6736(16)30512-8.
4. Babjuk M, Böhle A, Burger M, Capoun O, Cohen D, Compérat EM, et al. EAU guidelines on non-muscle-invasive urothelial carcinoma of the bladder: update 2016. Eur Urol. 2017;71:447–61. https://doi.org/10.1016/j.eururo.2016.05.041.
5. Kriegmair M, Baumgartner R, Knüchel R, Stepp H, Hofstädter F, Hofstetter A. Detection of early bladder cancer by 5-aminolevulinic acid induced porphyrin fluorescence. J Urol. 1996;155:105–9 (**discussion 9–10**).
6. Filbeck T, Roessler W, Knuechel R, Straub M, Kiel HJ, Wieland WF. Clinical results of the transurethreal resection and evaluation of superficial bladder carcinomas by means of fluorescence diagnosis after intravesical instillation of 5-aminolevulinic acid. J Endourol. 1999;13:117–21. https://doi.org/10.1089/end.1999.13.117.
7. De Dominicis C, Liberti M, Perugia G, De Nunzio C, Sciobica F, Zuccalà A, et al. Role of 5-aminolevulinic acid in the diagnosis and treatment of

superficial bladder cancer: improvement in diagnostic sensitivity. Urology. 2001;57:1059–62. https://doi.org/10.1016/s0090-4295(01)00948-7.
8. Zaak D, Kriegmair M, Stepp H, Stepp H, Baumgartner R, Oberneder R, et al. Endoscopic detection of transitional cell carcinoma with 5-aminolevulinic acid: results of 1012 fluorescence endoscopies. Urology. 2001;57:690–4. https://doi.org/10.1016/s0090-4295(00)01053-0
9. Naselli A, Introini C, Timossi L, Spina B, Fontana V, Pezzi R, et al. A randomized prospective trial to assess the impact of transurethral resection in narrow band imaging modality on non-muscle-invasive bladder cancer recurrence. Eur Urol. 2012;61:908–13. https://doi.org/10.1016/j.eururo.2012.01.018.
10. Kutwin P, Konecki T, Cichocki M, Falkowski P, Jabłonowski Z. Photodynamic diagnosis and narrow-band imaging in the management of bladder cancer: a review. Photomed Laser Surg. 2017;35:459–64. https://doi.org/10.1089/pho.2016.4217.
11. Grossman HB, Stenzl A, Fradet Y, Mynderse LA, Kriegmair M, Witjes JA, et al. Long-term decrease in bladder cancer recurrence with hexaminolevulinate enabled fluorescence cystoscopy. J Urol. 2012;188:58–62. https://doi.org/10.1016/j.juro.2012.03.007.
12. Nakai Y, Inoue K, Tsuzuki T, Shimamoto T, Shuin T, Nagao K, et al. Oral 5-aminolevulinic acid-mediated photodynamic diagnosis using fluorescence cystoscopy for non-muscle-invasive bladder cancer: a multicenter phase III study. Int J Urol. 2018;25:723–9. https://doi.org/10.1111/iju.13718.
13. Yamamoto S, Fukuhara H, Karashima T, Inoue K. Real-world experience with 5-aminolevulinic acid for the photodynamic diagnosis of bladder cancer: diagnostic accuracy and safety. Photodiagn Photodyn Ther. 2020;32: 101999. https://doi.org/10.1016/j.pdpdt.2020.101999.
14. Xiong Y, Li J, Ma S, Ge J, Zhou L, Li D, et al. A meta-analysis of narrow band imaging for the diagnosis and therapeutic outcome of non-muscle invasive bladder cancer. PLoS ONE. 2017;12: e0170819. https://doi.org/10.1371/journal.pone.0170819.
15. Babjuk M, Burger M, Capoun O, Cohen D, Comperat EM, Dominguez Escrig JL, et al. European Association of Urology Guidelines on Non-muscle-invasive Bladder Cancer (Ta, T1, and Carcinoma in Situ). Eur Urol. 2022;81:75–94. https://doi.org/10.1016/j.eururo.2021.08.010.
16. Naya Y, Oishi M, Yamada Y, Ueda T, Fujihara A, Nakanishi H, et al. Initial experience of combined use of photodynamic diagnosis and narrow band imaging for detection of flat urothelial lesion. Int J Clin Oncol. 2015;20:593–7. https://doi.org/10.1007/s10147-014-0748-5.
17. Drejer D, Béji S, Oezeke R, Nielsen AM, Høyer S, Bjerklund Johansen TE, et al. Comparison of white light, photodynamic diagnosis, and narrow-band imaging in detection of carcinoma in situ or flat dysplasia at transurethral resection of the bladder: the DaBlaCa-8 study. Urology. 2017;102:138–42. https://doi.org/10.1016/j.urology.2016.11.032.
18. Clavien PA, Barkun J, de Oliveira ML, Vauthey JN, Dindo D, Schulick RD, et al. The Clavien–Dindo classification of surgical complications: five-year experience. Ann Surg. 2009;250:187–96. https://doi.org/10.1097/SLA.0b013e3181b13ca2.
19. Yatabe T, Marie SL, Fukuhara H, Karashima T, Inoue K, Yokoyama M. 5-aminolevulinic acid-induced severe hypotension during transurethral resection of a bladder tumor: a case report. JA Clin Rep. 2019;5:58. https://doi.org/10.1186/s40981-019-0279-1.
20. Nohara T, Kato Y, Nakano T, Nakagawa T, Iwamoto H, Yaegashi H, et al. Intraoperative hypotension caused by oral administration of 5-aminolevulinic acid for photodynamic diagnosis in patients with bladder cancer. Int J Urol. 2019;26:1064–8. https://doi.org/10.1111/iju.14099.
21. Kanehira K, Yano Y, Hasumi H, Fukuhara H, Inoue K, Hanazaki K, et al. Fluorescence enhancement effect of TiO_2 nanoparticles and application for photodynamic diagnosis. Int J Mol Sci. 2019;20:3698. https://doi.org/10.3390/ijms20153698.

26

Protective role of intravesical BCG in COVID-19 severity

Héctor Gallegos[1†], Pablo A. Rojas[1,2†], Francisca Sepúlveda[3], Álvaro Zúñiga[1] and Ignacio F. San Francisco[1*]

Abstract

Objectives: To establish the role of BCG instillations in the incidence and mortality of COVID-19.

Patients and methods: NMIBC patients in instillations with BCG (induction or maintenance) during 2019/2020 were included, establishing a COVID-19 group (with a diagnosis according to the national registry) and a control group (NO-COVID). The cumulative incidence (cases/total patients) and the case fatality rate (deaths/cases) were established, and compared with the national statistics for the same age group. *T*-test was used for continuous variables and Fisher's exact test for categorical variables.

Results: 175 patients were included. Eleven patients presented CIS (11/175, 6.3%), 84/175 (48.0%) Ta and 68/175 (38.9%) T1. Average number of instillations = 13.25 ± 7.4. One hundred sixty-seven patients (95.4%) had complete induction. Forty-three patients (cumulative incidence 24.6%) were diagnosed with COVID-19. There is no difference between COVID-19 and NO-COVID group in age, gender or proportion of maintenance completed. COVID-19 group fatality rate = 1/43 (2.3%). Accumulated Chilean incidence 70–79 years = 6.3%. Chilean fatality rate 70–79 years = 14%.

Conclusions: According to our results, patients with NMIBC submitted to instillations with BCG have a lower case-fatality rate than the national registry of patients between 70 and 79 years (2.3% vs. 14%, respectively). Intravesical BCG could decrease the mortality due to COVID-19, so instillation schemes should not be suspended in a pandemic.

Keywords: COVID-19, Non-muscle invasive bladder cancer, Intravesical BCG

Introduction

The virus called severe acute respiratory syndrome coronavirus 2 (SARS-CoV-2), the cause of coronavirus disease 2019 (better known as COVID-19) has generated a pandemic never seen by mankind before [1]. Today, late July, at least 13 million people around the world have been diagnosed with COVID-19, and almost 5000 deaths are accounted daily due to the disease [2], exceeding 500 thousand deaths worldwide. In Chile, currently more than 300 thousand infected and 8 thousand deaths are described.

Major efforts focus on discovering a vaccine for the disease. In this context, the utility of Mycobacterium bovis Bacillus Calmette–Guérin (BCG) is proposed. BCG is a live attenuated vaccine for tuberculosis, and it has been described to provide protection against respiratory infections other than tuberculosis [3, 4], reducing its contagiousness, its severity and even mortality [5]. The mechanism by which BCG confers immunity to other infections is unknown [6], however, there is evidence that nonspecific protective effect is constituted by innate immune cells such as monocytes and natural killer cells, independent of T- and B-cell memory (called "trained inmmunity") [7, 8].

Various observational studies have shown that countries with BCG vaccination programs present lower mortality rates from COVID-19 than countries without vaccination [9]. Italy and USA, countries without

*Correspondence: isanfrancisco@med.puc.cl
†Héctor Gallegos and PabloA. Rojas have equal contribution
[1] Departamento de Urología, Facultad de Medicina, Pontificia Universidad Católica de Chile, Diagonal Paraguay 362, Santiago, Chile
Full list of author information is available at the end of the article

a vaccine program, have experienced higher mortality associated to COVID-19 than countries with long-standing universal BCG vaccination policies, such as South Korea and Japan [8]. Certainly, these relationships are observational and not necessarily causal.

Moreover, bladder instillations with BCG is a standard of care in patients with intermediate-high risk non-muscle invasive bladder cancer (NMIBC). BCG has shown a 32% reduction in bladder tumor recurrence risk and a 27% reduction in odds of progression [10].

The potential protective role of instillation of BCG in NMIBC against diagnosis and aggressiveness of COVID-19 has not been published or described in the current literature.

We aimed to observe whether intravesical BCG has protective role in terms of reduced infection by SARS-CoV-2, or, a less aggressive presentation of COVID-19 disease among NMIBC patients. We evaluated the incidence of COVID-19 and its severity in a cohort of patients with BCG bladder instillations.

Patients and methods

Patients

The study cohort included Chilean patients over 18 years, with histologic diagnose of NMIBC (CIS, Ta, T1) who underwent BCG treatment and had the diagnosis of COVID-19 after BCG instillations. This cohort of patients were treated with BCG instillations in 2019 and 2020 at Hospital Clínico de la Pontificia Universidad Católica de Chile. Patients were treated continuously with BCG bladder instillations and were receiving induction or maintenance at the time of the first case of COVID-19 was reported in Chile (March 3rd, 2020). Patients included were in induction or maintenance stages of their treatment as described by Morales et al. [11], with full dose (90 mg) or lower dose (30 mg) at least for 1-h intravesical instillation. Danish 1331 Mycobacterium bovis strain was used in every patient. We described all variables mentioned above and recurrence or BCG infection (BCGitis).

Patients with COVID-19 were diagnosed by real-time reverse transcription-PCR (RT-PCR) assays. The COVID-19 diagnosis notifications were obtained through the official Chilean national register ("Epivigila"), which performs immediate mandatory surveillance and notification of the COVID-19 diagnosis in all health centers in Chile.

We compared patients who underwent BCG treatment has COVID-19 diagnosis with patients without infection, to establish the influence of age, BCG dosis and induction or maintenance in reduce infection or less aggressiveness COVID-19.

Moreover, we compared our COVID-19 patients in BCG treatment with the overall population of the same age group (70–79 years), according to Chilean national register. National register of COVID-19 pandemic is complete and trustworthy [12].

Follow-up

Prospective follow-up of the patients was carried out from the start of the pandemic in Chile until February 2021. When one of our patients was diagnosed with COVID-19, a clinical follow-up of the evolution of the disease was carried out and, in case they survived the disease, they were contacted by telephone to define the consequences of the disease, such as severity, symptoms, need for mechanical ventilation. Informed consent was obtained from all subjects contacted.

Statistical analysis

Descriptive and analytic statistics were performed, expressing the numerical variables as measures of central tendencies and the categorical variables as percentages. Independent samples t-test (two tails) was used to compare continuous variables, Fisher's exact test or Chi-Square test to compare categorical variables. We define the cumulative incidence, as the ratio of the covid-19 infected cases within the cohort during the follow-up period (cases/total group), the case fatality rate was defined as deaths within the group of patients infected with covid-19 (death/COVID-19 infected patients). All data were analyzed with SPSS 22.0 software (IBM SPSS Software).

Statements

Ethics committee approval was granted by the Local Institutional Ethics Review Board. All procedures involving human participants were performed in accordance with the 1975 Helsinki declaration and its later amendments.

Results

A total of 175 patients were recruited in the study cohort. The main clinical-pathological and demographic characteristics of the group are described in Table 1.

During the study period, 43 patients (cumulative incidence = 24.6%) were diagnosed with COVID-19. There was no statistically significant difference between COVID-19 and No-COVID patients in age (72.9 years vs. 73.1 years, $p = 0.899$), Gender (83.7% vs. 72.0%, $p = 0.157$), and proportion of patients with maintenance therapy completed (62.8% vs. 75.0%, $p = 0.170$, respectively) (Table 2).

In the group of COVID-infected patients (43 patients), during follow-up only 1 patient died from the disease (Case Fatality Rate = 2.3%), only 2 patient (4.6%) required hospitalization, and only 2 patients (4.6%) had COVID

Table 1 Clinical-pathological characteristics

Characteristics	Covid-19 patients (n = 43)	All BCG patients (n = 175)
BCG dosage, mg ± SD	39.64 ± 22.9	44.3 ± 25.5
BCG instillations, n ± SD	12.20 ± 8.1	13.25 ± 7.4
Induction completed, % (n)	86.0% (37)	95.4% (167)
Maintenance completed, % (n)	62.8% (27)	65.1% (114)
Maintenance therapy time, years ± SD	1.48 ± 0.83	1.11 ± 0.98
T stage		
Cis, % (n)	9.3% (4)	6.3% (11)
Ta, % (n)	55.8% (24)	48.0% (84)
T1, % (n)	34.9% (15)	38.9% (68)
Previous relapse, % (n)	55.8% (24)	42.9% (75)
BCG infection ("BCGitis"), % (n)	25.6% (11)	18.9% (33)

Table 2 Univariate analysis between patients with COVID-19 and patients without infection

Characteristics	Covid group (n = 43)	No-covid group (n = 132)	*p* value
Mean age (years) ± SD	72.9 ± 10.9	73.1 ± 10.1	0.899
Male, % (n)	83.7% (36)	72.0% (95)	0.157
Full dose BCG, % (n)	16.3% (7)	22.0% (29)	0.518
Maintenance therapy, % (n)	62.8% (27)	75.0% (99)	0.170

pneumonia. Most patients only presented upper respiratory symptoms, compatible with a flu.

According official statistics of Chile [12], in the same period of time, control group (age group 70–79 years) had a cumulative incidence of COVID-19 infection of 6.3% (40.629 COVID-19 confirmed cases, 643.423 people in the 70–79 age group), and a case fatality rate of 14% (5.671 deaths due to COVID-19, 40.629 confirmed cases).

Discussion

As we showed previously, there are several studies that have compared the rates of infection and SARS-CoV-2 between different countries. Ozdemir et al. [7], in April 2020, demonstrated that mean cases per habitants is significantly lower in BCG-vaccinated countries than in BCG-non-vaccinated countries ($p < 0.0001$). Moreover, mean death is significantly lower in BCG-vaccinated countries compared to BCG-non-vaccinated countries ($p < 0.0001$). According to the evidence, BCG vaccination produces various pro- inflammatory cytokines, such as IL-1β, tumour necrosis factor and IL-6 [13], that explain the BCG vaccine's protective effect against other pathogens. Furthermore, there is an ongoing trial to use BCG to prevent COVID-19 (BCG Vaccination to Protect Healthcare Workers Against COVID-19 (BRACE) trial, NCT04327206).

Intravesical BCG not only generates a bladder inflammatory response; it induces a systemic effect with increased levels of IgG. The antibody response increased gradually at 3 months after instillations are completed [14]. According to Desouky, this can raise the question whether it is possible that intra-vesical BCG treatment for NMIBC patients provided them with a beneficial effect [15].

This manuscript is the first study that correlates intravesical BCG with less case fatality rate in a cohort of patients with NMIBC. It is interesting to note that this group of cancer patients undergoing BCG instillations had a lower-case fatality rate than general population of the same age group, even considering that cancer patients are basally more fragile. Our initial results are promising, but these data should be taken with caution, given that they are based on a limited number of infected patients.

It is striking that the infection rate in this cohort of instilled patients was not lower than the rate of the general population in the same age group, it was even higher. This could indicate that perhaps the immunity associated with BCG could influence the severity of the disease more than preventing infection.

Recent evidence suggests that patients with cancer are at higher risk of infection for SARS-CoV-2 and may have poorer outcomes [16]. Thus, it has been proposed to defer instillations with BCG by at least 3 weeks due to the risk of increasing severity in patients with COVID-19 [17]. However, according to our data, intravesical BCG would be beneficial in case of infection, since it would decrease the illness' severity (and mortality).

This study has some limitations. First, this is a cohort study with a reduced number of patients and a limited total number of infected (43 patients), which could not allow definitive conclusions to be made. Second, we cannot assure that the patients present an infection rate due to their intravesical BCG instillations or because the patients are in lockdown. The mean age was 73 years old, and most of these patients are in mandatory quarantine. Therefore, our best conclusions are in relation to the case fatality rate, since it begins with a point in common (confirmatory diagnosis of COVID-19).

Conclusion

According to our results, patients with NMIBC in BCG bladder instillations had lower case fatality rate than same age overall population (2.3% vs. 14%, respectively), but had more cumulative incidence (24.6% to NMIBC and 6.3% to overall population). Intravesical BCG could protect against aggressive presentation of COVID-19. More studies are needed in order to confirm our findings.

Acknowledgements

Not applicable.

Authors' contributions

HG: conception, design of the work, data acquisition, data analysis, interpretation of data, drafted the work, substantively revised the manuscript. PR: conception, design of the work, data acquisition, data analysis, interpretation of data, drafted the work, substantively revised the manuscript. FS: data acquisition, drafted the work. AZ: data analysis, interpretation of data, substantively revised the manuscript. ISF: conception, data analysis, interpretation of data, substantively revised the manuscript. *All authors have approved the submitted version.

Author details

[1] Departamento de Urología, Facultad de Medicina, Pontificia Universidad Católica de Chile, Diagonal Paraguay 362, Santiago, Chile. [2] Servicio de Urología, Hospital Sótero del Río, Santiago, Chile. [3] Escuela de Pregrado, Facultad de Medicina, Pontificia Universidad Católica de Chile, Santiago, Chile.

References

1. O'Neill LAJ, Netea MG. BCG-induced trained immunity: can it offer protection against COVID-19? Nat Rev Immunol. 2020;20(6):335–7.
2. Roser M, Ritchie H, Ortiz-Ospina E, Hasell J. Coronavirus pandemic (COVID-19). https://ourworldindata.org/coronavirus (Online Resource). Accessed 20 Feb 2021.
3. Pollard AJ, Finn A, Curtis N. Non-specific effects of vaccines: plausible and potentially important, but implications uncertain. Arch Dis Child. 2017;102:1077–81.
4. Goodridge HS, Ahmed SS, Curtis N, et al. Harnessing the beneficial heterologous effects of vaccination. Nat Rev Immunol. 2016;16:392–400.
5. Biering-Sorensen S, Aaby P, Lund N, et al. Early BCG-Denmark and neonatal mortality among infants weighing < 2500 g: a randomized controlled trial. Clin Infect Dis. 2017;65:1183–90.
6. Curtis N, Sparrow A, Ghebreyesus TA, Netea MG. Considering BCG vaccination to reduce the impact of COVID-19. Lancet. 2020;395(10236):1545–6.
7. Ozdemir C, Kucuksezer UC, Tamay ZU. Is BCG vaccination affecting the spread and severity of COVID-19? Allergy. 2020;75(7):1824–7.
8. Redelman-Sidi G. Could BCG be used to protect against COVID-19? Nat Rev Urol. 2020;17(6):316–7.
9. Miyasaka M. Is BCG vaccination causally related to reduced COVID-19 mortality? EMBO Mol Med. 2020;12(6):e12661.
10. Babjuk M, Burger M, Compérat EM, et al. European association of urology guidelines on non-muscle-invasive bladder cancer (TaT1 and carcinoma in situ)—2019 update. Eur Urol. 2019;76(5):639–57.
11. Morales A, Eidinger D, Bruce AW. Intracavitary bacillus Calmette–Guérin in the treatment of superficial bladder tumors. J Urol. 1976;116:180–3.
12. Ministerio de ciencias. Reporte epidemiológico de Ministerio de Salud Febrero 2021. https://www.gob.cl/coronavirus/cifrasoficiales/ (Online Resource). Accessed 23 Feb 2021.
13. Kleinnijenhuis J, van Crevel R, Netea MG. Trained immunity: consequences for the heterologous effects of BCG vaccination. Trans R Soc Trop Med Hyg. 2015;109(1):29–35.
14. Zlotta A, Drowart A, Huygen K, et al. Humoral response against heat shock proteins and other mycobacterial antigens after intravesical treatment with BCG in patients with superficial bladder cancer. Clin Exp Immunol. 1997;109:157–65.
15. Desouky E. BCG versus COVID-19: impact on urology. World J Urol. 2020;16:1–5.
16. Liang W, Guan W, Chen R, et al. Cancer patients in SARS-CoV-2 infection: a nationwide analysis in China. Lancet Oncol. 2020;21:335–7.
17. Lenfant L, Seisen T, Loriot Y, Rouprêt M. Adjustments in the use of intravesical instillations of bacillus Calmette–Guérin for high-risk non-muscle-invasive bladder cancer during the COVID-19 pandemic. Eur Urol. 2020;78(1):1–3.

27

Transvaginal closure of urinary bladder opening and Mitrofanoff technique in a neurologically impaired female with chronic indwelling catheter

Athanasios Zachariou[1,6*], Minas Paschopoulos[2], Aris Kaltsas[1], Fotios Dimitriadis[3], Athanasios Zikopoulos[1], Charalampos Mamoulakis[4], Atsushi Takenaka[5] and Nikolaos Sofikitis[1]

Abstract

Background: Chronic catheterization remains the only attractive option in specific circumstances, especially in neurologically impaired patients. Complications produced by the indwelling catheters, like patulous urethra and bladder neck destruction, usually lead to severe incontinence and significant nursing difficulties. Here, we describe a rare case, a urinary bladder opening representing massive and extensive destruction of the urethra and bladder sphincter due to an indwelling catheter.

Case presentation: We present a 46-year-old paraplegic woman complaining of recurrent febrile urinary tract infections and severe urinary incontinence. She suffered from persistent malodorous urine and skin breakdowns from constant urine leakage. The vaginal examination revealed extensive destruction of the urethra and a 10 cm opening permitting the urinary bladder wall to prolapse into the vagina. The patient underwent a combined surgical approach; a transvaginal bladder closure with anterior colporrhaphy and a Mitrofanoff procedure to ensure a continent stoma for future clean intermittent self-catheterization (CISC). The patient is compliant with CISC and, remains continent twelve years after surgery.

Conclusion: This case demonstrates that in the era of CISC, there are still neurologically impaired females suffering from rare but critical adverse effects of indwelling catheters. The urethra and bladder neck erosion represent a demanding treatment assignment. The Mitrofanoff procedure for continent stoma and the transvaginal closure of urinary bladder opening produced a lifesaving potential treatment.

Keywords: Urethral damage, Indwelling catheter, Transvaginal urethral closure, Mitrofanoff, Case report

Background

Clean intermittent self-catheterization (CISC) has become generally accepted during the last decades as the gold standard for the management of neurogenic bladder. The principles of CISC are to empty the bladder efficiently, to avoid complications and to improve storage function [1]. The main reason for the institution of an indwelling catheter is the challenge in controlling urinary incontinence in female patients. Chronic catheterization remains an attractive option only in specific conditions. These are the impaired upper limb function in high cervical spine injury patients, the absence of a caregiver to perform clean intermittent catheterization and the lack

*Correspondence: zahariou@otenet.gr
[1] Urology Department, Medical School, University of Ioannina, Ioannina, Greece
Full list of author information is available at the end of the article

of satisfactory external collection device in the females [2].

There are several reports in the literature describing the complications of long term indwelling catheterization. These include bladder and peritoneal perforation [3], urinary infections [4], bladder calculi and catheter encrustations [5], catheter complications like blockage [6], urethral stenosis, urethral damage and malignancy associated with chronic infection [7]. In a multicenter cohort study of 2076 adults with an indwelling urethral catheter, 57% of patients reported at least 1 complication because of the catheter, and noninfectious complications (55%) were 5 times as common as infectious complications (11%) [8].

One of the most challenging problems in the management of women with neurogenic bladders is incontinence around their indwelling catheter. Anticholinergics, β_3-adrenoceptor agonist and a larger catheter, resolve urinary leakage for a limited time. The use of larger caliber catheters, can produce patients facing acute adverse effects [9]. For example, pressure necrosis from long-term indwelling catheters and extrusion of a Foley catheter during sudden movements damage the urethra. Complications produced by the catheters, like patulous urethra and bladder neck destruction, usually lead to significant nursing difficulties. Severe incontinence increases the depression of these patients, who are often bedridden or wheelchair-bound and may also be suffering from coexisting pressure sores.

In the present study, a rare case is described; a urinary bladder opening representing massive and extensive destruction of the urethra and bladder sphincter due to indwelling catheter in a neurologically impaired woman. The combined use of two surgical approaches, the transvaginal closure of bladder opening and the Mitrofanoff technique, produced a urinary bladder with a continent stoma. Furthermore, the reason to publish our case now was that there is a long term evaluation of the proposed therapy since more than a decade has passed since the procedures. Finally, emphasis should be given to the fact that in the era of CISC, there are still unusual critical complications concerning indwelling catheters and a combination of rehabilitation surgical techniques are always crucial for radical treatment.

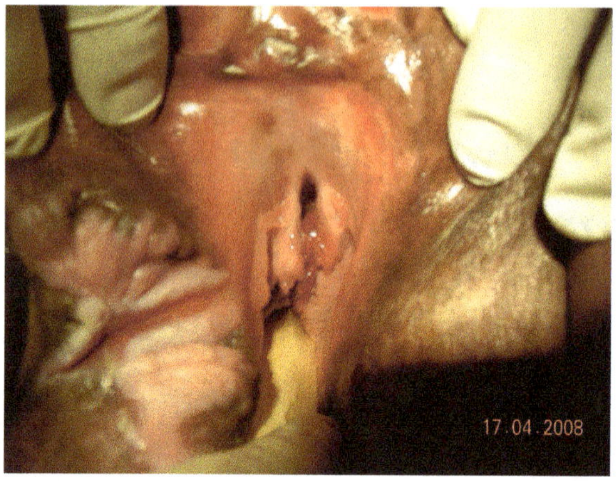

Fig. 1 The vaginal examination revealed destruction of the urethra

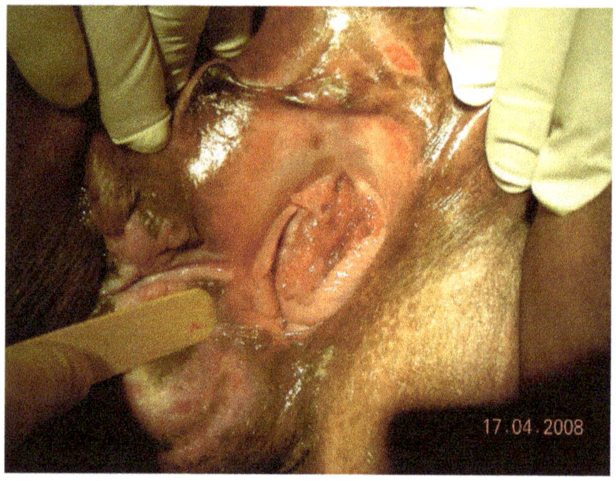

Fig. 2 The vaginal examination revealed a 10 cm opening permitting the urinary bladder wall to prolapse into the vagina

Case presentation

A 46-year-old paraplegic woman presented to the outpatient urology department, complaining of recurrent febrile urinary tract infections and severe urinary incontinence for 2 years. She suffered from persistent malodorous urine and skin breakdowns from constant urine leakage. She typically used long-term urethral catheters, which had resulted in dilatation and pressure necrosis of the urethra with subsequent severe incontinence.

The vaginal examination revealed destruction of the urethra and a 10 cm opening permitting the urinary bladder wall to prolapse into the vagina (Figs. 1, 2). Three fingers could be easily inserted into the urethra, and the bladder wall could practically be observed from the outside. A diffuse scar tissue area had replaced bladder trigone, and ureteral orifices were visible through the bladder opening. An intravenous urography was performed to check the anatomy of the upper urinary tract, which was within normal limits. The computed tomography (CT) scan did not assist in the diagnosis because of the artifacts caused by the bilateral total hip replacements.

The patient underwent a combined transvaginal urethral closure with anterior colporrhaphy and a

Mitrofanoff procedure to ensure a continent stoma for future CISC. The patient was placed initially in the dorsal lithotomy position, and a retractor was placed in the vagina. The labia were retracted laterally with stay sutures. The damaged bladder wall was circumcised, and an anterior vaginal flap was raised. Special care was taken to entirely free the lateral part of the bladder base and the attachments of the pubic bone. There was extensive destruction of pubourethral ligaments, and that allowed a complete mobilization of the bladder wall from the symphysis pubis. The opening was closed with a 2/0 polyglactin (Vicryl™) suture. A second layer, using the same suture, was applied to invaginate further the bladder opening to ensure an excellent postoperative result. An anterior colporrhaphy was accomplished to push anteriorly further the bladder (third layer). Finally, the anterior vaginal flap was advanced to cover the area where the previous urethra and bladder neck were present, forming the last (fourth) layer of closure.

A laparotomy followed immediately after that, and an appendicectomy was done, maintaining its blood supply. The tip of the appendix was transected, and a catheter was introduced to ensure patency. A Mitrofanoff procedure was performed, and the appendix brought out through umbilicus. A small cystostomy was made, and the bladder mucosa was prepared to accomplish an appendico-vesical anastomosis. Recovery from this procedure took six weeks. Initially, the Mitrofanoff channel was not used for draining urine. During this time, a suprapubic catheter was inserted to drain urine. The suprapubic catheter was removed once CISC through the Mitrofanoff channel started. The suprapubic catheter opening closed easily.

During the initial postoperative period, the patient received oxybutynin for three months. The patient is compliant with CISC and remains continent twelve years after surgery. She has a normal renal function with no upper tract dilatation on ultrasonography. The woman underwent evaluation recently, and she is still dry with no urinary fistula reported (Fig. 3).

The patient reported complications concerning recurrent urinary tract infections and urine leakage when delays the emptying. She performs four CISC per day and undergoes annual evaluation with an ultrasound examination to ensure that any stones that may have formed are removed.

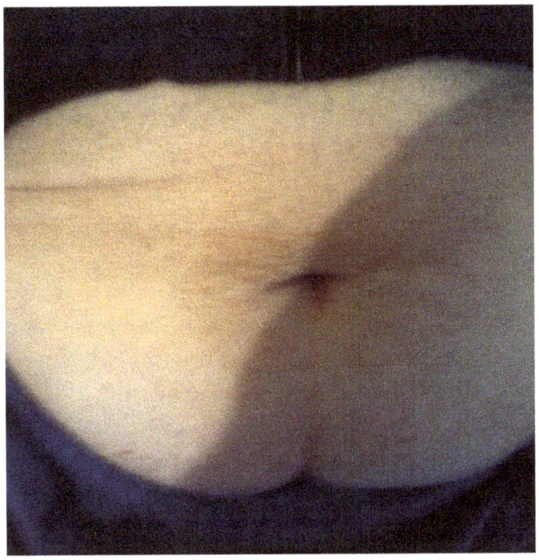

Fig. 3 The Mitrofanoff continent stoma

Discussion and conclusion

Long- term urethral catheters in neurologically impaired female patients result in dilatation of the urethra and severe incontinence. Patients presenting urine leakage are usually treated with a larger catheter, anticholinergics and/or β_3 adrenoceptor agonists. Conventional management of this condition has been urethral closure (abdominal or vaginal) and the simultaneous placement of a suprapubic catheter. Postoperative detrusor spasms represent a significant concern because they could probably increase the rate of fistula formation and postoperative incontinence. During the initial postoperative period, it is critical to continue the treatment with anticholinergics and/or β_3 adrenoceptor agonists [10, 11]. The transvaginal closure of urethra and anterior colporrhaphy ensure low morbidity and high success rates. The complete mobilization of bladder opening prevents high rates of a postoperative urinary fistula. At long-term follow-up of this procedure, 50% of the women were dry after the initial operation. Other complications encountered were bladder stones (21%), leakage around the catheter (17%), recurrent catheter blockage (10%), and urinary tract infections [11].

The functional urethral closure with pubovaginal sling [12], tension-free vaginal tape (TVT) [13], or a modified endoscopic colposuspension where sutures are tied more closely than for patients with genuine stress incontinence [14], represent alternative proposals. Careful patient selection for the aforementioned surgical methods is necessary because females with a completely eroded bladder neck and proximal urethra are not candidates for this procedure. They represent pilot studies with small number of patients and success rates up to 70%.

Because patients with advanced neurological conditions are at high surgical risk, the transvaginal approach may be the ideal option. It provides a good exposure, excellent tolerance and low morbidity. It can perform in obese patients and the very unfit disabled patients even under local anaesthetic. However, there are very few reports about the optimal treatment of a large bladder opening in female patients who are neurologically impaired.

For patients who do not desire or are unable to perform regular intermittent catheterization, the options include bladder neck closure done in conjunction with ileovesicostomy or construction of an ileal conduit. The main reason for choosing a conduit over ileovesicostomy is determined by the stoma site. Patients who use a wheelchair benefit from a stoma in a higher position on the abdominal wall and this may be difficult to reach for an ileovesicostomy [15].

Umbilical location is an ideal position for cosmetic reasons, especially for patients willing to perform CISC. Mitrofanoff appendicovesicostomy represents a convenient way to construct a continent abdominal, urinary stoma [16]. The advantages of appendix diversion include maintaining complete continence, easy catheterization; excellent body image; and rarity of post-surgical complications such as dermatitis and urinary tract infection. Regarding the length of appendix, the cutaneous stoma can be placed in the umbilicus or the lower right abdominal quadrant [17, 18]. The submucosal tunnel and abdominal wall muscles are critical factors concerning the success rate of continence according to Yang et al. [19].

Continent catheterizable stomas display high rates of complications, including stomal stenosis requiring revision or conversion to an alternative channel (12–30% of cases). Usually, an ileal conduit is the alternative stoma, but a stomal appliance is a significant drawback for resource-deprived families [20].

We performed an anterior colporrhaphy to ensure the transposition of the bladder gap to a new position, high behind the symphysis pubis. The multiple layers and the special care for the underlying layers without apposition of the suture lines diminish the rates of fistula. We used the Mitrofanoff technique, usually presented in children, to create a continent catheterizable stoma as an adjunct to continent urinary tract reconstruction.

This case demonstrates that in the era of CISC, there are still neurologically impaired females suffering from rare but critical adverse effects of indwelling catheters. The urethra and bladder neck erosion represent a demanding treatment assignment. The combined use of two surgical approaches (Mitrofanoff technique for continent stoma and transvaginal closure of urethra with anterior colporrhaphy) represent rare but lifesaving potential treatment.

Abbreviations

CISC: Clean intermittent self-catheterization; CT: Computed tomography; TVT: Tension-free vaginal tape.

Acknowledgements

Not applicable.

Authors' contributions

AZ drafted the manuscript and reviewed the literature. AZ, FD, AK, CM helped with the draft. AT, NS, MP revised the manuscript. All authors read and approved the final manuscript.

Author details

[1]Urology Department, Medical School, University of Ioannina, Ioannina, Greece. [2]Department of Obstetrics and Gynaecology, Medical School, University of Ioannina, Ioannina, Greece. [3]Urology Department, Medical School, Aristotle University of Thessaloniki, Thessaloniki, Greece. [4]Urology Department, Medical School, University of Crete, Heraklion, Greece. [5]Urology Department, Medical School, Tottori University, Yonago, Japan. [6]3 Spyridi Street, 38221 14 Volos, Greece.

References s

1. Shamout S, Biardeau X, Corcos J, et al. Outcome comparison of different approaches to self-intermittent catheterization in neurogenic patients: a systematic review. Spinal Cord. 2017;55:629–43.
2. Andrews HO, Shah PJR. Surgical management of urethral damage in neurologically impaired femal patients with chronic indwelling catheters. Br J Urol. 1998;82:820–4.
3. Zachariou A, Kolynou A, Filiponi M. Rectal perforation: a rare complication of indwelling urethral catheterization. Hippokratia. 2017;21:58.
4. Murphy C, Cowan A, Moore K, et al. Managing long term indwelling urinary catheters. BMJ. 2018;363:3711.
5. Norsworthy A, Pearson M. From catheter to kidney stone: the uropathogenic lifestyle of Proteus mirabilis. Trends Microbiol. 2017;4:304–15.
6. Milo S, Nzakizwanayo J, Hathaway H, et al. Emerging medical and engineering strategies for the prevention of long-term indwelling catheter blockage. Proc Inst Mech Eng [H]. 2018;1:68–83.
7. Gui-Zhong L, Li-Bo M. Bladder cancer in individuals with spinal cord injuries: a meta-analysis. Spinal Cord. 2017;55:341–5.
8. Saint S, Trautner BW, Fowler KE, Colozzi J, Ratz D, Lescinskas E, Hollingsworth JM, Krein S. A multicenter study of patient-reported infectious and noninfectious complications associated with indwelling urethral catheters. JAMA. 2018;178(8):1078–85.
9. Linsenmeyer TA. Catheter-associated urinary tract infections in persons with neurogenic bladders. J Spinal Cord Med. 2018;41(2):132–41.
10. Zimmern P, Hadley R, Leach G, Raz S. Tranvaginal closure of the bladder neck and placement of a suprapubic catheter for destroyed urethra after long-term indwelling catheterization. J Urol. 1985;134:554–6.
11. Kubai U, Arunkalaivanan S, Baptiste M. Transvaginal closure of urethra and correction of uterovaginal prolapse in neurologically impaired patient with chronic indwelling catheter. Int Urogynecol J. 2009;20:991–3.
12. Chancellor M, Erhard M, Kiilholma P, Karasick S, Rivas D. Functional urethral closure with pubovaginal sling for destroyed female urethra after long-term urethral catheterization. Adult Urology. 1994;43:499–505.
13. Poddar A, Jackson S. Intentional urethral closure with a TVT (tension-free vaginal tape) for intractable urinary incontinence: a preliminary report of three cases. Int Urogynecol J Pelvic Floor Dysfunct. 2007;18:195–7.
14. Wedderburn AW, Adamson AS. Management of the incompetent urethra in the chronically debilitated female patient: an alternative to urethral closure. BJU Int. 1999;84:727–8.
15. Ginsberg D. Management of the neurogenic bladder in the female patient. Curr Bladder Dysfunct Rep. 2006;1:65–70.
16. Cain MP, Casale AJ, King SJ, Ring RC. Appendicovesicostomy and newer alternatives for the Mitrofanoff procedure: results in the last 100 patients at Riley Children's Hospital. J Urol. 1999;1999(162):1749.
17. Abedi AR, Ghiasy S, Fallah-karkan M, Hojjati SA, Hosseini J. Appendicovesicostomy as an alternative procedure for patients with complex urethral distraction defect. Urol J. 2020;17(4):386–90.

18. Hakenberg OW, Ebermayer J, Manseck A, Wirth MP. Application of the Mitrofanoff principle for intermittent self-catheterization in quadriplegic patients. Urology. 2001;58:38–42.
19. Yang W-H. Yang needle tunneling technique in creating antireflux and continent mechanisms. J Urol. 1993;150:830–4.
20. Liard A, Seguier-Lipszyc E, Mathiot A, Mitrofanoff P. The Mitrofanoff procedure: 20 years later. J Urol. 2001;165:2394–8.

Permissions

All chapters in this book were first published by BioMed Central; hereby published with permission under the Creative Commons Attribution License or equivalent. Every chapter published in this book has been scrutinized by our experts. Their significance has been extensively debated. The topics covered herein carry significant findings which will fuel the growth of the discipline. They may even be implemented as practical applications or may be referred to as a beginning point for another development.

The contributors of this book come from diverse backgrounds, making this book a truly international effort. This book will bring forth new frontiers with its revolutionizing research information and detailed analysis of the nascent developments around the world.

We would like to thank all the contributing authors for lending their expertise to make the book truly unique. They have played a crucial role in the development of this book. Without their invaluable contributions this book wouldn't have been possible. They have made vital efforts to compile up to date information on the varied aspects of this subject to make this book a valuable addition to the collection of many professionals and students.

This book was conceptualized with the vision of imparting up-to-date information and advanced data in this field. To ensure the same, a matchless editorial board was set up. Every individual on the board went through rigorous rounds of assessment to prove their worth. After which they invested a large part of their time researching and compiling the most relevant data for our readers.

The editorial board has been involved in producing this book since its inception. They have spent rigorous hours researching and exploring the diverse topics which have resulted in the successful publishing of this book. They have passed on their knowledge of decades through this book. To expedite this challenging task, the publisher supported the team at every step. A small team of assistant editors was also appointed to further simplify the editing procedure and attain best results for the readers.

Apart from the editorial board, the designing team has also invested a significant amount of their time in understanding the subject and creating the most relevant covers. They scrutinized every image to scout for the most suitable representation of the subject and create an appropriate cover for the book.

The publishing team has been an ardent support to the editorial, designing and production team. Their endless efforts to recruit the best for this project, has resulted in the accomplishment of this book. They are a veteran in the field of academics and their pool of knowledge is as vast as their experience in printing. Their expertise and guidance has proved useful at every step. Their uncompromising quality standards have made this book an exceptional effort. Their encouragement from time to time has been an inspiration for everyone.

The publisher and the editorial board hope that this book will prove to be a valuable piece of knowledge for researchers, students, practitioners and scholars across the globe.

List of Contributors

Athanasios Zachariou, Maria Filiponi, Aris Kaltsas and Nikolaos Sofikitis
Urology Department, Medical School, University of Ioannina, 3 Spyridi Street, 38221 Vólos, Greece

Fotios Dimitriadis
1st Urology Department, Medical School, Aristotle University of Thessaloniki, Thessaloníki, Greece

Rong Lv, Chongrui Jin and Huiquan Shu
Department of Urology, Shanghai Jiao Tong University Affiliated Sixth People's Hospital, Shanghai, China

Lin Wang
Department of Urology, Shanghai Jiao Tong University Affiliated Sixth People's Hospital, Shanghai, China
Department of Urology, Shanghai Children's Hospital, Shanghai Jiao Tong University, Shanghai, China

Yinglong Sa
Department of Urology, Shanghai Jiao Tong University Affiliated Sixth People's Hospital, Shanghai, China
Shanghai Eastern Institute of Urologic Reconstruction, Shanghai, China

Elijah P. Ward and Sarah N. Bartolone
Department of Urology, Beaumont Health System, 3811 W. 13 Mile Road, Suite 504, Royal Oak, MI 48073, USA

Michael B. Chancellor, Kenneth M. Peters and Laura E. Lamb
Department of Urology, Beaumont Health System, 3811 W. 13 Mile Road, Suite 504, Royal Oak, MI 48073, USA
Oakland University William Beaumont School of Medicine, Rochester, MI, USA

Peter Ella-Tongwiis and Stephen Fôn Hughes
North Wales Clinical Research Centre, Betsi Cadwaladr University Health Board (BCUHB), Wrexham Maelor Hospital, Wrexham, Wales, UK
Faculty of Social and Life Sciences, Wrexham Glyndwr University, Wrexham, UK

Rebecca May Lamb
Department of Biological Sciences, University of Chester, Chester, UK

Alexander Makanga
Department of Histopathology, Ysbyty Glan Clwd, Betsi Cadwaladr University Health Board (BCUHB), Wrexham, UK

Iqbal Shergill
North Wales Clinical Research Centre, Betsi Cadwaladr University Health Board (BCUHB), Wrexham Maelor Hospital, Wrexham, Wales, UK
Faculty of Social and Life Sciences, Wrexham Glyndwr University, Wrexham, UK
Department of Urology, BCUHB Wrexham Maelor Hospital, Wrexham, Wales, UK

Yafei Ding, Peng Li, Tao Wang and Siyuan He
Department of Urology, Zhengzhou University First Affiliated Hospital, Zhengzhou 450052, China

Bowen Liu, Zhankui Jia and Jinjian Yang
Department of Urology, Zhengzhou University First Affiliated Hospital, Zhengzhou 450052, China
Zhengzhou Institute of Urology, Zhengzhou University First Affiliated Hospital, Zhengzhou 450052, China

Mozhdeh Amiri
Department of Epidemiology and Biostatistics, Faculty of Medicine, Kurdistan University of Medical Sciences, Sanandaj, Iran

Sofimajidpour Heshmatollah
Department of Urology, Faculty of Medicine, Kurdistan University of Medical Sciences, Sanandaj, Iran

Nader Esmaeilnasab, Ebrahim Ghaderi and Daem Roshani
Social Determinants of Health Research Center, Research Institute for Health Development, Kurdistan University of Medical Sciences, Sanandaj, Iran

Jamshid Khoubi
Environmental Health Research Center, Research Institute for Health Development, Kurdistan University of Medical Sciences, Sanandaj, Iran

Alejandro Majerson
Departamento de Urología, Escuela de Medicina, Pontificia Universidad Católica de Chile, Diagonal Paraguay 362, Santiago, Chile

Cristián González
División de Ginecología y Obstetricia, Escuela de Medicina, Pontificia Universidad Católica de Chile, Santiago, Chile

Gonzalo P. Mendez
Departamento de Anatomía-Patológica, Escuela de Medicina, Pontificia Universidad Católica de Chile, Santiago, Chile

Dayin Chen, Liang Cheng, Huifeng Cao and Wensi Liu
Department of Urology, The First Affiliated Hospital of Jiamusi University, No. 348, Dexiang Street, Jiamusi 154002, Heilongjiang, People's Republic of China

Kiren Gill and Rajvinder Khasriya
Women's Health, Whittington Health NHS Trust, Magdala Avenue, London N19 5FN, UK

Harry Horsley
Bladder Infection and Immunity Group (BIIG), Department of Renal Medicine, Division of Medicine, University College London, Royal Free Hospital Campus, Rowland Hill Street, London NW3 2PF, UK

Sheela Swamy
Women's Health, St Thomas' Hospital, Westminster Bridge Road, London SE1 7EH, UK

James Malone-Lee
Bladder Infection and Immunity Group (BIIG), Department of Renal Medicine, Division of Medicine, University College London, 10 Harley Street, London W1G 9PF, UK

James Gross and Joel M. Vetter
Division of Urologic Surgery, Department of Surgery, Washington University School of Medicine, 4960 Children's Place, Campus, St Louis, MO 63110, USA

H. Henry Lai
Division of Urologic Surgery, Department of Surgery, Washington University School of Medicine, 4960 Children's Place, Campus, St Louis, MO 63110, USA
Department of Anesthesiology, Washington University School of Medicine, St Louis, MO, USA

Li Chen and Jiwei Wang
Department of Ultrasound, The Second Affiliated Hospital of Nanchang University, Nanchang 330006, Jiangxi, China

Bin Lai
Department of Gastrointestinal Surgery, The Second Affiliated Hospital of Nanchang University, No1 Mingde Road, Nanchang 330006, Jiangxi, China

Xiaoyan Su
Department of Pathology, The Second Affiliated Hospital of Nanchang University, Nanchang 330006, Jiangxi, China

Reza Yahyazadeh
Department of Urology, Shariati Hospital, Tehran University of Medical Sciences, Tehran, Iran

Davood Bashash and Ava Safaroghli-Azar
Department of Hematology and Blood Banking, School of Allied Medical Sciences, Shahid Beheshti University of Medical Sciences, Tehran, Iran

Parisa Ghaffari, Saeid Kord and Seyed H. Ghaffari
Hematology, Oncology and Stem Cell Transplantation Research Center, School of Medicine, Shariati Hospital, Tehran University of Medical Sciences, Tehran, Iran

Shusuke Akamatsu and Osamu Ogawa
Department of Urology, Faculty of Medicine, Kyoto University Graduate School of Medicine, 54 Shogoinkawahara-cho, Sakyo-ku, Kyoto 606-8507, Japan

Satoshi Funada
Department of Urology, Faculty of Medicine, Kyoto University Graduate School of Medicine, 54 Shogoinkawahara-cho, Sakyo-ku, Kyoto 606-8507, Japan
Department of Health Promotion and Human Behavior, Kyoto University School of Public Health, Kyoto, Japan

Yan Luo and Toshi A. Furukawa
Department of Health Promotion and Human Behavior, Kyoto University School of Public Health, Kyoto, Japan

Takashi Yoshioka
Center for Innovative Research for Communities and Clinical Excellence (CiRC2LE), Fukushima Medical University, Fukushima City, Fukushima, Japan
Department of Healthcare Epidemiology, Kyoto University Graduate School of Medicine and School of Public Health, Kyoto, Japan

Kazuya Setoh, Yasuharu Tabara and Fumihiko Matsuda
Center for Genomic Medicine, Faculty of Medicine, Kyoto University Graduate School of Medicine, Kyoto, Japan

Hiromitsu Negoro
Department of Urology, University of Tsukuba, Ibaraki, Japan

Koji Yoshimura
Department of Urology, Shizuoka General Hospital, Shizuoka, Japan

Orestis Efthimiou
Institute of Social and Preventive Medicine, University of Bern, Bern, Switzerland
Department of Psychiatry, University of Oxford, Oxford, UK

Aldhabi Mokhtar, Chuize Kong, Zhe Zhang and Yan Du
Department of Urology, The First Hospital of China Medical University, 155 Nanjing North Street, Shenyang, Liaoning 110001, P.R. China

Xi Tu, Neng Zhang, Shulian Chen and Xu Luo
Department of Urology, Affiliated Hospital of Zunyi Medical University, Zunyi 563000, Guizhou, China

Xiyao Zhuang
Department of Internal Medicine, Chengdu Shuangliu Hospital of Traditional Chinese Medicine, Chengdu, Sichuan, China

Ben-zheng Zhou and Ye Zhang
Department of Urology, Xiangyang No.1 People's Hospital, Hubei University of Medicine, Xiangyang, Hubei, People's Republic of China

Qin Luo
Department of Gynaecoogy and Obstetrics, Xiangyang No.1 People's Hospital, Hubei University of Medicine, Xiangyang, Hubei, People's Republic of China

Hyun Bin Shin and Hyun Sik Park
Department of Urology, Eulji University Hospital, Eulji University School of Medicine, Daejeon, Korea

Joo Heon Kim
Department of Pathology, Eulji University Hospital, Eulji University School of Medicine, Daejeon, Korea

Jinsung Park
Department of Urology, Eulji University Hospital, Eulji University School of Medicine, Daejeon, Korea
Department of Urology, Uijeongbu Eulji Medical Center, Eulji University School of Medicine, 712, Dongil-ro, Uijeongbu-si, Gyeonggi-do 11759, Republic of Korea

Ae-Ri Ahn, Ho Sung Park, Myoung Ja Chung, Woo Sung Moon, Kyu Yun Jang and Myoung Jae Kang
Department of Pathology, Jeonbuk National University Medical School, Jeonju, Republic of Korea

Sang Jae Noh and Ho Lee
Department of Forensic Medicine, Jeonbuk National University Medical School, Jeonju, Republic of Korea

Usama Khamis Hussein
Department of Pathology, Jeonbuk National University Medical School, Jeonju, Republic of Korea
Faculty of Science, Beni-Suef University, Beni-Suef, Egypt

Hyung Jin Kim
Department of Urology, Jeonbuk National University Medical School, Jeonju, Republic of Korea

Na Ri Lee
Department of Internal Medicine, Jeonbuk National University Hospital-Jeonbuk National University Medical School, Jeonju, Republic of Korea

Kyoung Min Kim
Department of Pathology, Jeonbuk National University Medical School, Jeonju, Republic of Korea
Research Institute of Clinical Medicine of Jeonbuk National University-Biomedical Research Institute of Jeonbuk National University Hospital, Jeonju, Republic of Korea

Ramzi Shawahna
Department of Physiology, Pharmacology and Toxicology, Faculty of Medicine and Health Sciences, An-Najah National University, New Campus, Building: 19, Office: 1340, Nablus, Palestine
An-Najah BioSciences Unit, Centre for Poison Control, Chemical and Biological Analysis, An-Najah National University, Nablus, Palestine

Hatim Hijaz
Department of Medicine, Faculty of Medicine and Health Sciences, An-Najah National University, Nablus, Palestine
An- Najah National University Hospital, An-Najah National University, Nablus, Palestine

Khaled Jallad, Mohammad Abushamma and Mothana Sawafta
Department of Medicine, Faculty of Medicine and Health Sciences, An-Najah National University, Nablus, Palestine

Hidetoshi Tabata, Nobuo Shinkai, Koji Ichihara and Naoya Masumori
Department of Urology, Sapporo Medical University School of Medicine, Sapporo 060-8556, Japan

Masanori Sasaki and Osamu Honmou
Department of Neural Regenerative Medicine, Research Institute for Frontier Medicine, Sapporo Medical University School of Medicine, Sapporo, Hokkaido 060-8556, Japan
Department of Neurology, Yale University School of Medicine, New Haven, CT 06510, USA
Center for Neuroscience and Regeneration Research, VA Connecticut Healthcare System, West Haven, CT 06516, USA

Yuko Kataoka-Sasaki
Department of Neural Regenerative Medicine, Research Institute for Frontier Medicine, Sapporo Medical University School of Medicine, Sapporo, Hokkaido 060-8556, Japan

Jeffery D. Kocsis
Department of Neurology, Yale University School of Medicine, New Haven, CT 06510, USA
Center for Neuroscience and Regeneration Research, VA Connecticut Healthcare System, West Haven, CT 06516, USA

Shijie Li, Xuefeng Liu and Xiaonan Chen
Department of Urology, Shengjing Hospital of China Medical University, 36 Sanhao Street, Shenyang 110004, Liaoning, People's Republic of China

Ali Hashemi Gheinani
Functional Urology Research Group, Department for BioMedical Research DBMR, University of Bern, Bern, Switzerland
Urological Diseases Research Center, Boston Children's Hospital, Boston, MA, USA
Department of Surgery, Harvard Medical School, Boston, MA, USA
Broad Institute of MIT and Harvard, Cambridge, MA, USA

Akshay Akshay, Mustafa Besic and Katia Monastyrskaya
Functional Urology Research Group, Department for BioMedical Research DBMR, University of Bern, Bern, Switzerland

Annette Kuhn
Department of Gynaecology, Inselspital University Hospital, 3010 Bern, Switzerland

Irene Keller and Rémy Bruggmann
Interfaculty Bioinformatics Unit, University of Bern, Bern, Switzerland

Hubert Rehrauer
Functional Genomics Center Zurich, ETH Zurich/ University of Zurich, Zurich, Switzerland

Rosalyn M. Adam
Urological Diseases Research Center, Boston Children's Hospital, Boston, MA, USA
Department of Surgery, Harvard Medical School, Boston, MA, USA
Broad Institute of MIT and Harvard, Cambridge, MA, USA

Fiona C. Burkhard
Department of Urology, Inselspital University Hospital, 3010 Bern, Switzerland

Gang Xu, Shouhua Pan, Zhirong Zhu and Junlong Li
Department of Urology, Shaoxing People's Hospital (Shaoxing Hospital, Zhejiang University School of Medicine), No. 568, Zhongxing North Road, Shaoxing 312000, Zhejiang, China

Yuxin Li, Xiong Chen, Dongjie Li, Zhiming Yang, Yao Bai, Sheng Hu and Zhenyu Liu
Department of Geriatric Urology, Xiangya International Medical Center, Xiangya Hospital, Central South University, Changsha, Hunan 410008, People's Republic of China
National Clinical Research Center for Geriatric Disorders, Xiangya Hospital, Central South University, Changsha, Hunan 410008, People's Republic of China

Jie Gu
Department of Geriatric Urology, Xiangya International Medical Center, Xiangya Hospital, Central South University, Changsha, Hunan 410008, People's Republic of China
National Clinical Research Center for Geriatric Disorders, Xiangya Hospital, Central South University, Changsha, Hunan 410008, People's Republic of China
Martini-Klinik Prostate Cancer Center, University Hospital Hamburg-Eppendorf, Hamburg, Germany

XiaoBo Zhang
Department of Geriatric Urology, Xiangya International Medical Center, Xiangya Hospital, Central South University, Changsha, Hunan 410008, People's Republic of China
National Clinical Research Center for Geriatric Disorders, Xiangya Hospital, Central South University, Changsha, Hunan 410008, People's Republic of China
Urolithiasis Institute of Central South University, Changsha, Hunan 410008, People's Republic of China

Hiroki Hagimoto, Noriyuki Makita, Yuta Mine, Hidetoshi Kokubun, Shiori Murata, Yohei Abe, Masashi Kubota, Naofumi Tsutsumi, Toshinari Yamasaki and Mutsushi Kawakita
Department of Urology, Kobe City Medical Center General Hospital, 2-1-1 Minatojima-Minamimachi, Chuo-ku, Kobe, Hyogo 650-0047, Japan

Héctor Gallegos, Álvaro Zúñiga and Ignacio F. San Francisco
Departamento de Urología, Facultad de Medicina, Pontificia Universidad Católica de Chile, Diagonal Paraguay 362, Santiago, Chile

Pablo A. Rojas
Departamento de Urología, Facultad de Medicina, Pontificia Universidad Católica de Chile, Diagonal Paraguay 362, Santiago, Chile
Servicio de Urología, Hospital Sótero del Río, Santiago, Chile

Francisca Sepúlveda
Escuela de Pregrado, Facultad de Medicina, Pontificia Universidad Católica de Chile, Santiago, Chile

Minas Paschopoulos
Department of Obstetrics and Gynaecology, Medical School, University of Ioannina, Ioannina, Greece

Charalampos Mamoulakis
Urology Department, Medical School, University of Crete, Heraklion, Greece

Atsushi Takenaka
Urology Department, Medical School, Tottori University, Yonago, Japan

Athanasios Zachariou
Urology Department, Medical School, University of Ioannina, Ioannina, Greece
3 Spyridi Street, 38221 14 Volos, Greece

Index

www.ingramcontent.com/pod-product-compliance
Lightning Source LLC
LaVergne TN
LVHW081034210926
848485LV00004B/1017
* 9 7 8 1 6 3 9 2 7 9 3 6 4 *